The illustrated lecture

Neurology and Psychiatry

The *illustrated* lecture series

Neurology and Psychiatry	P. N. Plowman
Endocrinology and Metabolic Diseases	P. N. Plowman
Nephrology, Electrolyte Pathophysiology and Poisoning	P. N. Plowman
Haematology and Immunology	P. N. Plowman
Cardiology	T. J. Phillips, P. N. Plowman
Respiratory Medicine	P. N. Plowman
Alimentary Medicine and Tropical Diseases	P. N. Plowman, T. J. Phillips, S. J. Rose

In Preparation

Surgery
Anatomy
Obstetrics and Gynaecology
Pathology
Physiology
Ophthalmology

The illustrated lecture series

Neurology and Psychiatry

P. N. Plowman MA MD (Cantab) MRCP FRCR
Consultant Physician
St Bartholomew's Hospital and Medical College
London EC1 UK

A Wiley-Phoenix Publication

JOHN WILEY & SONS
Chichester · New York · Brisbane · Toronto · Singapore

Copyright©1987 by John Wiley & Sons Ltd.

Distributors in United States and Canada:
Medical Examination Publishing Company,
A Division of Elsevier Science Publishing Co. Inc., New York

All rights reserved.

No part of this book may be reproduced by any means, or transmitted, or
translated into a machine language without
the written permission of the publisher

British Library Cataloguing in Publication Data:

Plowman, P. N.
  Neurology and psychiatry.—(The
  illustrated lecture series).
  1. Nervous system—Diseases
  I. Title II. Series
  616.8   RC346
  ISBN 0 471 91450 9

Printed and bound in Great Britain

Contents

Preface	ix
Publisher's Note	xi

Neurology

Higher Functions	4
Examination/Assessment of Higher Cerebral Functions	13
Cranial Nerve Functions	16
The Pupil	29
Nystagmus	35
Cranial Nerve Functions (continued)	39
The Peripheral Motor System	58
The Peripheral Sensory System	67
Spinal Cord Compression	69
Lumbago	75
The Cerebrospinal Fluid (CSF)	79
Brain Tumours	99
Intracranial Haemorrhage	109
Occlusive Cerebrovascular Disease	117
Venous Sinus Thrombosis	123
Epilepsy—Classification	124

Contents

Epilepsy—Treatment	133
Multiple Sclerosis (MS, Disseminated Sclerosis)	137
Parkinsonism	143
Abnormal Movement Disorders	147
Headache	150
Tension Headache (Psychogenic Headache)	151
Migraine	151
Other Vascular Causes of Headache	156
Headache due to Raised Intracranial Pressure	158
Other Causes of Headache	158
Coma	159
Brain Death	163
Syringomyelia	163
Motor Neurone Disease	167
Diseases of Peripheral Nerves	169
Mononeuropathy	169
Mononeuritis Multiplex	171
Polyneuropathy	172
Acute Infectious Polyneuritis (Guillain-Barré Syndrome)	177
Vitamins B_1 and B_{12} Deficiency	178
Myasthenia Gravis	181
Myopathies	186
Muscular Dystrophy	187

Pseudohypertrophic Muscular Dystrophy (Duchenne type)	188
Limb-Girdle Muscular Dystrophy	190
Myotonic Dystrophy	191
Acquired Myopathies	192
Polymyositis	194

Psychiatry

Classification of Psychiatric Disorders	200
Psychiatric History and Examination	202
The Neuroses	206
Classification of Depressive States and Reactive Depression	216
Functional Psychoses	222
Schizophrenia	235
Organic Psychoses	249
Delirium	249
Dementia	250
Alcoholism	256
Index	**261**

Preface

Neurology is one of the most fascinating branches of medicine and yet this subject is found notoriously difficult to comprehend by those in training. Organic lesions in the central nervous system and their clinical sequelae lend themselves well to illustration and in this book hundreds of illustrations, side by side with the text, serve to teach the subject in perhaps the most explicit way to date. In this particular volume of the Illustrated Lecture Series it has been considered logical to partner the clinical study and treatment of organic disorders of the central nervous system (neurology) with that of psychiatric disorders; indeed, it is absolutely essential that the clinician be able to distinguish and not confuse the two. Psychiatry is a most vital subject to understand as the proportion of our patients presenting with psychiatric complaints forms a large fraction of our total workload and may be predicted to increase. The attention paid in this book to the psychiatric history-taking, before the logical descriptions of the complaints, is important to the understanding and practice of psychiatry.

Whilst readers will use this new teaching concept in different ways to learn the subject, it is suggested that reading the text on a page is followed by a study of the figures and, lastly, by the reading of the labels that surround the figure, which provide reinforcement of the facts and their visual demonstration. Space for extra notes is available on each page and so allows the book to become personalised by the reader's own experience in addition to the printed facts.

P. N. Plowman

Publisher's Note

Modern medicine is now more interesting and challenging than ever before. Unfortunately, the subject is now so large that it presents a formidable task for students to encompass and for the practising physician to maintain an up-to-date knowledge.

This series of illustrated books represents an entirely new concept which we believe will open up a new method of medical teaching, adding an extra dimension which will keep the reader's interest alive and active throughout the whole syllabus of general medicine.

The most important feature of the book is the linkage and locking of prose with figures in such a way that illustrations (with repeated key phrases) reinforce the comprehension of the text at all stages as one proceeds through the pages. The content of the series also differs from many standard works in that not only does it bring in new sections on subjects such as coma, brain death, blood transfusion reactions, etc. omitted in older texts, but it also recognises that certain diseases (e.g. tertiary syphilis) no longer merit extensive description whilst other subjects (e.g. current successes in oncology) merit a more generous coverage.

This series, when completed and collected together, should comprise a uniquely illustrated textbook for the entire medical curriculum. Although primarily intended for the undergraduate student, these books should also prove substantially helpful to nurses, paramedics and social workers who are academically inclined, and offer a refresher course to the busy practitioner.

We have tried to make academic life for the student easier. We shall welcome criticisms, comments and suggestions from academics, students and other readers since we feel sure that these will help us to improve future editions.

Neurology

A **good history** is essential for a certain neurological diagnosis. A full account of the patient's symptoms must be recorded before the clinician enquires a little more carefully into the order, periodicity, time span of symptoms and exactly what the patient means by 'numbness', 'giddiness', 'pain' etc. The clinician must always elicit the nature of progression of symptoms. For example, was a neurological deficit of sudden onset and then gradually improved, (as in cerebrovascular disease), or were the symptoms gradually and relentlessly progressive, (eg. cerebral tumour), or were they relapsing and remitting (eg. multiple sclerosis). The clinician must document the location of symptoms, their exact nature, timing, character, exacerbating and relieving factors. A history from a relative may be useful. A thorough past medical history may elicit birth injury, convulsions in childhood, past meningitis etc., and such events may be relevant or confusing to the current complaint; a family history of nervous diseases and an occupational history may also occasionally be pertinent.

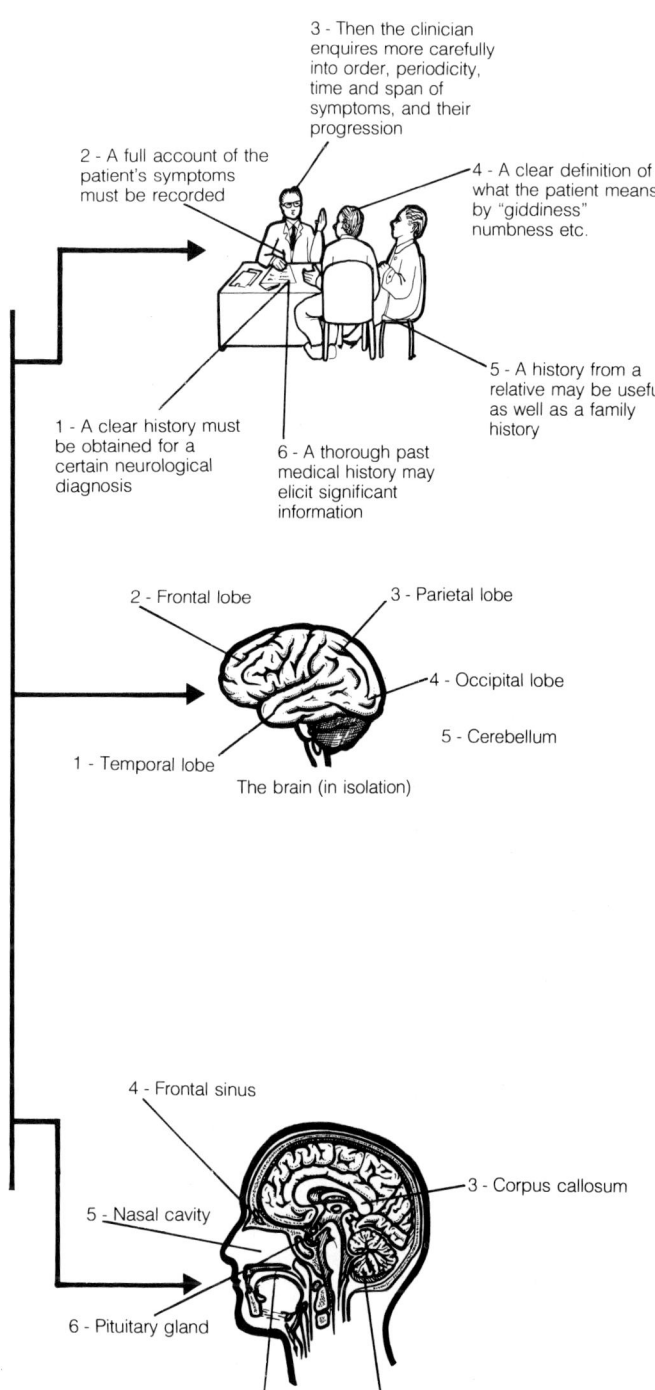

The **examination** of the nervous system is also essential for accurate neurological diagnosis and the secret is in a methodical approach. By such an approach it is possible to localise a lesion in the central nervous system (CNS) or to discriminate several lesions at different CNS locations:

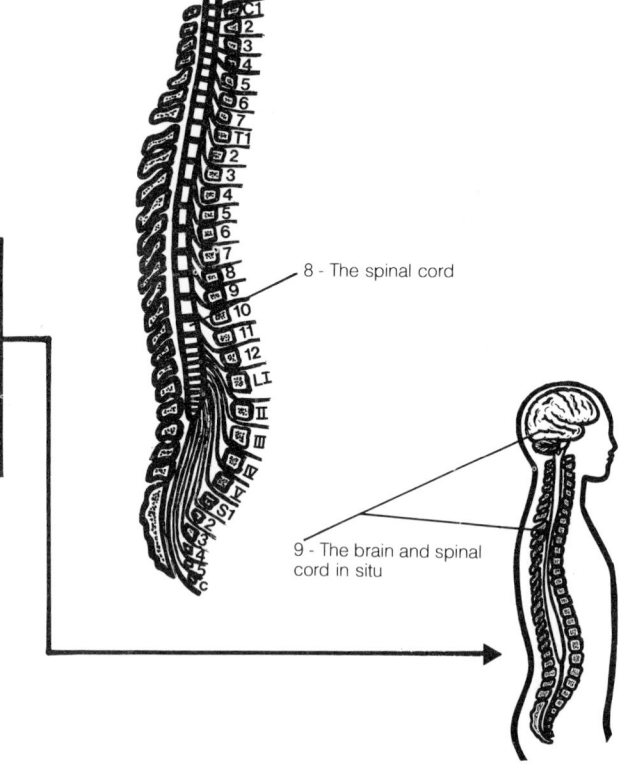

8 - The spinal cord

9 - The brain and spinal cord in situ

HIGHER FUNCTIONS

Frontal lesions – Lesions in the frontal lobe may be clinically silent but usually produce changes in personality, (dulling of intellect, apathy, altered personality, irrational jocularity or sadness, loss of inhibitions and social etiquette etc.). Involvement of contralateral motor pathways may occur if the lesion extends posteriorly and if the primary motor cortex is involved, then a profound paresis may occur; a grasp reflex is a classic feature of frontal lobe lesion affecting contralateral motor paths. Frontal

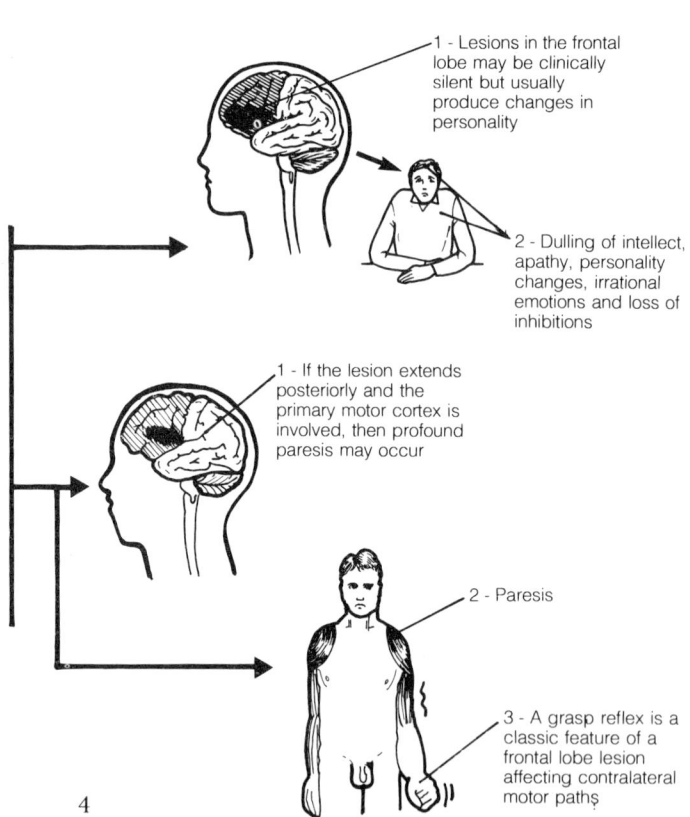

1 - Lesions in the frontal lobe may be clinically silent but usually produce changes in personality

2 - Dulling of intellect, apathy, personality changes, irrational emotions and loss of inhibitions

1 - If the lesion extends posteriorly and the primary motor cortex is involved, then profound paresis may occur

2 - Paresis

3 - A grasp reflex is a classic feature of a frontal lobe lesion affecting contralateral motor paths

Higher Functions

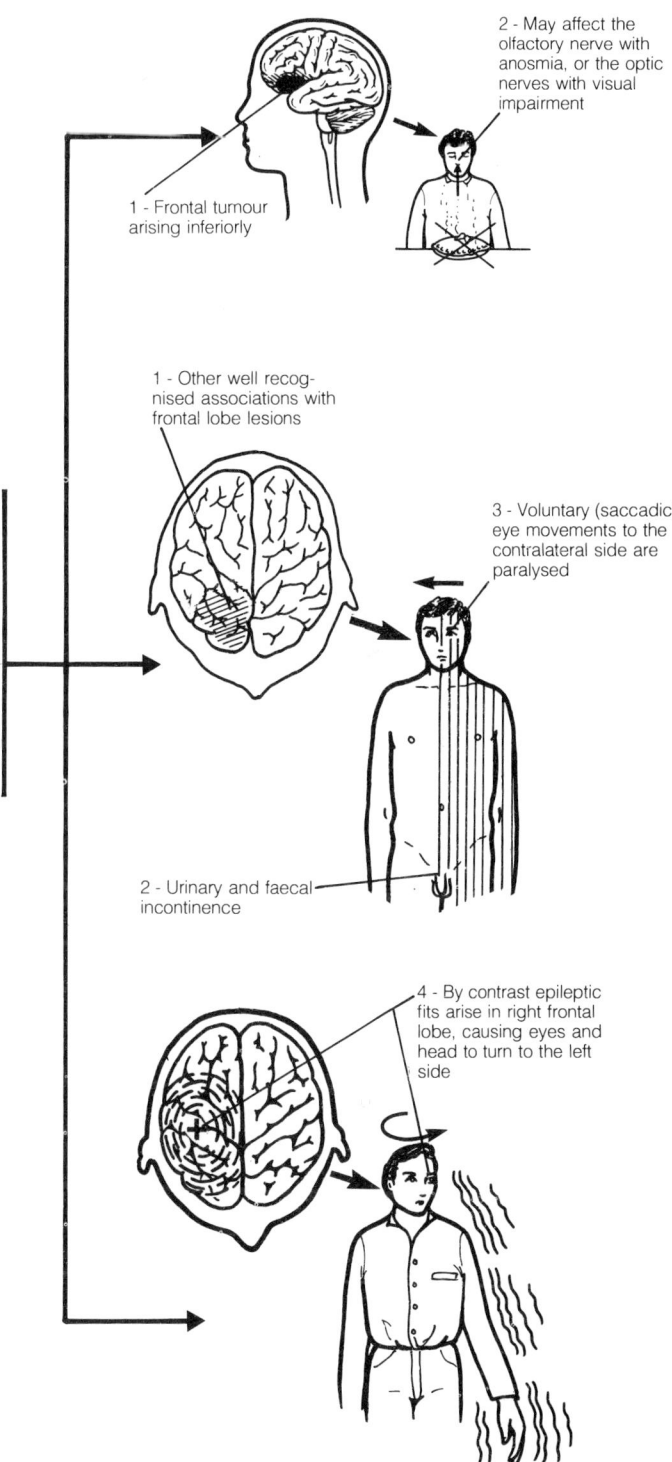

tumours arising inferiorly may affect the olfactory nerve with anosmia or the optic nerves with visual impairment. Other well recognised associations with frontal lobe lesions are urinary or even faecal incontinence and loss of voluntary (saccadic) eye movements to the contralateral side. By contrast, epileptic fits that arise in one frontal lobe may cause the eyes (and head) to turn to the opposite side.

Higher Functions

The posterior part of the inferior frontal gyrus of the dominant (usually left) hemisphere contains **Broca's area**, the motor speech centre. Motor aphasia or dysphasia or that particular inability to name objects (nominal aphasia) may result from damage to this region and adjacent temporal lobe. Damage in this region may also cause ideomotor apraxia (see below).

Lesions in the non-dominant frontal lobe may cause similar 'neglect' phenomena as with non-dominant parietal lobe lesions (eg. the neglect of a paralysed limb). It is for this reason that patients with non-dominant hemisphere lesions causing hemiparesis may mobilise less well than patients with similar lesions affecting the dominant hemisphere.

Disorders of Speech The disorders of the cortical control of speech (dysphasias) must be distinguished from the disorders of the peripheral mechanism of speech articulation (dysarthrias) and both these groups must be themselves distinguished from disorders preventing the production of a normal volume of sound (dysphonias) and lastly the lack of any attempt to speak (mutism).

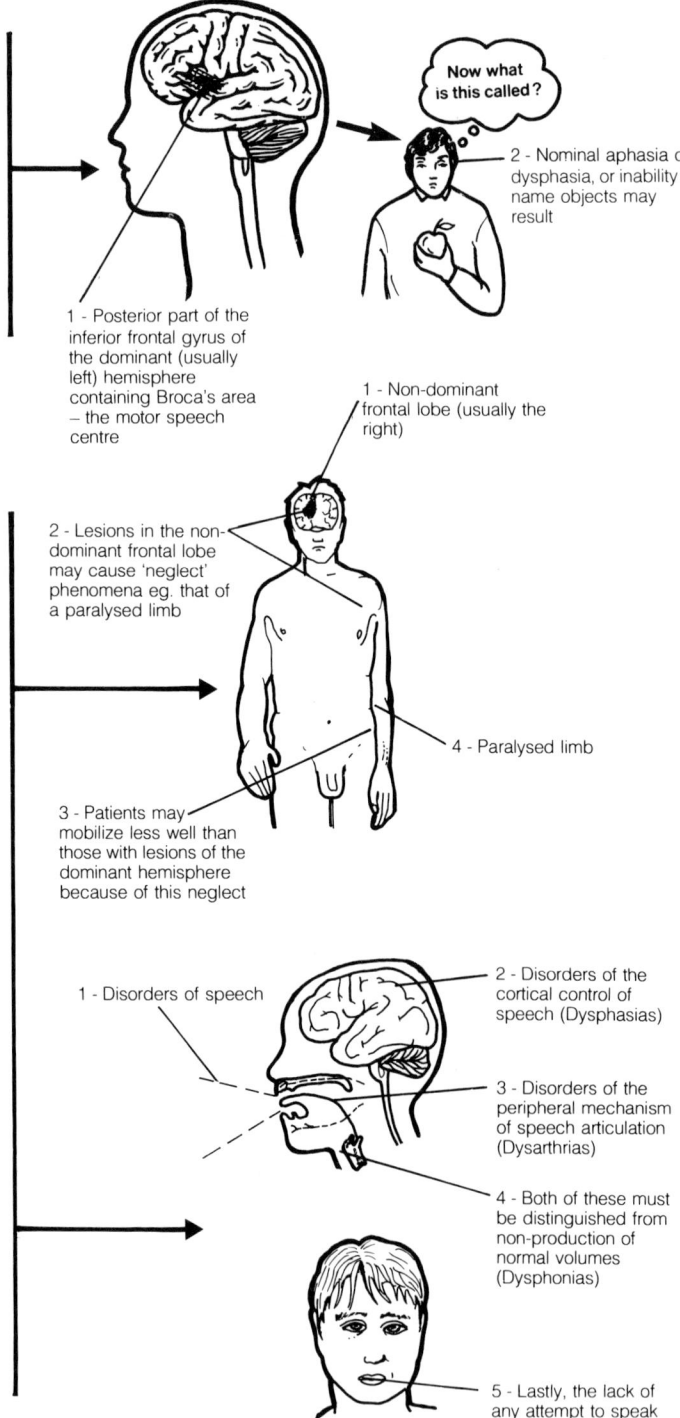

Dysphasia is associated with a lesion in the dominant hemisphere, (which is the left cerebral hemisphere in all but 30% of left-handed people). Although the dysphasia usually contains a mixture of the two components, it is usual for either the expressive (motor) or the receptive (sensory) component to dominate.

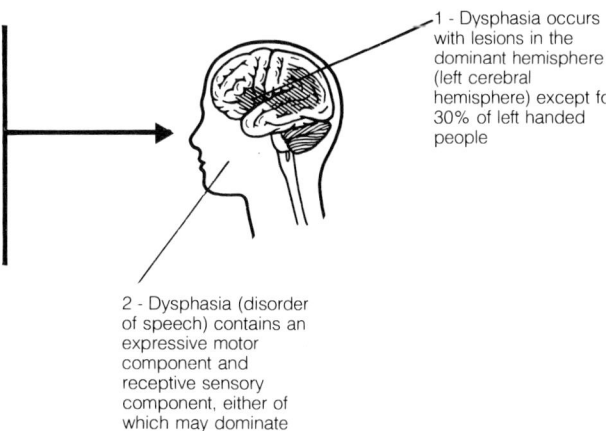

1 - Dysphasia occurs with lesions in the dominant hemisphere (left cerebral hemisphere) except for 30% of left handed people

2 - Dysphasia (disorder of speech) contains an expressive motor component and receptive sensory component, either of which may dominate

Motor or Expressive dysphasias usually arise from lesions more anteriorly placed and here the patient is unable to express his thoughts in words. At first, he will use words that are not quite correct saying 'cloche' (instead of clock) or 'leppuce' (not lettuce) – paraphasias. Later, he will invent a word that is wrong in at least two syllables (neologism) and then he may not produce a word at all, circumlocuting to explain some thing. The inability to find the names of persons or articles is termed nominal

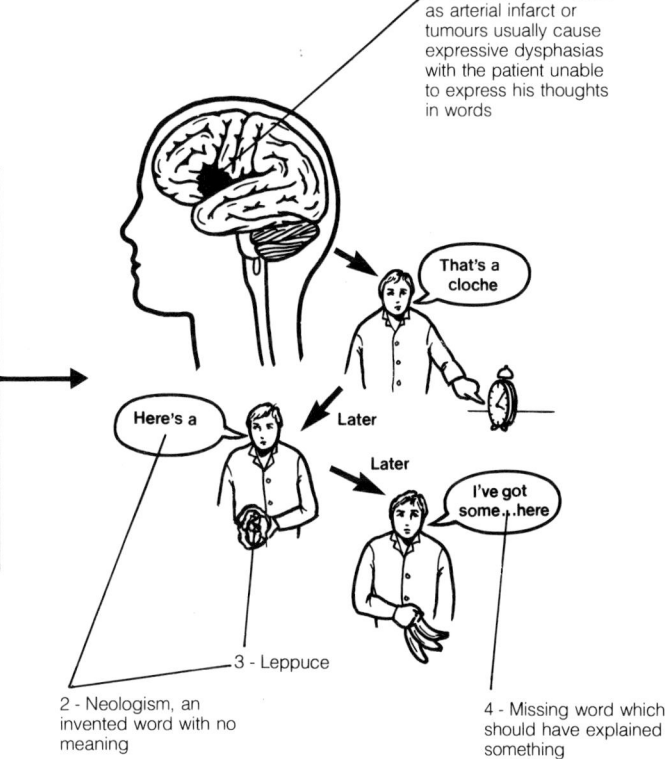

1 - Anterior lesions such as arterial infarct or tumours usually cause expressive dysphasias with the patient unable to express his thoughts in words

2 - Neologism, an invented word with no meaning

3 - Leppuce

4 - Missing word which should have explained something

Higher Functions

dysphasia/aphasia. More posteriorly placed dominant hemisphere lesions are likely to produce sensory dysphasias where the patient may produce a comprehensible soliloquy but is unable to understand or 'process' what is said to him by others. Sometimes, these patients are unable to 'process' what they themselves are saying and so are unable to correct their speech mistakes. When this happens, their dialogue deteriorates into verbal rubbish, (jargon dysphasia).

1 - Posteriorly placed dominant hemisphere lesions may produce sensory dysphasia

2 - The patient produces a comprehensible soliloquy

3 - The patient is unable to understand what is said to him by others

4 - Sometimes these patients are unable to process their speech which is therefore fluent, but full of mistakes — a mere rubbish

1 - Testing for speech disturbances must include:

2 - Test for abnormality in reading (Dyslexia)

3 - Test for abnormality in writing (Dysgraphia)

4 - Test for abnormality in calculating (Dyscalculia)

The testing for speech disturbances must include tests for abnormalities in reading (dyslexia), writing (dysgraphia) and calculation (dyscalculia) as these capabilities are frequently affected together.

Higher Functions

Disorders of praxis – Apraxia (dyspraxia) is the inability, (impaired ability) to carry out a purposive action (ie. an integrated series of fluent movements), the nature of which the patient understands, in the absence of severe motor paralysis, sensory loss or ataxia. Simple actions such as combing one's hair, loading a tooth-brush and cleaning one's teeth, lighting a cigarette – all test praxis. Lesions in the dominant parietal lobe are likely to produce bilateral apraxia, (due to connections through the corpus callosum with the other cortex).

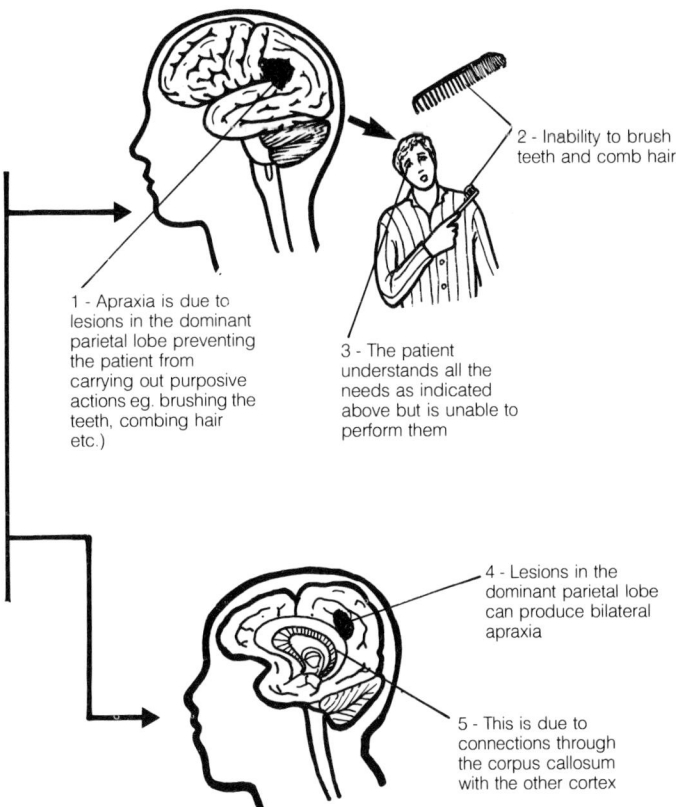

Parietal lobe

Left parietal lobe lesions are more likely to cause dysphasias of sensory type when they are more posteriorly situated and may be accompanied by dyslexia and dysgraphia. Bilateral apraxia occurs with lesions of the dominant supramarginal gyrus. A classic symptom complex occurring with lesions of the dominant angular gyrus includes dysgraphia, dyscalculia, finger agnosia (see below) and left-right disorientation (**Gerstmann's syndrome**).

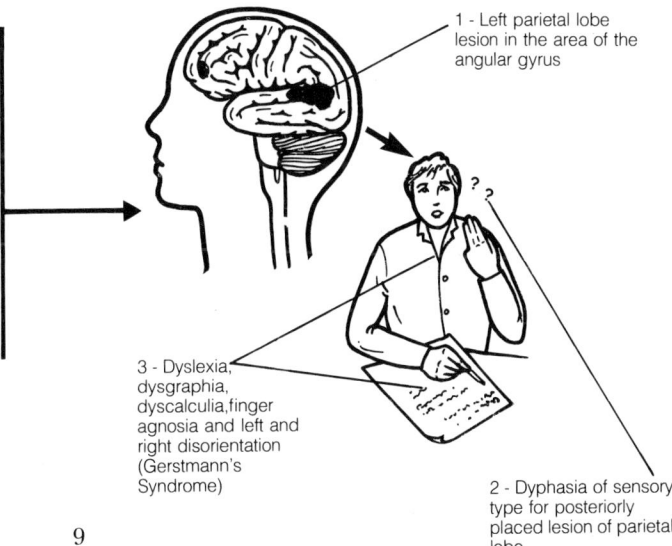

Higher Functions

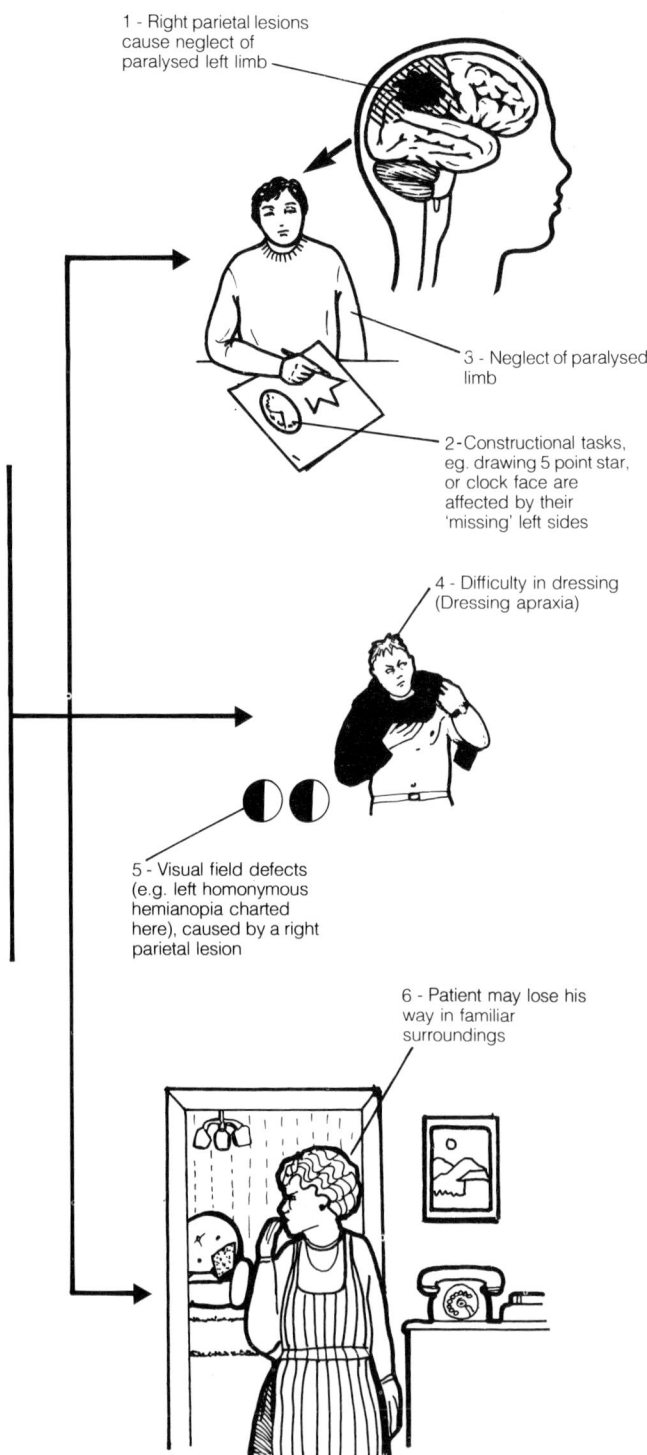

Right parietal lesions cause neglect of paralysed left limbs or the denial of a problem with the left side. There may be difficulty in dressing, (dressing apraxia), and the patient may lose his way in familiar surroundings. Constructional tasks or copying patterns, (eg. drawing a five-pointed star or copying a clock face) may be performed poorly and the patient may omit detail from the left side of drawings (eg. cramming all the numbers into the right side of a clock face). Visual field defects (homonymous hemianopias) may occur with parietal lobe lesions due to interruption of fibres in the optic radiation.

Higher Functions

Disorders of Gnosis – When a stimulus, (visual, auditory or tactile) is received by the brain, it is normally processed by various cortical association pathways so that a familiar object is recognised. A patient suffering from visual agnosia fails to recognise common objects although they are seen; (usually this is due to a left parieto-occipital lesion). Various forms of agnosia exist, for example auto-topagnosia, where a patient fails to recognise part of his body as his own.

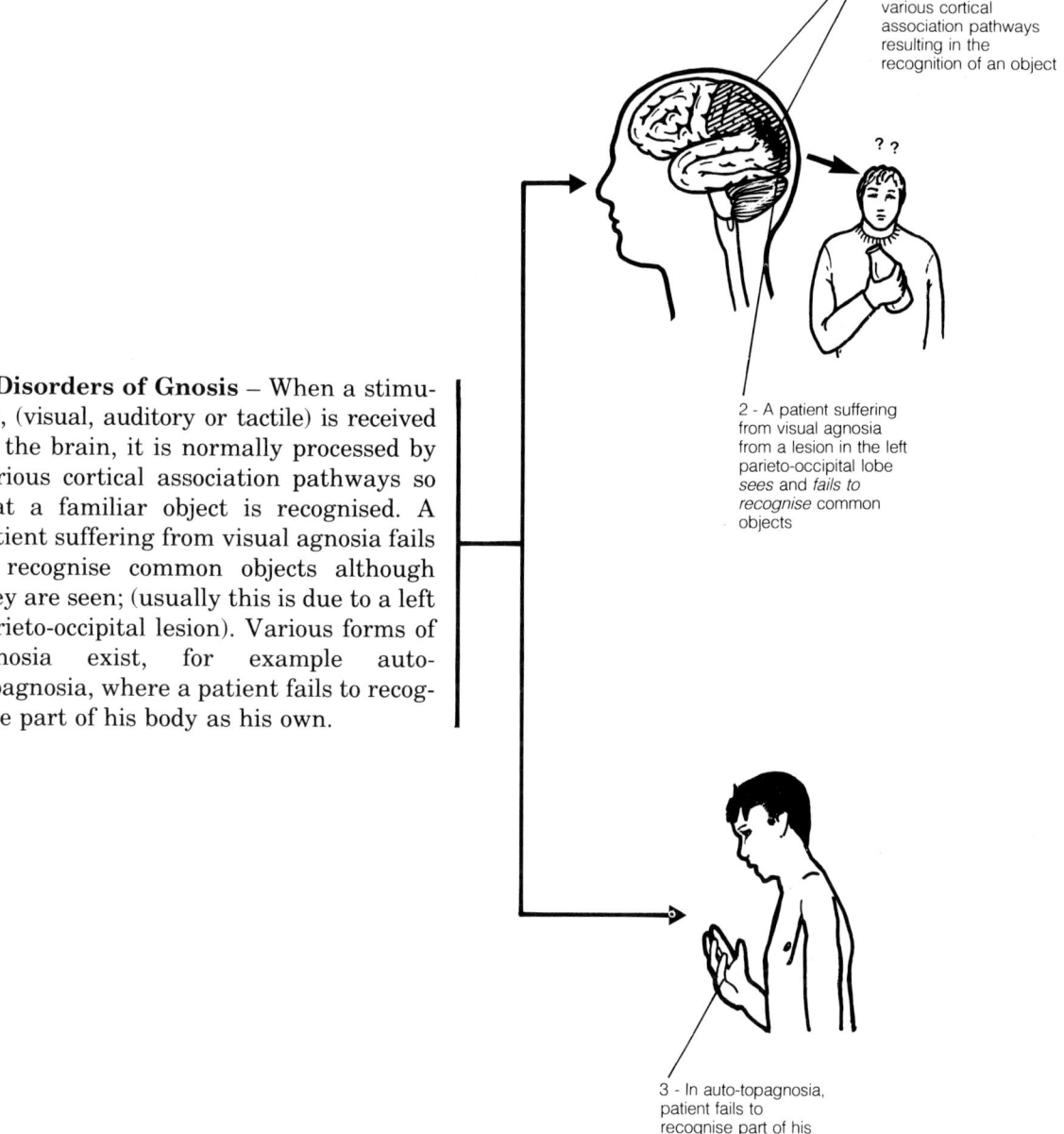

1 - All stimuli, visual, auditory or tactile received by the brain are processed by various cortical association pathways resulting in the recognition of an object

2 - A patient suffering from visual agnosia from a lesion in the left parieto-occipital lobe *sees* and *fails to recognise* common objects

3 - In auto-topagnosia, patient fails to recognise part of his own body

Temporal lobe

The main manifestations of lesions in the temporal lobes are temporal lobe epilepsy, visual field defects, (due to involvement of the lower part of the optic radiation) and amnesia. Amnesia is a disturbance of memory which spares both immediate recall for events and memory from the distant past; it does not significantly affect intelligence testing.

1 - Temporal lobe lesions may result in temporal lobe epilepsy and visual field defects (due to involvement of lower part of optic radiation) causing upper homonymous quadrantanopia as shown

2 - Amnesia affects the memory of immediate events and of the distant past, but not intelligence testing

2 - Spoken words

1 - Wernicke's aphasia is a form of sensory aphasia occuring in lesions of the dominant superior temporal gyrus. The patient is unable to understand any spoken words

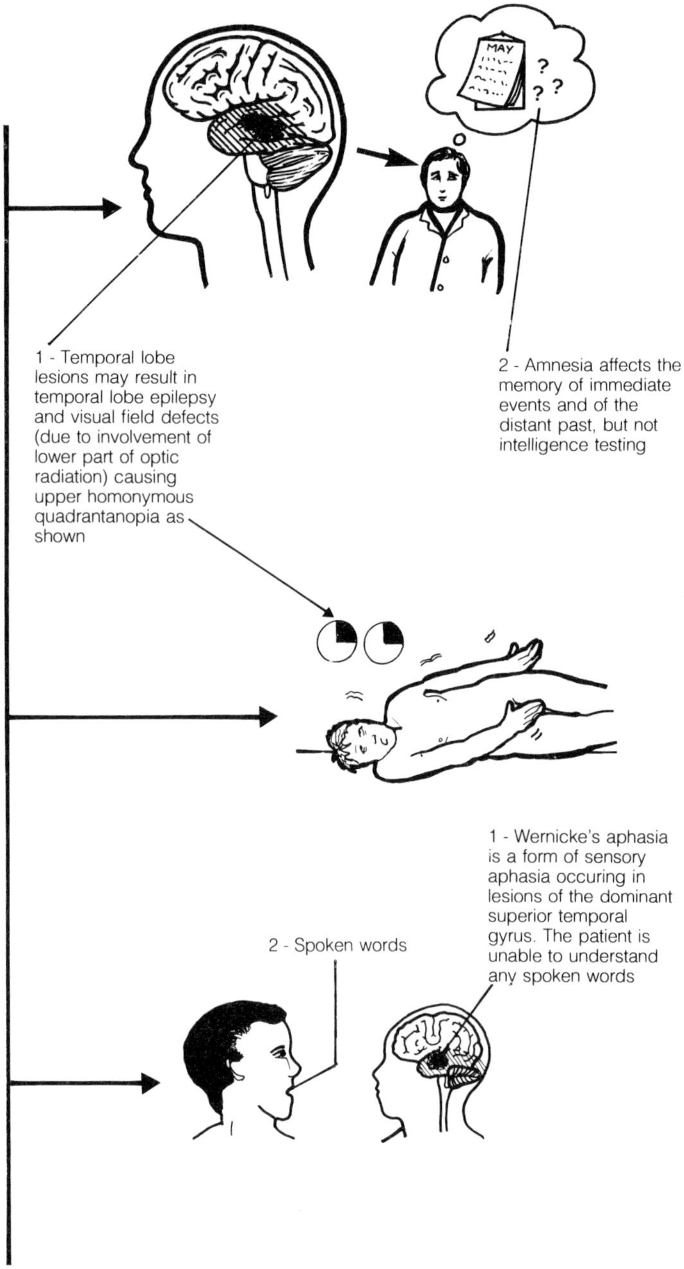

A particular form of sensory aphasia with severely impaired comprehension occurs with dominant, superior temporal gyrus lesions, situated posteriorly – Wernicke's aphasia.

Occipital lobe

Lesions in an occipital lobe cause disturbances in the contralateral visual field of varying severity up to a homonymous hemianopia. Discrete lesions may cause other (eg. central) field defects or distortion of vision and parieto-occipital lesions may lead to visual agnosia.

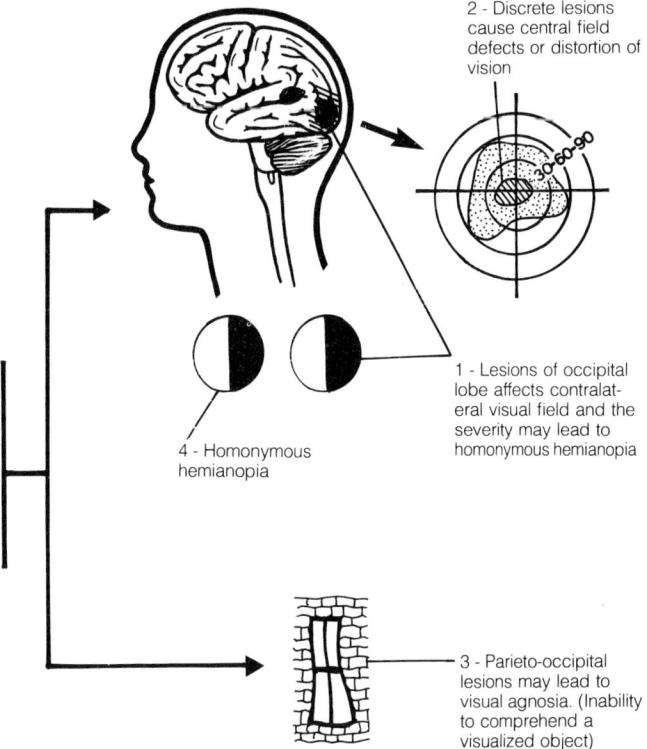

2 - Discrete lesions cause central field defects or distortion of vision

1 - Lesions of occipital lobe affects contralateral visual field and the severity may lead to homonymous hemianopia

4 - Homonymous hemianopia

3 - Parieto-occipital lesions may lead to visual agnosia. (Inability to comprehend a visualized object)

EXAMINATION/ASSESSMENT OF HIGHER CEREBRAL FUNCTIONS

The first objective is to assess the conscious level (eg. alert, attentive and co-operative or obtunded, even comatose). The patient having been engaged in conversation, the language he uses is noted – the fluency and articulation of speech and conversely the obvious comprehension of what is said to him. Direct tests of

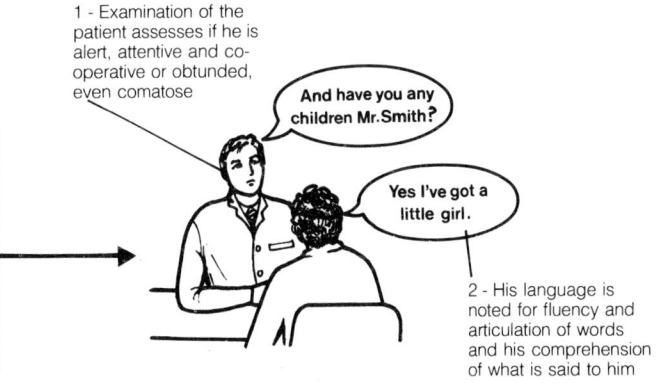

1 - Examination of the patient assesses if he is alert, attentive and co-operative or obtunded, even comatose

2 - His language is noted for fluency and articulation of words and his comprehension of what is said to him

Examination/Assessment of Higher Cerebral Functions

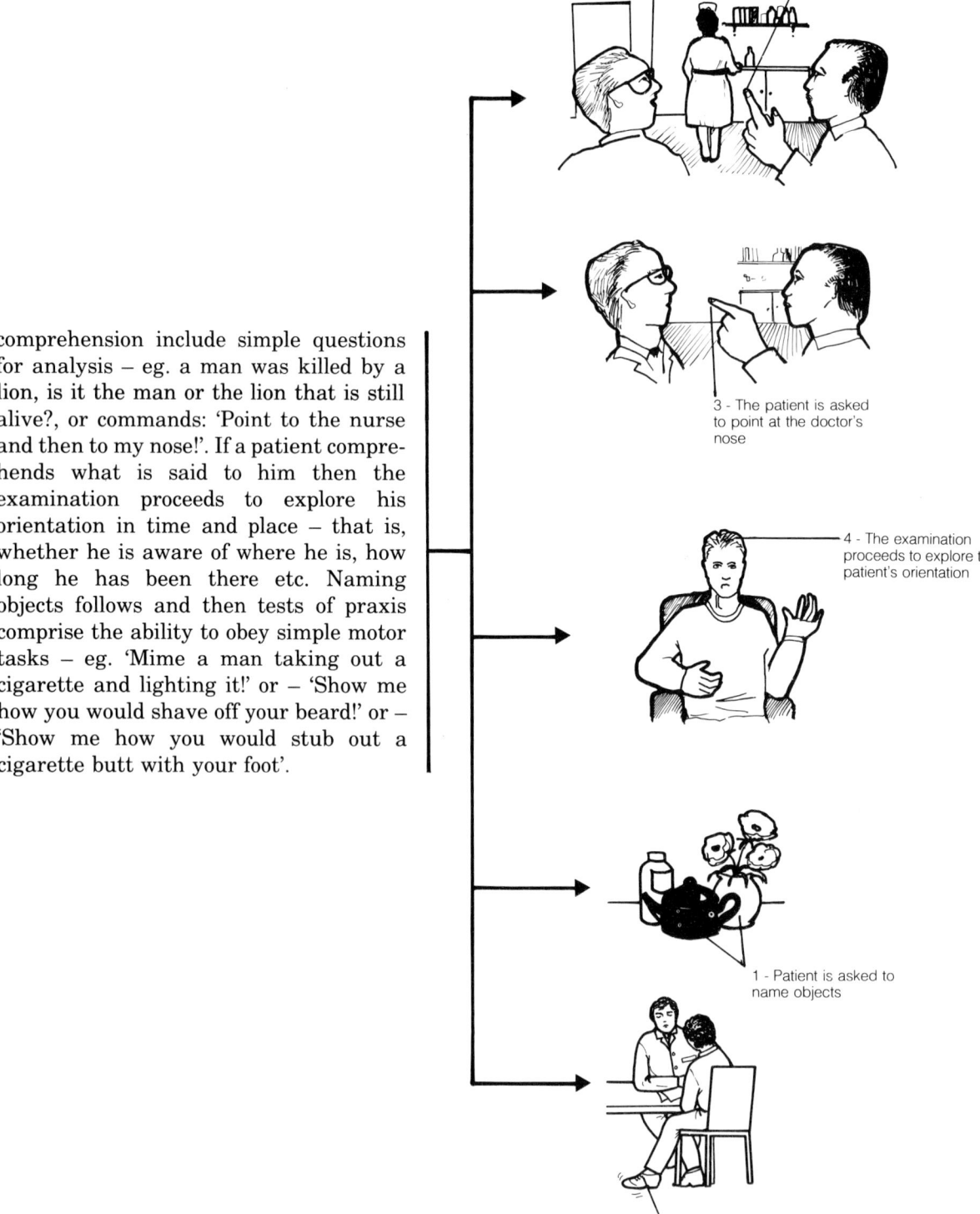

1 - Direct tests of comprehension performed by asking simple questions

2 - The patient is asked to point to the nurse

3 - The patient is asked to point at the doctor's nose

4 - The examination proceeds to explore the patient's orientation

1 - Patient is asked to name objects

2 - Mime tests: Stamp out a cigarette stub

comprehension include simple questions for analysis – eg. a man was killed by a lion, is it the man or the lion that is still alive?, or commands: 'Point to the nurse and then to my nose!'. If a patient comprehends what is said to him then the examination proceeds to explore his orientation in time and place – that is, whether he is aware of where he is, how long he has been there etc. Naming objects follows and then tests of praxis comprise the ability to obey simple motor tasks – eg. 'Mime a man taking out a cigarette and lighting it!' or – 'Show me how you would shave off your beard!' or – 'Show me how you would stub out a cigarette butt with your foot'.

Examination/Assessment of Higher Cerebral Functions

Tests of gnosis, drawing and constructional tasks, dressing, topographical orientation may all follow in appropriate patients and memory should always be tested – good simple tests includes questiong the patient as to how long he has been in hospital and the name of the ward. Good tests of recent memory include the ability to recall three or four unrelated words, (eg. pen, clock, bed, free).

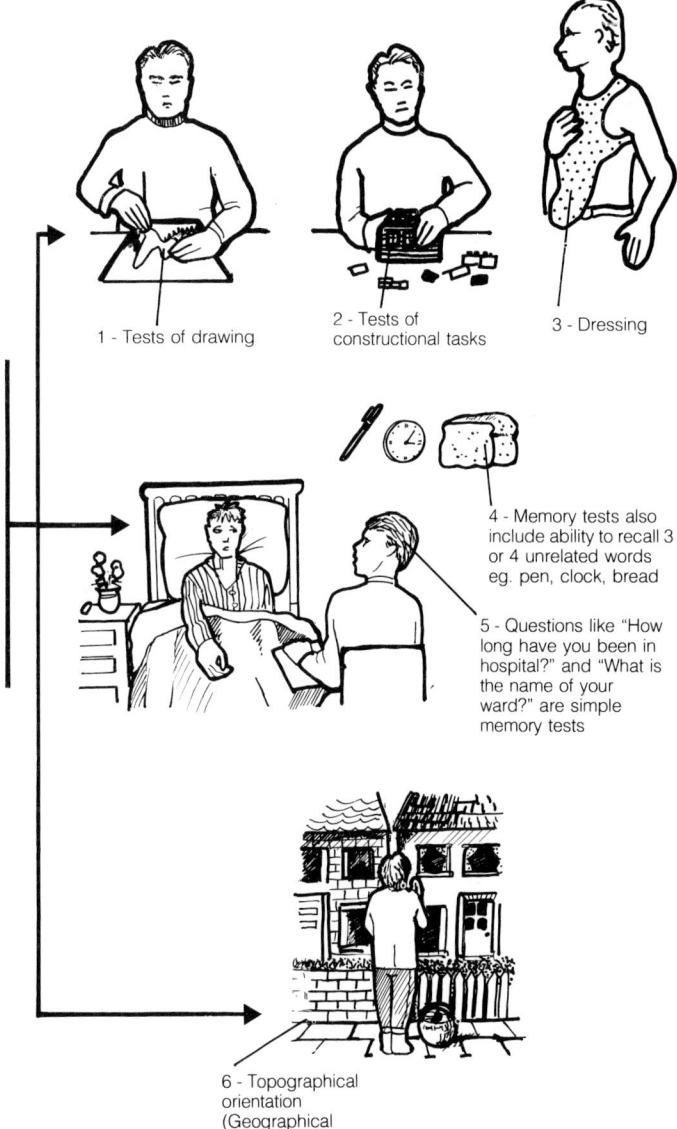

1 - Tests of drawing

2 - Tests of constructional tasks

3 - Dressing

4 - Memory tests also include ability to recall 3 or 4 unrelated words eg. pen, clock, bread

5 - Questions like "How long have you been in hospital?" and "What is the name of your ward?" are simple memory tests

6 - Topographical orientation (Geographical orientation) are tested

CRANIAL NERVE FUNCTIONS

The Olfactory Nerve (I) – The smell receptors in the nasal mucosa lead to the olfactory bulb, from which the olfactory tract stretches along the floor of the anterior cranial fossa to the uncus. Bilateral anosmia is most commonly due to head trauma. Unilateral anosmia occurs due to an olfactory groove or frontal lobe lesion. Smell is tested – one nostril at a time – with various musks, or more traditional smells (eg. coffee, peppermint, almond).

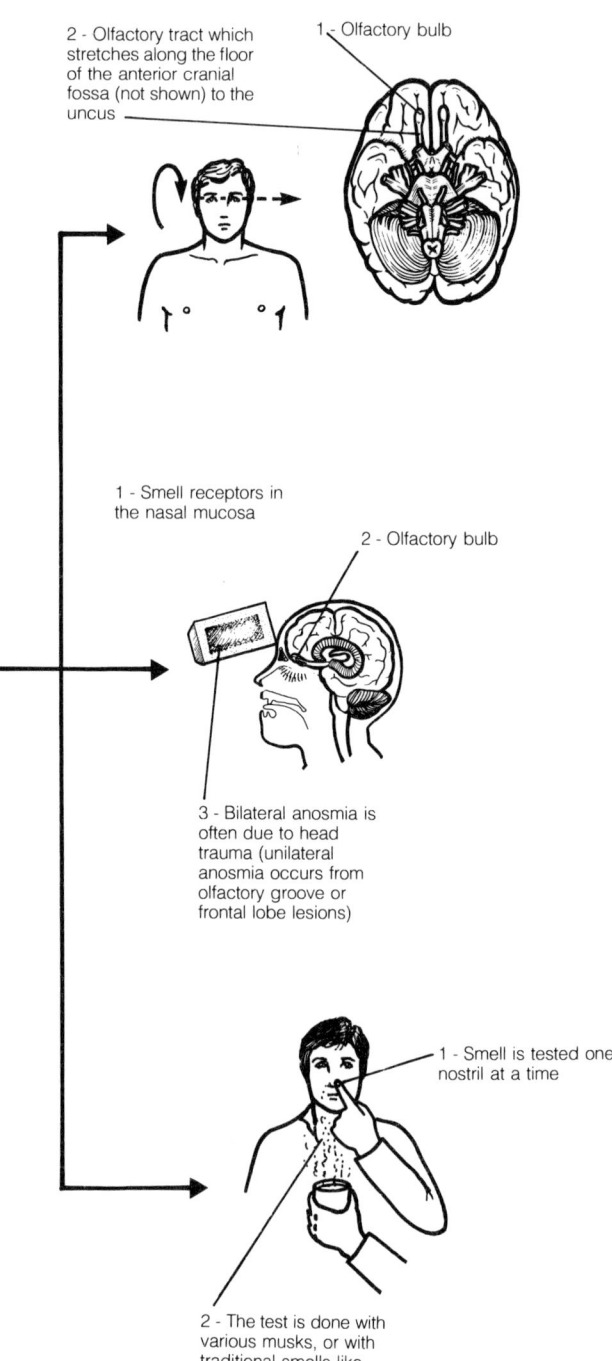

The Optic Nerve (II) – The nerve fibres originate in the retina, and those arising from the upper quadrants of the retina also lie superiorly in the optic nerve bundle. There is a partial decussation of the fibres from each optic nerve at the chiasm such that those from the nasal halves of each retina cross over to join those from the temporal half of the other retina. Each optic tract then leads to the lateral geniculate body from which the optic radiation takes impulses to the visual cortex in the occipital lobe. The result of the decussation is that visual stimuli from the contralateral half visual field pass to one visual cortex. The consequences of this are that optic nerve leions may lead to ipsilateral field defects (scotomata) or blindness; chiasmal lesions lead to bitemporal hemianopia and tract radiation or visual cortex lesions lead to homonymous hemianopia (or quadrantanopsia).

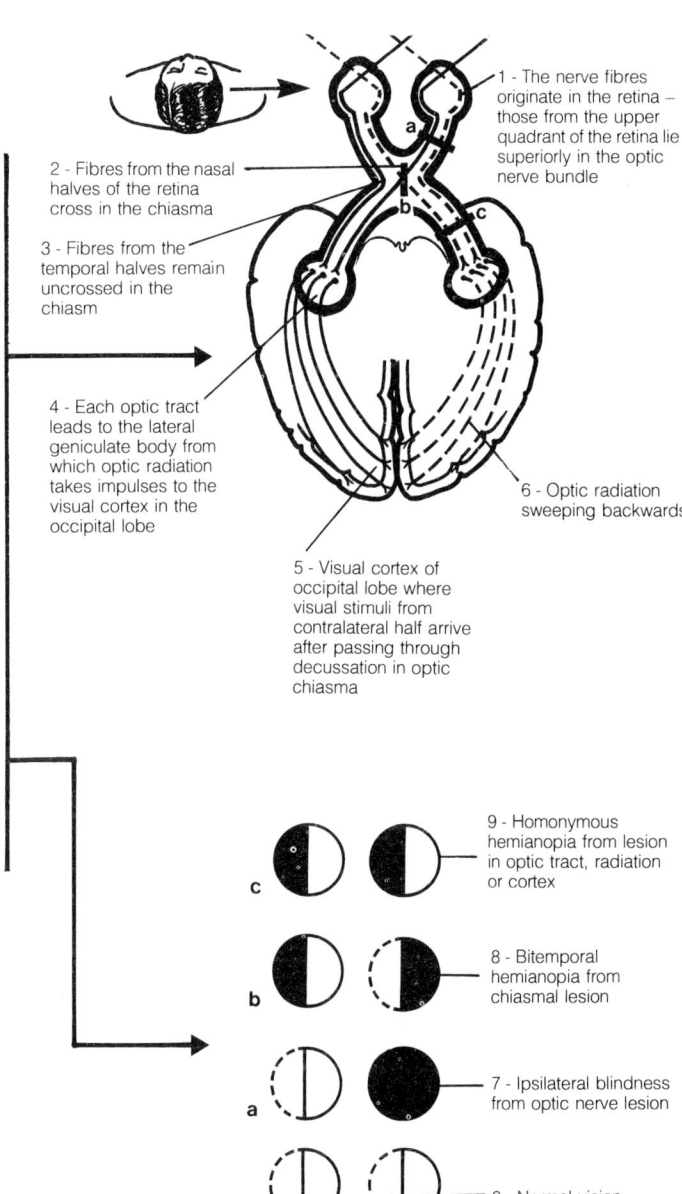

1 - The nerve fibres originate in the retina – those from the upper quadrant of the retina lie superiorly in the optic nerve bundle

2 - Fibres from the nasal halves of the retina cross in the chiasma

3 - Fibres from the temporal halves remain uncrossed in the chiasm

4 - Each optic tract leads to the lateral geniculate body from which optic radiation takes impulses to the visual cortex in the occipital lobe

5 - Visual cortex of occipital lobe where visual stimuli from contralateral half arrive after passing through decussation in optic chiasma

6 - Optic radiation sweeping backwards

9 - Homonymous hemianopia from lesion in optic tract, radiation or cortex

8 - Bitemporal hemianopia from chiasmal lesion

7 - Ipsilateral blindness from optic nerve lesion

8 - Normal vision

Cranial Nerve Functions

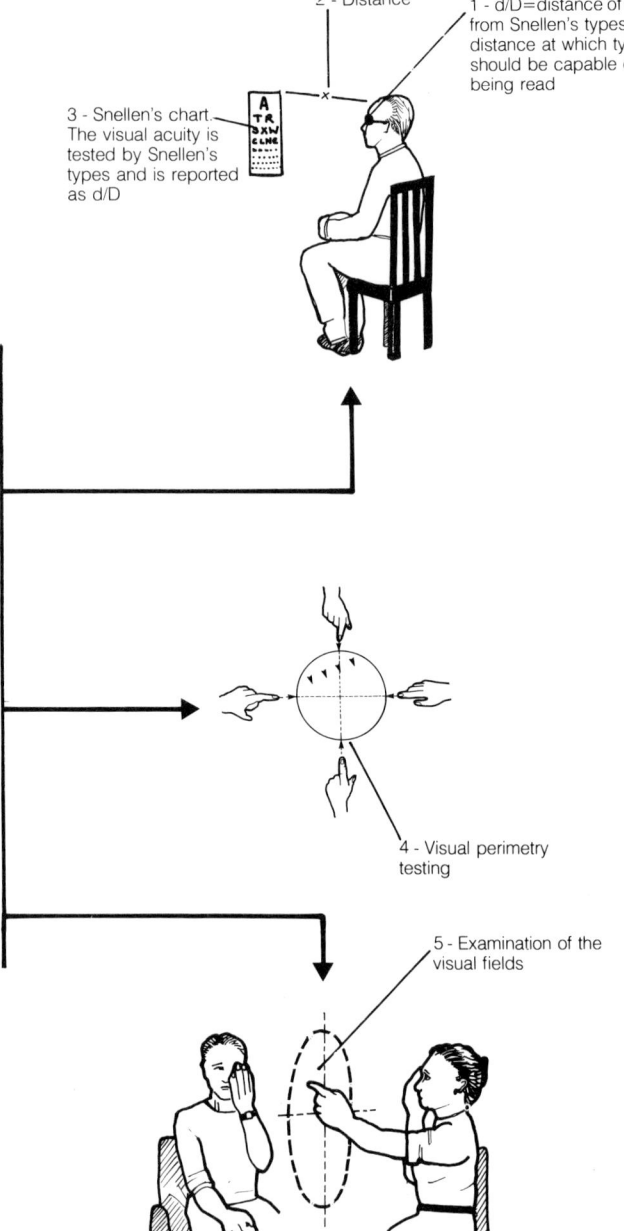

Examination of the visual pathways comprises tests of visual acuity, visual fields, and colour. The visual acuity is tested by Snellen's types and is reported as d/D = distance of eye from Snellen's types/distance at which type should be capable of being read. The visual fields are tested with the clinician sitting opposite the patient and holding the lid of one eye closed. Then the other eye is tested:- a test object, (usually a 5mm white pin head), is brought in from the four cardinal directions along an arc and matched against the clinician's own perimetry. The procedure is repeated for the other eye. More formal plotting of the visual fields (perimetry) is performed with a special screen. Perimetry does not detect scotomas within the visual fields, for which a Bjerrum screen is used.

Ophthalmoscopy– Examination of the fundus of the eye is part of the examination of the IInd nerve but can be of great general importance in neurology. The normal optic disc is pink but paler than the surrounding retina; it has distinct edges and the blood vessels can be clearly traced emanating out from its centre. In **papilloedema** (swelling of the disc), there is at first an engorgement of the veins and a pinker colour of the disc. Next, the nasal edge of the disc becomes blurred, after which the whole disc swells, no edges are apparent and circumferential haemorrhages may occur. Papilloedema classically occurs in raised intracranial pressure of which it is a very important diagnostic sign.

However, papilloedema also occurs in retinitis, retrobulbar neuritis, central retinal vein thrombosis, conditions of raised CSF protein (eg. Guillain Barré syndrome, macroglobulinaemia), hypocalcaemia and certain other conditions.

Optic atrophy is another important diagnostic observation that may relate to pathology beyond the optic nerve. In optic atrophy the disc is very pale in colour or white and usually flat. In primary optic atrophy, the optic disc becomes atrophic without any obvious preceding changes.

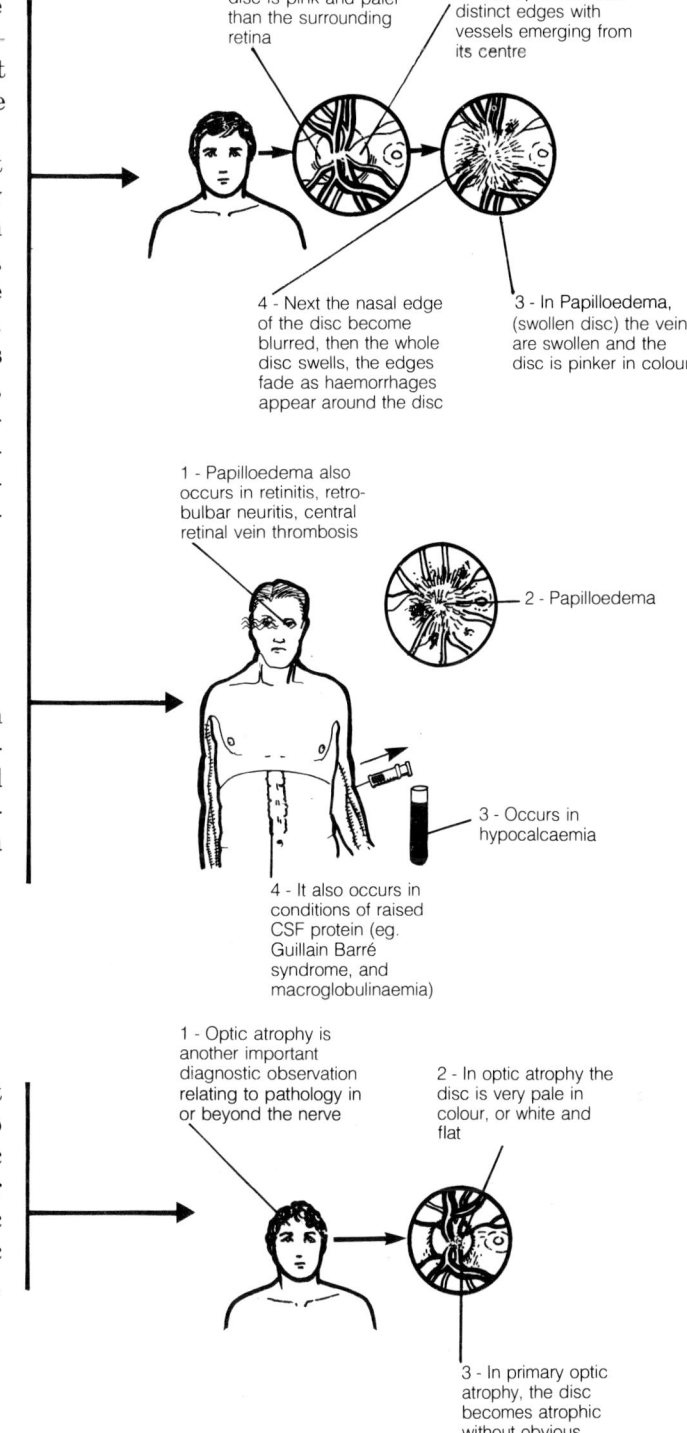

Cranial Nerve Functions

Primary optic atrophy may follow pressure on the optic nerve (eg. by tumour or trauma). Primary optic atrophy may also follow a vascular occlusive lesion of the optic nerve, (eg. cerebrovascular disease due to diabetes, old age or cranial arteritis). Less common causes include neurosyphilis, vitamin B_{12} deficiency, poisonings (eg. methanol, lead, arsenic). Secondary optic atrophy occurs after prolonged papilloedema; the disc swelling lessens as pallor and vascular atrophy set in. Consecutive optic atrophy resembles the optic disc in primary atrophy except that it is consequent upon retinal disease (eg. retinitis pigmentosa).

Whilst the optic disc yields the most valuable diagnostic information at fundoscopy, other diagnostic clues are sometimes available. Thus miliary tubercles in the choroid give the diagnosis of tuberculosis, a subhyaloid haemorrhage is an important clue in subarachnoid haemorrhage etc.

2 - e.g. by tumour or trauma

1 - Primary optic atrophy may follow pressure on the optic nerve

3 - It may also follow a vascular occlusive lesion of the optic nerve

6 - Vitamin B12 deficiency is a less common cause

4 - e.g. cerebrovascular disease due to diabetes, old age or cranial arteritis

5 - Less common causes include: neurosyphilis

7 - Poisoning is a rarer cause eg. by methanol, lead or arsenic

1 - Secondary optic atrophy after prolonged papilloedema

2 - The disc swelling lessens as pallor and vascular atrophy set in

1 - Other diagnostic clues are available from the optic disc

2 - Miliary tubercles in the choroid give the diagnosis of TB

3 - A subhyaloid haemorrhage is an important clue to subarachnoid haemorrhage

The Oculomotor (III) the Trochlear (IV) the Abducent (VI) Nerves

These three cranial nerves supply the six muscles that move the eye. The superior oblique muscle is supplied by the trochlear nerve (IV), the lateral rectus by the abducent nerve (VI) and all the others by the oculomotor nerve (III). Due to the direction of pull of these muscles, the oblique muscles act as pure elevators and depressors of the eye in adduction (inferior oblique to elevate, superior oblique to depress), whereas the superior and inferior recti act as pure elevators and depressors of the abducted eye, (superior rectus to elevate, inferior rectus to depress). This is all explicable on simple mechanics, remembering that a muscle acts most efficiently when stretched along its direction of pull. In central gaze both obliques and recti contribute to elevation and depression. The lateral and medial recti are simple abductors and adductors of the eye.

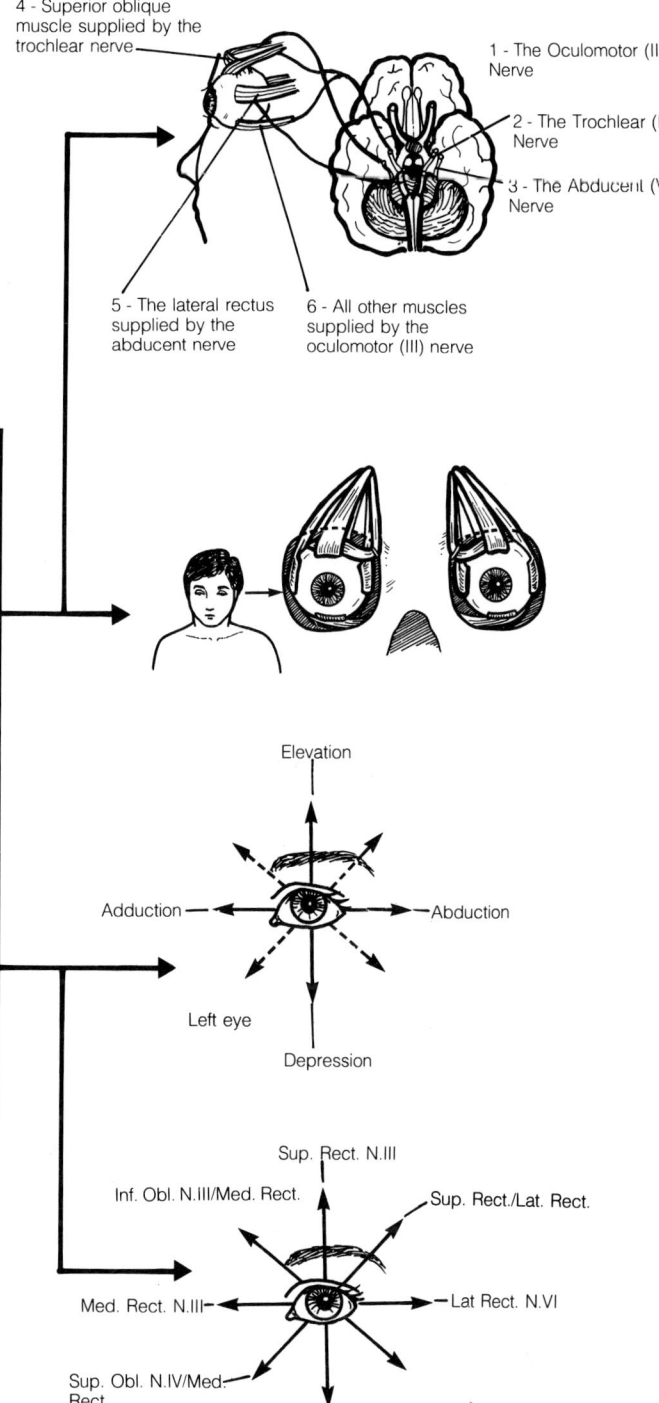

Cranial Nerve Functions

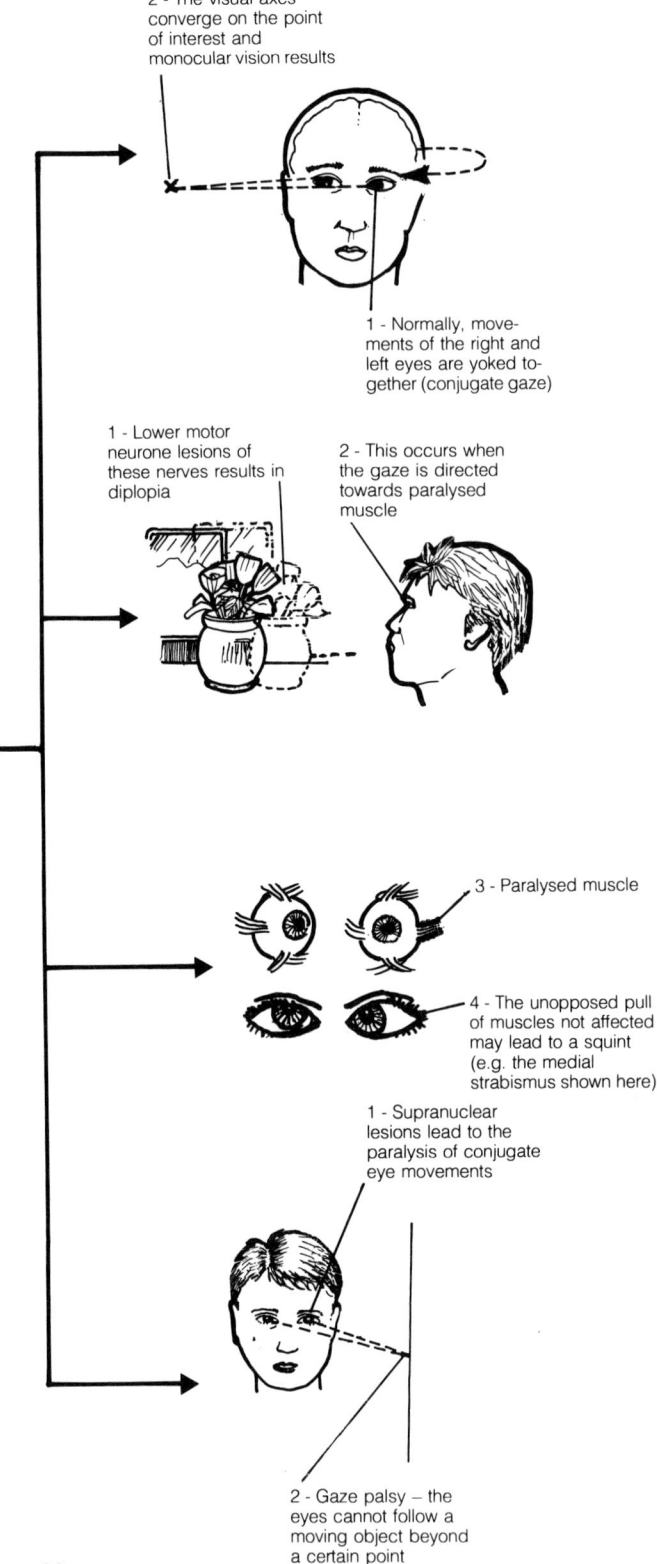

Normally, movements of the right and left eyes are yoked together (conjugate gaze), so that the visual axes converge on the point of interest and monocular vision results. Infranuclear (lower motor neurone) lesions of III, IV or VI lead to paralysis of individual eye muscles, often with double vision (diplopia) on attempted gaze in the direction of pull of the paralysed muscle; the unopposed pull of the muscles not affected by the paralysis may lead to a squint. Supranuclear lesions lead to the paralysis of conjugate eye movement (gaze

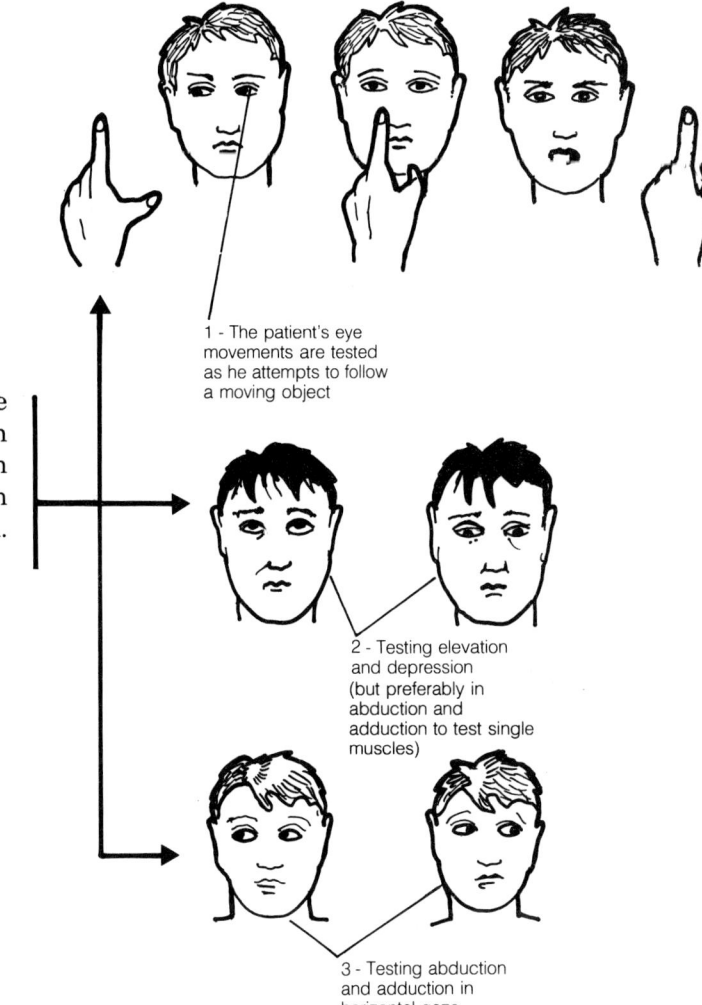

1 - The patient's eye movements are tested as he attempts to follow a moving object

2 - Testing elevation and depression (but preferably in abduction and adduction to test single muscles)

3 - Testing abduction and adduction in horizontal gaze

palsies). The patient's eye movements are tested when he attempts to follow an object – testing abduction and adduction in horizontal gaze and testing elevation and depression in abduction and adduction. The patient is asked to report diplopia.

IIIrd Nerve Palsy – The IIIrd nerve emerges from the ventrolateral aspect of the midbrain lateral to the basilar artery and passes between the posterior cerebral and superior cerebellar arteries and close to the posterior communicating artery. Arterial aneurysms at these sites may compress the IIIrd nerve. The IIIrd nerve passes in the wall of the cavernous sinus to gain access to the orbit through the superior orbital fissure.

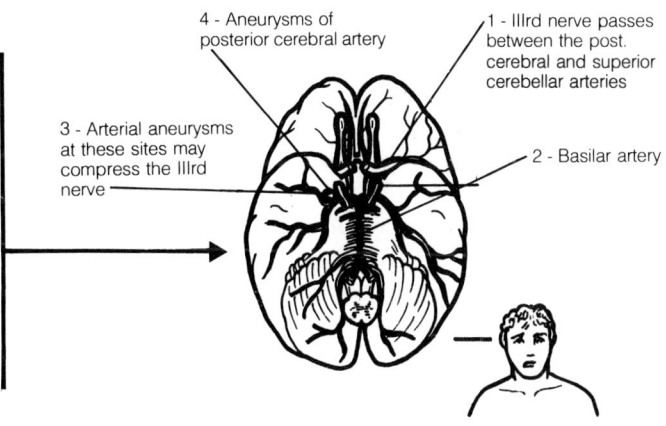

1 - IIIrd nerve passes between the post. cerebral and superior cerebellar arteries

2 - Basilar artery

3 - Arterial aneurysms at these sites may compress the IIIrd nerve

4 - Aneurysms of posterior cerebral artery

The most obvious feature of IIIrd nerve palsy is ptosis (drooped lid), and when the eyelid is lifted the eye is looking down and out, due to the unopposed lateral rectus and superior oblique actions. When the patient attempts to look down and in, the superior oblique produces intorsion of the eye as visible evidence to the clinician that the IVth nerve function is intact.

3 - This is due to unopposed lateral rectus, and superior oblique actions

1 - Ptosis (drooped lid) is the most obvious feature of IIIrd nerve palsy

2 - When the eyelid is lifted the eye is looking down and out

1 - Aneurysm, especially of the posterior communicating artery is a common cause of IIIrd nerve palsy

Common causes of IIIrd nerve palsy include aneurysms, (especially of the posterior communicating artery), trauma, basal meningitides (infective, malignant or granulomatous sarcoid), diabetes, collagen disease (especially temporal arteritis), tumours (eg. nasopharyngeal carcinoma or tumours of the tip of the petrous temporal bone or even parapituitary region), cavernous sinus lesions (eg. thrombosis). Lesions tending to compress the

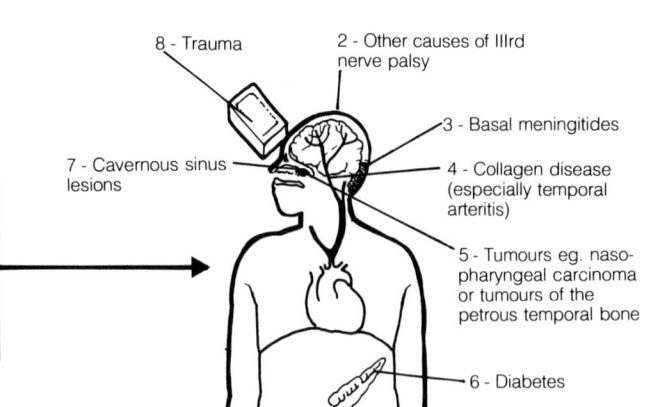

8 - Trauma
2 - Other causes of IIIrd nerve palsy
7 - Cavernous sinus lesions
3 - Basal meningitides
4 - Collagen disease (especially temporal arteritis)
5 - Tumours eg. nasopharyngeal carcinoma or tumours of the petrous temporal bone
6 - Diabetes

IIIrd nerve (eg. aneurysms) may cause pain and changes in the pupil, whilst the medical causes of IIIrd nerve palsy tend to spare the pupil. Many palsies of the IIIrd nerve are partial – only some muscles being affected.

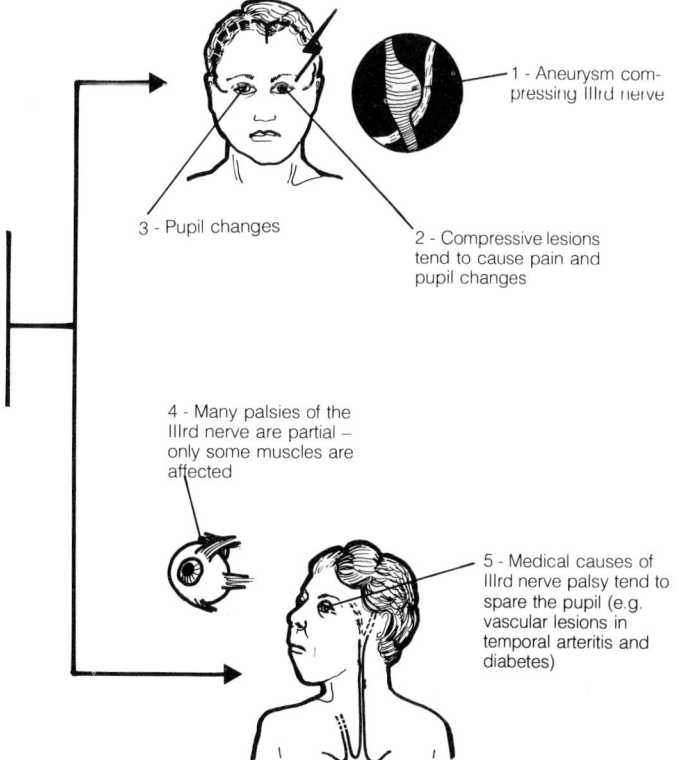

IVth Nerve Palsy – The left IVth nerve nucleus in the midbrain supplies the right superior oblique and vice versa, due to a decussation of the IVth nerves in the superior medullary velum, immediately after leaving the brainstem. As pineal tumours may compress this area, these are one cause of bilateral IVth nerve palsies.

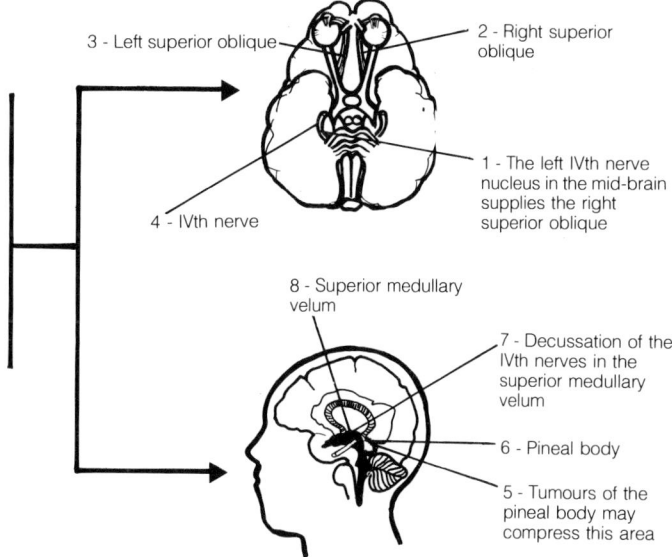

Cranial Nerve Functions

The main symptom of IVth nerve palsy is diplopia on looking downwards and inwards – eg. a patient may complain of diplopia on looking to find his way down a flight of stairs.

1 - The main symptom of IVth nerve palsy is diplopia on looking downwards and inwards. (eg. when walking down stairs)

2 - Failure to depress and adduct right eye due to right IVth nerve palsy

VIth Nerve Palsy – The VIth nerve emerges from the ponto-medullary junction and ascends to reach the middle temporal fossa by a near right-angle bend over the the petrous apex. It is here that it is so liable to compression in raised intracranial pressure. It then lies free in the cavernous sinus to gain access to the orbit through the superior orbital fissure. The IVth and VIth nerves are liable to many of the causes of paralysis enumerated for the IIIrd nerve but the VIth nerve is particularly vulnerable in raised intracranial pressure.

3 - It is very liable to compression in raised intracranial pressure

2 - It ascends to reach the middle temporal fossa by a near 90° bend over the petrous apex

1 The VIth nerve emerges from the ponto-medullary junction

4 - Failure to abduct right eye due to right VIth nerve palsy

Cranial Nerve Functions

The patient with VIth nerve palsy usually has an easily visible squint (medial strabismus) and diplopia worst in lateral gaze.

When testing the eye movements of a patient complaining of diplopia, certain 'rules' apply which help to define the paralysed muscle:

1) False images are consistently peripheral ones.

2) The peripheral images are always seen by the affected eye.

3) Separation of images is always maximal in the direction of pull of the paralysed muscle.

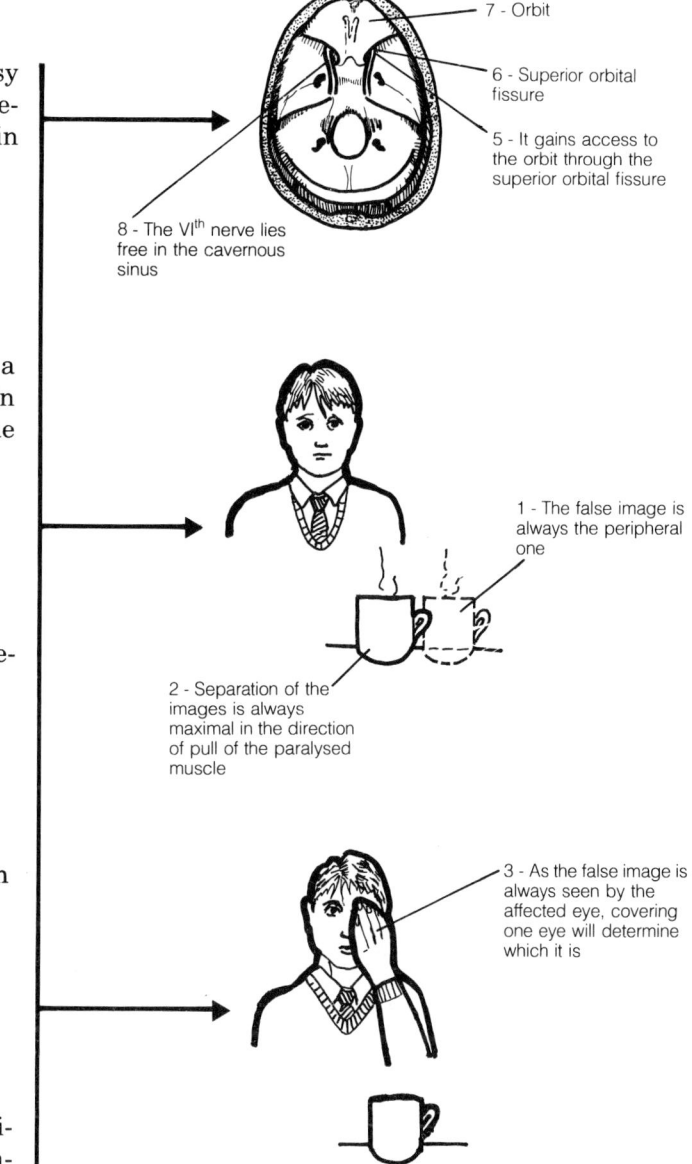

7 - Orbit

6 - Superior orbital fissure

5 - It gains access to the orbit through the superior orbital fissure

8 - The VIth nerve lies free in the cavernous sinus

1 - The false image is always the peripheral one

2 - Separation of the images is always maximal in the direction of pull of the paralysed muscle

3 - As the false image is always seen by the affected eye, covering one eye will determine which it is

Brainstem lesions causing oculomotor palsies – Various discrete brainstem lesions may produce ocular palsies associated with other focal neurological signs. For example, when there is a lesion (eg. infarct) of the IIIrd nerve fibres where they pass through the red nucleus (a synapse station for contralateral cerebellar fibres) there may be a IIIrd nerve palsy and ataxia in the contralateral arm (**Benedikt's syndrome**). When the IIIrd nerve is locally damaged as it emerges from the midbrain cerebral peduncle, a 'crossed' (i.e. contra-lateral) hemiplegia due to pyramidal tract damage here may be associated with the IIIrd nerve lesion (**Weber's syndrome**).

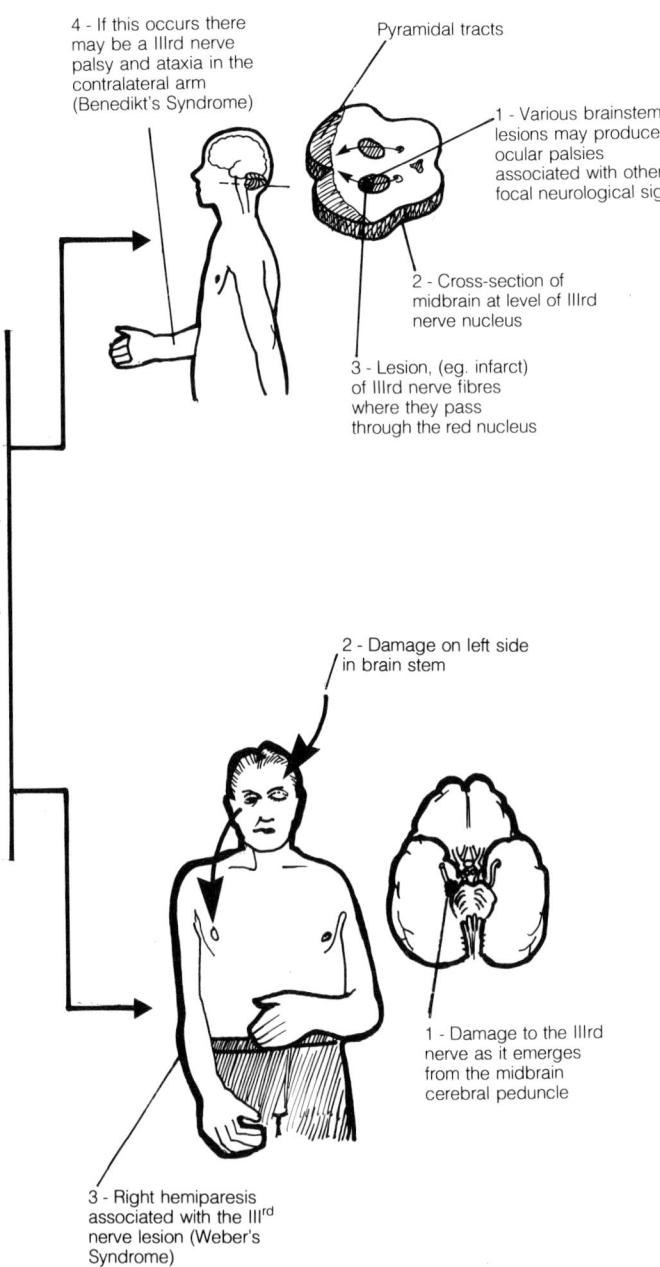

4 - If this occurs there may be a IIIrd nerve palsy and ataxia in the contralateral arm (Benedikt's Syndrome)

Pyramidal tracts

1 - Various brainstem lesions may produce ocular palsies associated with other focal neurological signs

2 - Cross-section of midbrain at level of IIIrd nerve nucleus

3 - Lesion, (eg. infarct) of IIIrd nerve fibres where they pass through the red nucleus

2 - Damage on left side in brain stem

1 - Damage to the IIIrd nerve as it emerges from the midbrain cerebral peduncle

3 - Right hemiparesis associated with the IIIrd nerve lesion (Weber's Syndrome)

Ophthalmoplegia due to muscle disorders – In the differential diagnosis of all the foregoing causes of ocular muscle weakness come the muscular disorders that may give rise to opthalmoplegias – notably myasthenia gravis, (fatiguable weakness responding to Tensilon) and exophthalmic ophthalmoplegia.

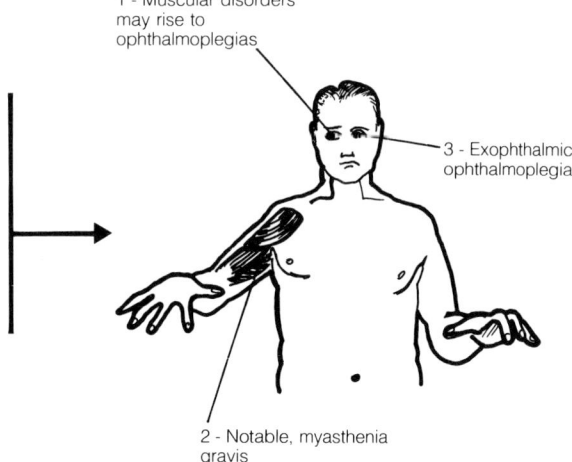

THE PUPIL

The pupil consists of a ring of constrictor fibres controlled by the parasympathetic pathways, (the 'pupillo-constrictor centre' being a relay station in the IIIrd nerve nuclear complex in the midbrain and synapsing in the ciliary ganglion before postganglionic fibres pass to the eye); the sympathetic dilator fibres are radially arranged. (See also **The Pupil** in **Illustrated Lecture Series on Ophthalmology**).

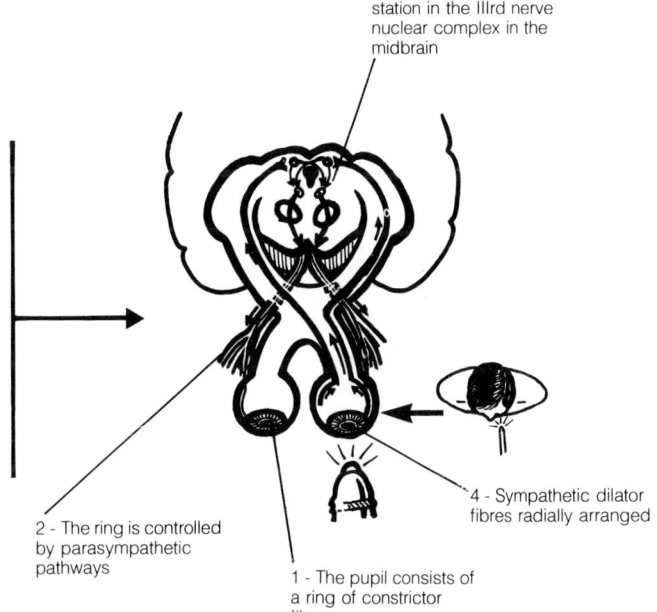

The Pupil

These dilator fibres can be identified as passing from the hypothalamus via the brainstem and passing caudally to D1 level where they leave the CNS to synapse in the paravertebral sympathetic ganglia; the post-ganglionic fibres then ascend into the cranium as a meshwork of nerve fibres in the carotid bundle (the carotid nerve). Sympathetic fibres are then transferred to the IIIrd nerve, (thence to levator palpebrae superioris), and to the nasociliary branch of the Vth nerve, the pupillary supply being given off as the long ciliary nerves.

1 - Dilator fibres passing from the hypothalamus via the brainstem

2 - They pass to DI level

3 - At DI level they leave the CNS to synapse in the paravertebral sympathetic ganglia

4 - They ascend into the cranium as a meshwork of nerve fibres in the carotid bundle

5 - Sympathetic fibres are then transferred to the IIIrd nerve

Paralysis of the parasympathetic fibres produces a fixed dilated pupil due to unopposed sympathetic tone; and a sympathetic paralysis produces pupilloconstriction and ptosis, (together with slight enophthalmos and absent sweating on the ipsilateral side of the face – Horner's syndrome).

1 - Paralysis of the parasympathetic fibres produces a fixed dilted pupil due to unopposed sympathetic tone

2 - Sympathetic paralysis produces pupillo constriction and ptosis

3 - Sweat test shows absent sweating on the ipsilateral side of the face in Horner's Syndrome

Horner's syndrome   Normal pupil

The pupils of the two eyes are normally equal in size; absolute size is largely determined by the ambient illumination. A light shone in one eye produces bilateral pupillary constriction due to bilateral transmission of afferent stimuli (concensual reaction). The reflex activity of the pupils is tested to light (there should be a brisk contraction of both pupils in response to a light stimulus to one or both retinae), and then to accommodation – there should be bilateral pupillary constriction as a patient looks from a distant to a near object.

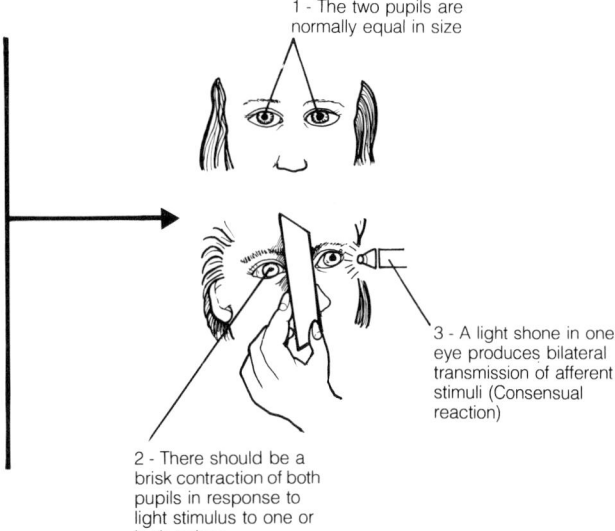

A patient who is bilaterally blind due to occipital lobe disease will still have normal pupillary reflexes as these are subserved at brainstem level. Lesions in the midbrain (pretectal area) may lead to fixed dilated pupils and this is often coupled with an impairment of upward gaze – Parinaud's syndrome. A patient

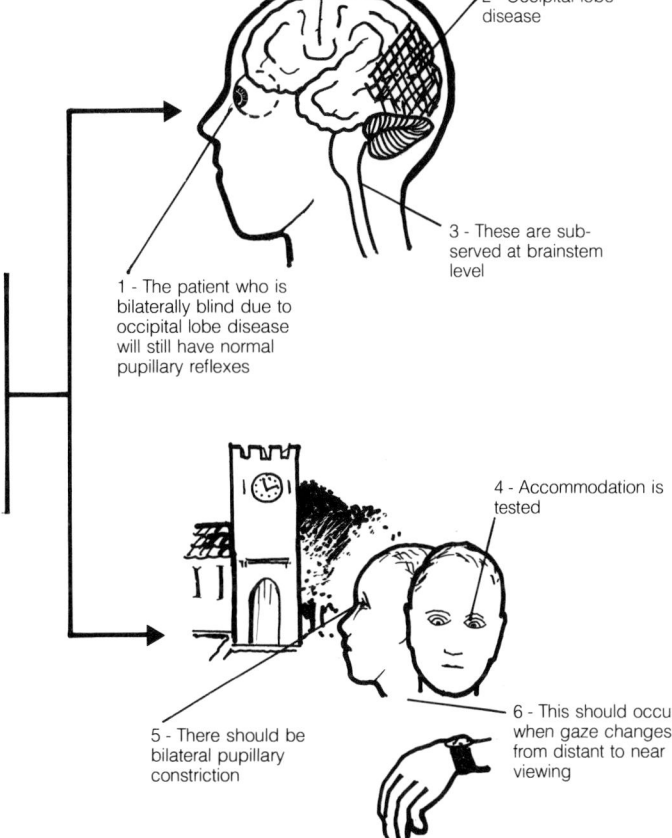

The Pupil

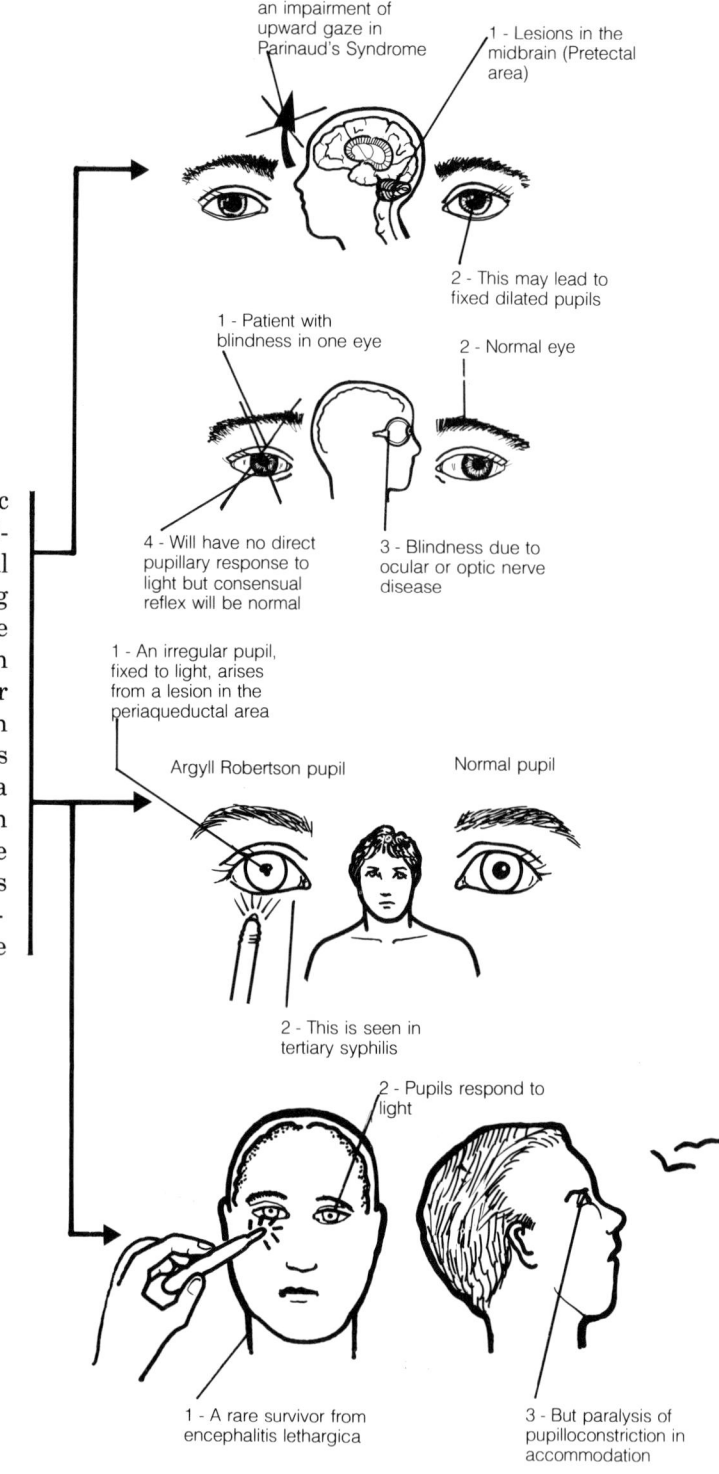

blind in one eye due to ocular or optic nerve disease will have no direct pupillary response to light but the concensual reflex will be normal. Other interesting pupillary abnormalities include the **Argyll Robertson** (AR) pupil – seen in tertiary syphilis, where an irregular pupil, fixed to light, arises from a lesion in the periaqueductal area. The nowadays rare survivor from encephalitis lethargica had paralysis of pupilloconstriction in accommodation but not to light, (reverse AR pupil). Compressive IIIrd nerve lesions (especially tentorial pressure cones), Posterior communicating aneurysms, ridge meningiomas, etc) also affect the pupil-leading to pupil dilation. A rare degenerative condition of the ciliary ganglion leading to a fixed, dilated pupil occurs in young adult women and may be associated with depressed deep tendon reflexes and rarely depressed sweating (**Holmes-Adie pupil**). Actually prolonged gazing at a near object or prolonged bright light will induce pupilloconstriction in these women.

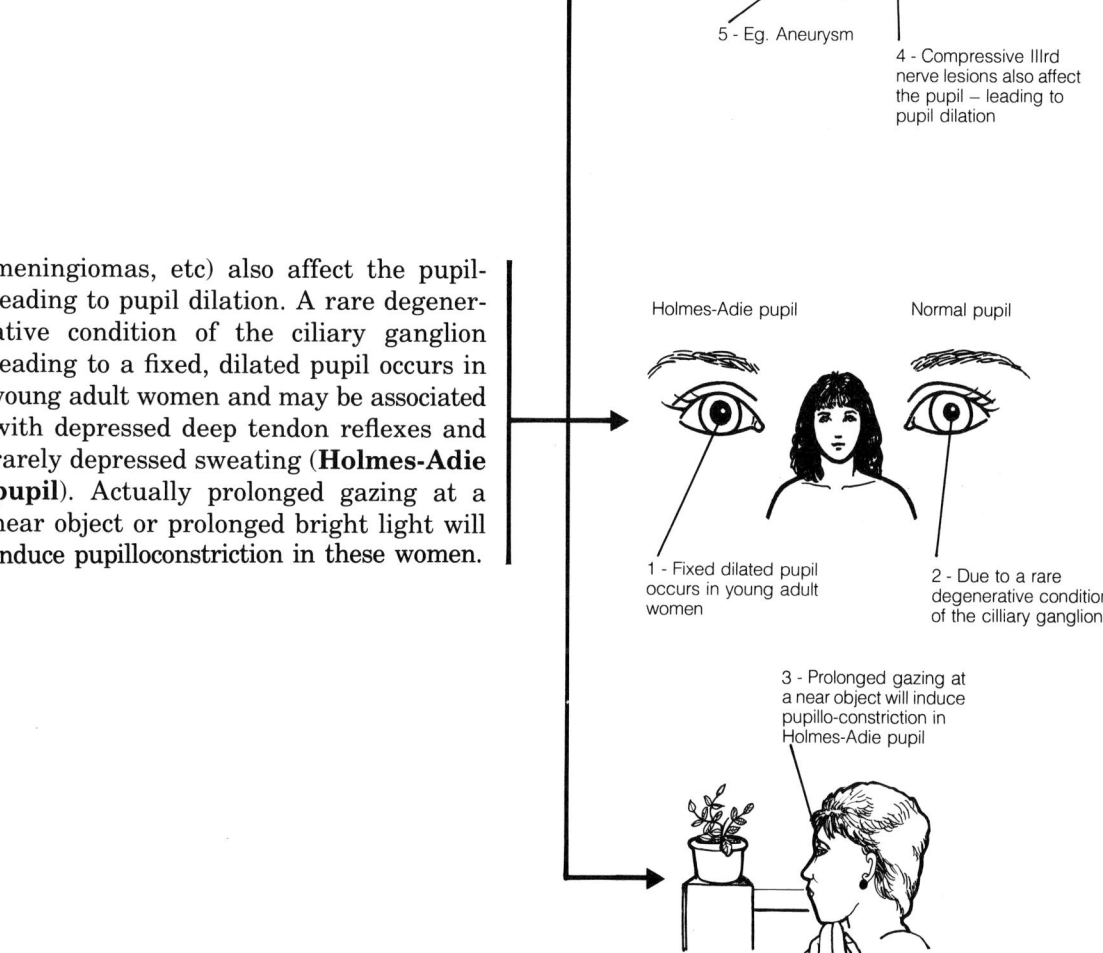

5 - Eg. Aneurysm

4 - Compressive IIIrd nerve lesions also affect the pupil – leading to pupil dilation

Holmes-Adie pupil   Normal pupil

1 - Fixed dilated pupil occurs in young adult women

2 - Due to a rare degenerative condition of the cilliary ganglion

3 - Prolonged gazing at a near object will induce pupillo-constriction in Holmes-Adie pupil

The Pupil

The **symptom complex** called **Horner's syndrome** has already been mentioned. This is caused by interruption of the sympathetic supply to one side of the head. The lesion may be in the hypothalamus, brainstem or cervical cord, or in the spinal root of T1 and T2, or in the ascending sympathetic nerve chain in the neck or base of skull.

For example, an apical carcinoma of bronchus may infiltrate the T1 nerve root causing a Horner's syndrome, (as well as a T1 root lesion). A CNS cause of Horner's syndrome may be distinguished from a post-synaptic (post-ganglionic) lesion because of the phenomenon of post-denervation hypersensitivity. Adrenaline 1:1000 eye drops are too weak to induce pupillary dilation in normal eyes or those with Horner's due to central causes; however, in the post-synaptic group of lesions, the pupil dilates.

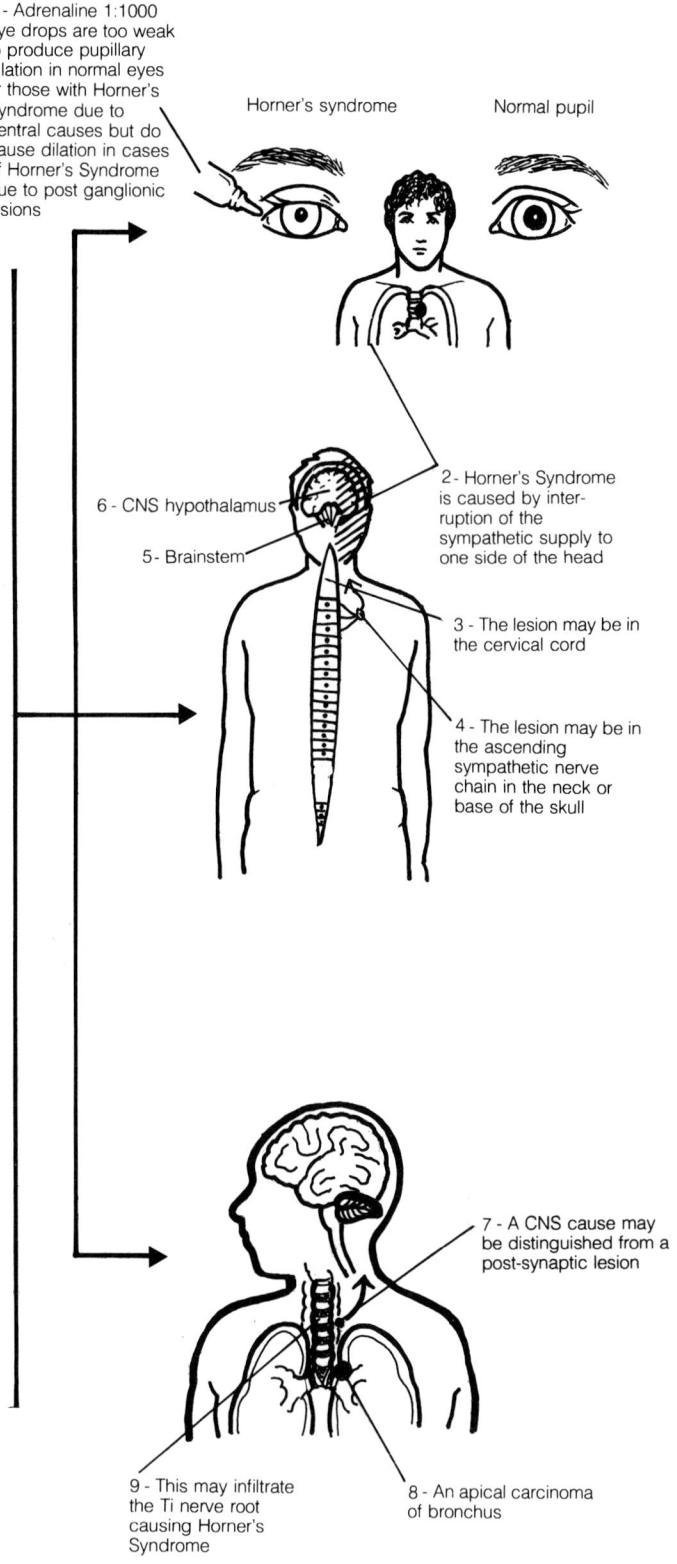

1 - Adrenaline 1:1000 eye drops are too weak to produce pupillary dilation in normal eyes or those with Horner's Syndrome due to central causes but do cause dilation in cases of Horner's Syndrome due to post ganglionic lesions

2 - Horner's Syndrome is caused by interruption of the sympathetic supply to one side of the head

3 - The lesion may be in the cervical cord

4 - The lesion may be in the ascending sympathetic nerve chain in the neck or base of the skull

5 - Brainstem

6 - CNS hypothalamus

7 - A CNS cause may be distinguished from a post-synaptic lesion

8 - An apical carcinoma of bronchus

9 - This may infiltrate the Ti nerve root causing Horner's Syndrome

In the comatose patient, detection of pupillary inequality is probably the single most vital physical sign. Until proven otherwise, the fixed dilated pupil indicates a tentorial pressure cone on that side of the head, (i.e. pressure prolapse of the temporal lobe through the tentorium with IIIrd nerve palsy). This finding requires an immediate neurosurgical opinion.

Bilateral fixed pupils are one of the physical signs of death.

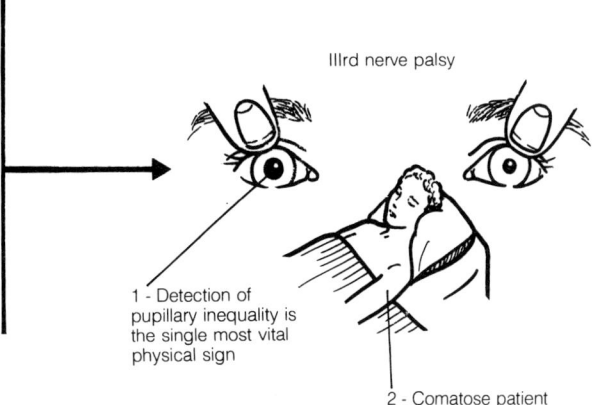

1 - Detection of pupillary inequality is the single most vital physical sign

2 - Comatose patient

NYSTAGMUS

Nystagmus is caused by a weakness in conjugate deviation of both eyes or an imbalance of the postural control of ocular movements. There is a tendency for the eyes to drift back slowly to the central position, (and this is the abnormal movement), before they deviate again with a

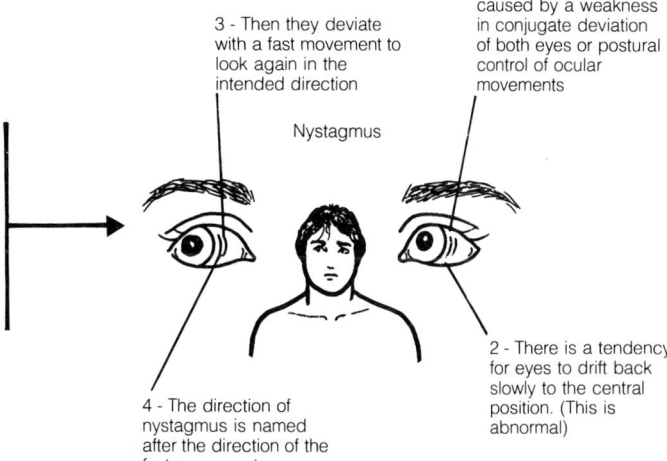

1 - Nystagmus — caused by a weakness in conjugate deviation of both eyes or postural control of ocular movements

2 - There is a tendency for eyes to drift back slowly to the central position. (This is abnormal)

3 - Then they deviate with a fast movement to look again in the intended direction

4 - The direction of nystagmus is named after the direction of the fast movement

Nystagmus

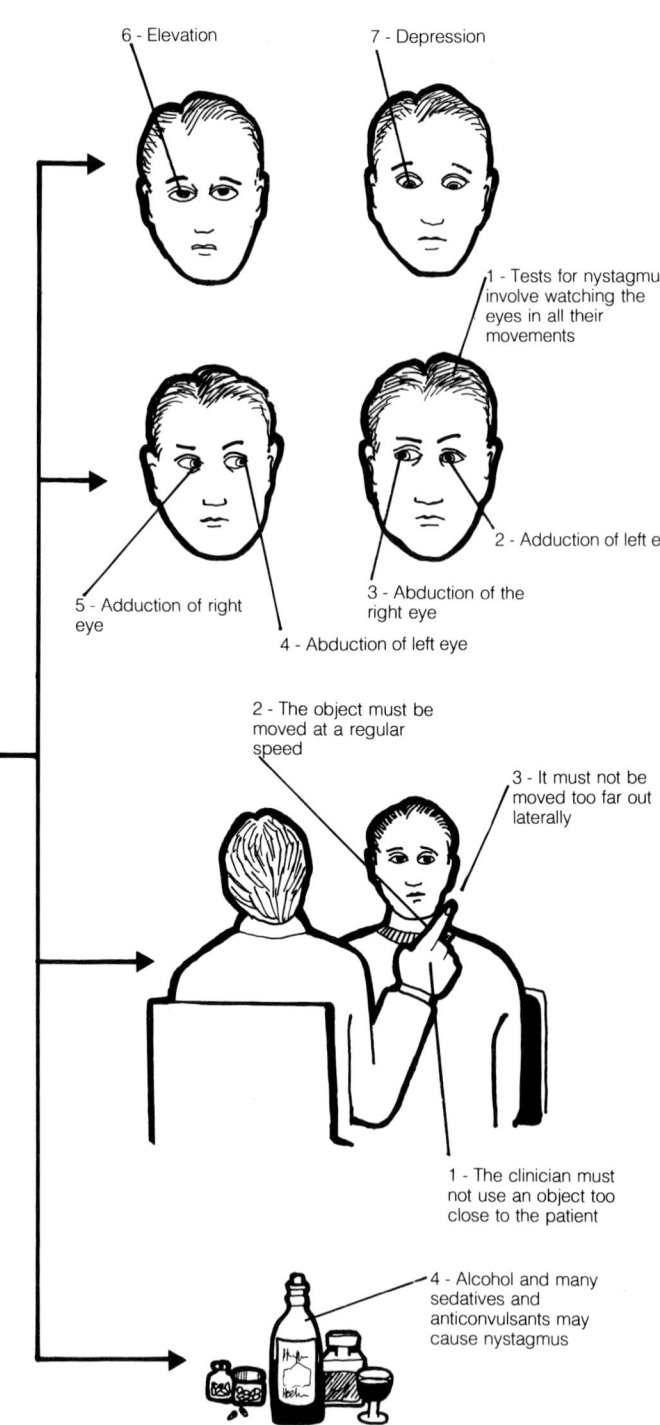

fast movement to look again in the intended direction; the direction of nystagmus is named after the direction of the fast movement. Tests for nystagmus involve watching the eyes as they abduct and adduct, elevate and depress. The clinician must not use an object for fixation that is too close to the patient nor move it too far out laterally, nor move it too fast, as all these procedures may provoke minor degrees of nystagmus in normal people. Alcohol and many sedative and anticonvulsant drugs may cause nystagmus.

There are certain congenital forms of nystagmus which tend to be continuous and pendular (i.e no slow and no fast components); this 'pendular' type of nystagmus may also be provoked by bright light in albinos and miners.

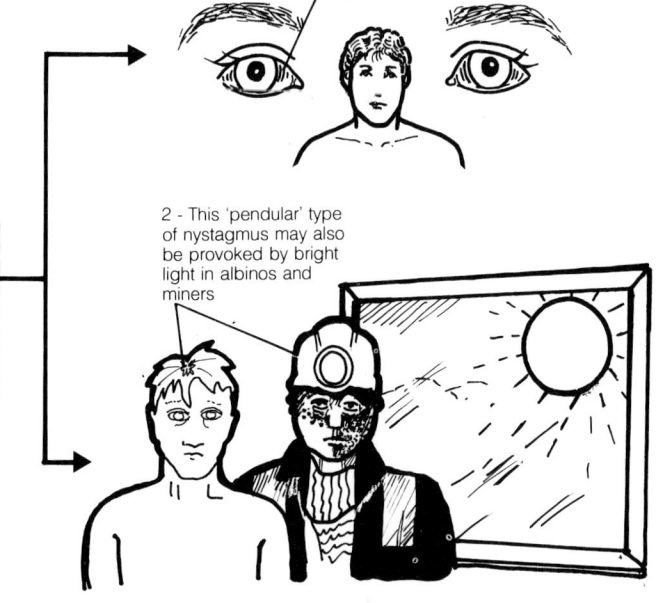

Any lesion affecting the vestibular nerve or semicircular canals will disrupt the 'push-pull' vestibular control of eye movements and lead to vestibular nystagmus. Vestibular nystagmus is precipitated by sudden movements of the head and the eye movements are "jerky". If damage occurs in the right vestibular apparatus which tends to turn the eyes to the left, then on attempted gaze to the left the eyes drift slowly back towards central gaze before a fast, jerky 'flick' again turns them to the left (left horizontal nystagmus). When the lesion is in the periphery,

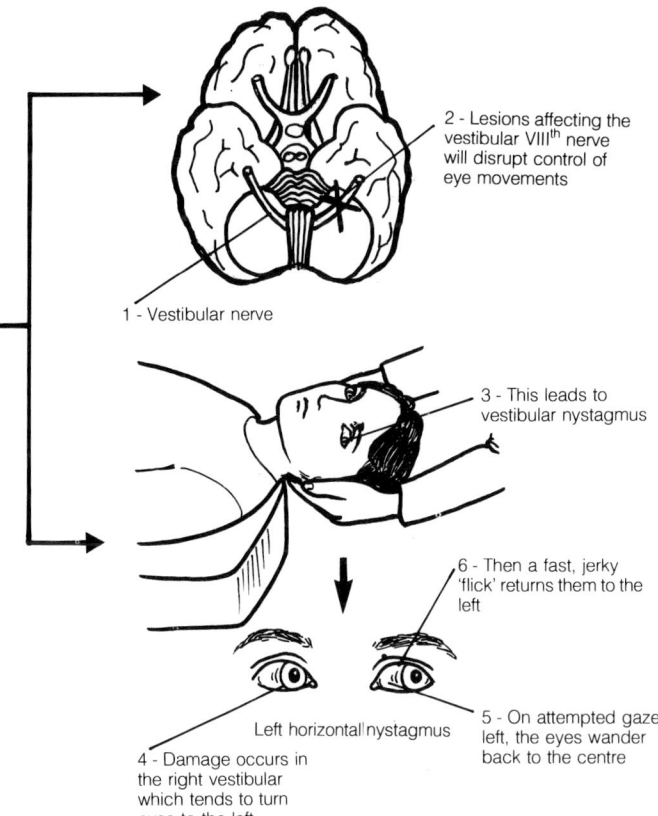

(e.g. late **Menière's disease**, acoustic neuroma), compensation may occur and the nystagmus reduces with time; when the lesion is centrally sited in the brain-stem (e.g. multiple sclerosis, cerebrovascular accident, glioma, syringobulbia – affecting central vestibular pathways), the nystagmus is persistant. Central lesions may produce vertical nystagmus as well as horizontal nystagmus.

Cerebellar nystagmus is a poorly understood type of nystagmus that may be interconnected with cerebellar-vestibular links. In cerebellar nystagmus the fast jerk component of nystagmus is towards the damaged cerebellar hemisphere.

A distinctive type of nystagmus (ataxic nystagmus) is classically associated with multiple sclerosis. This condition tends to affect the medial longitudinal fasciculus – a brainstem nerve fibre bundle connecting the IIIrd, IVth and VIth nuclei; the consequence is that the medial recti fail to contract with the lateral recti on attempted lateral gaze to either side. There is marked nystagmus of the abducting eye.

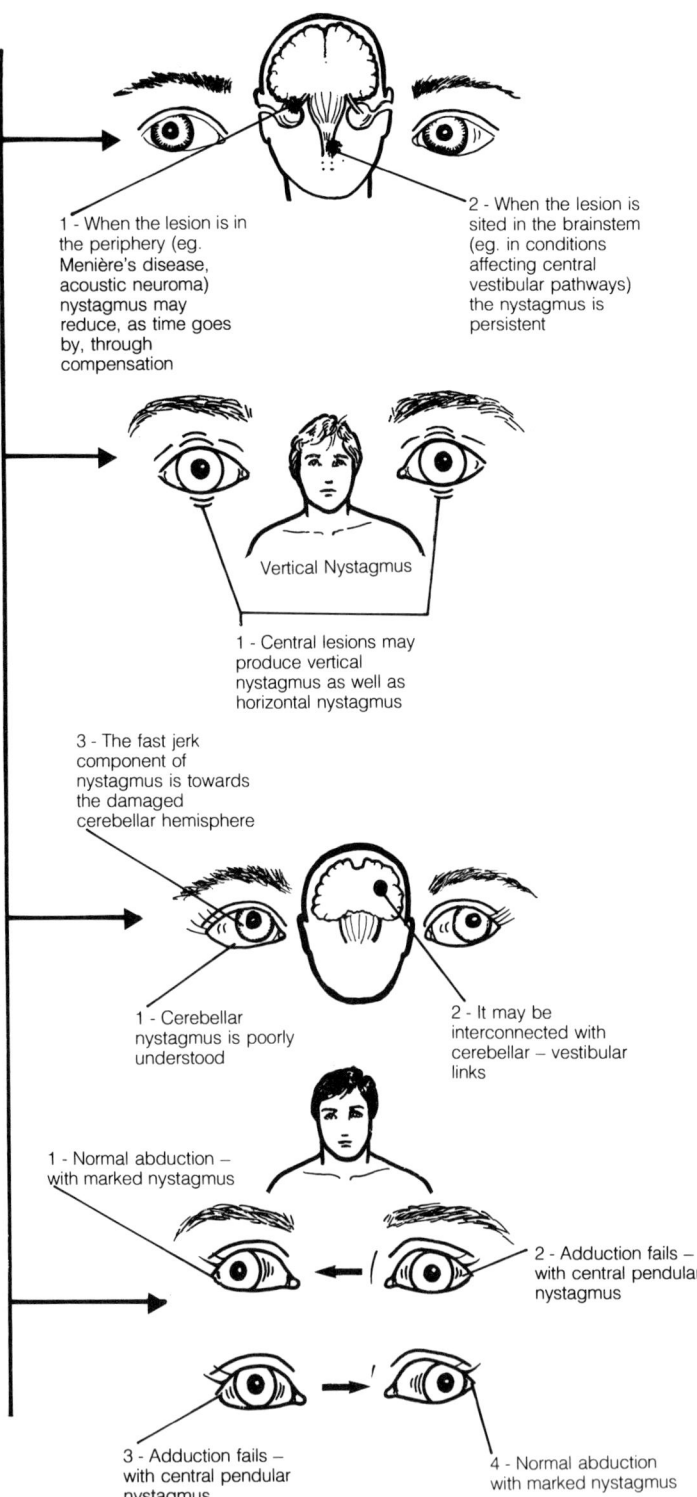

CRANIAL NERVE FUNCTIONS (continued)

The Trigeminal Nerve (V)

The Vth nerve carries sensation from the face and anterior scalp, mouth and nasal passages. It also provides motor innervation to the muscles of mastication, and the corneal and jaw jerks are dependent on Vth nerve function. The Vth nerve emerges as distinct sensory and motor roots from the ventrolateral aspect of the pons. The roots pass anteriorly towards the tip of the petrous temporal bone where the sensory root expands into the Gasserian (semilunate) ganglion before giving off the three main sensory divisions. The ophthalmic division (Va) supplies the skin of the forehead, anterior scalp and eyeball. The maxillary division (Vb) supplies the infraorbital region of the cheek, upper lip and mucous membrane of the upper gum. The mandibular division (Vc) supplies the skin overlying the mandible, lower lip, lower gum and ordinary (somatic) sensation to the anterior two-thirds of the tongue and floor of mouth.

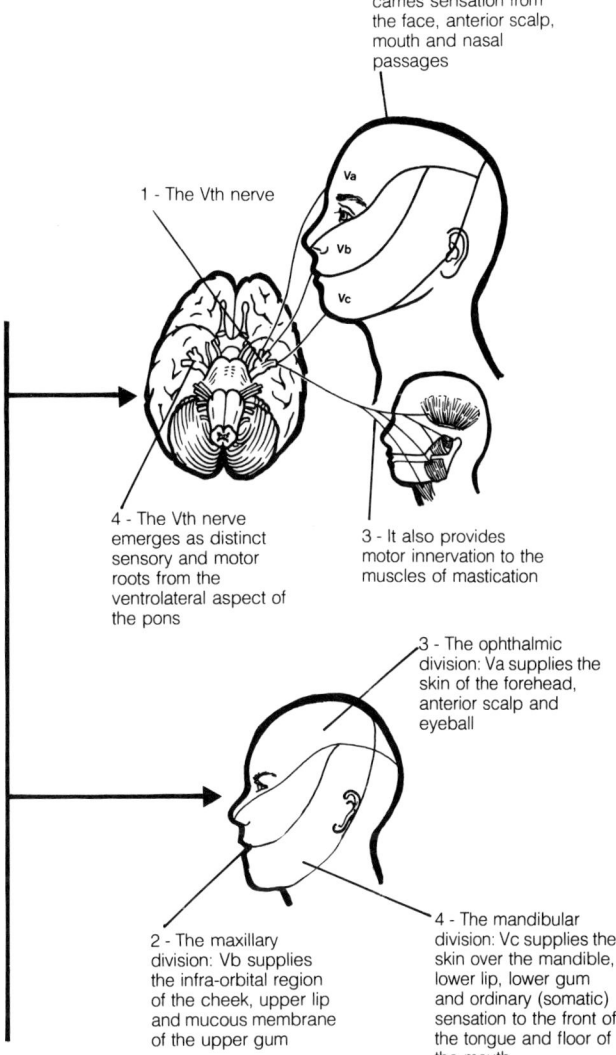

Cranial Nerve Functions (continued)

The major muscles innervated by V are temporalis, masseter, medial and lateral pterygoids and tensor veli palatini. When there is paralysis due to a unilateral Vth motor root lesion, there is deviation of the jaw towards the paralysed side on mouth opening due to the unopposed lateral pterygoid contraction, and masseter and temporalis, (both of which are wasted) may be felt to remain slack on biting. The jaw jerk is tested with the jaw hanging limply open on the clinician's forefinger whilst a patella hammer gives a brisk downward blow to the mandible, (transmitted throught the clinician's thumb).

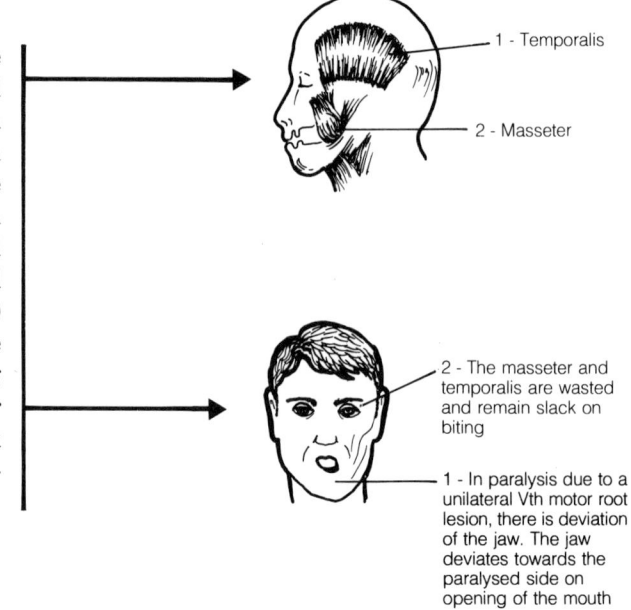

1 - Temporalis
2 - Masseter

2 - The masseter and temporalis are wasted and remain slack on biting

1 - In paralysis due to a unilateral Vth motor root lesion, there is deviation of the jaw. The jaw deviates towards the paralysed side on opening of the mouth

The jaw jerk is pathologically brisk in bilateral upper motor neurone lesions. The jaw jerk may help in the determination of the level of neurological damage in spastic tetraplegia.

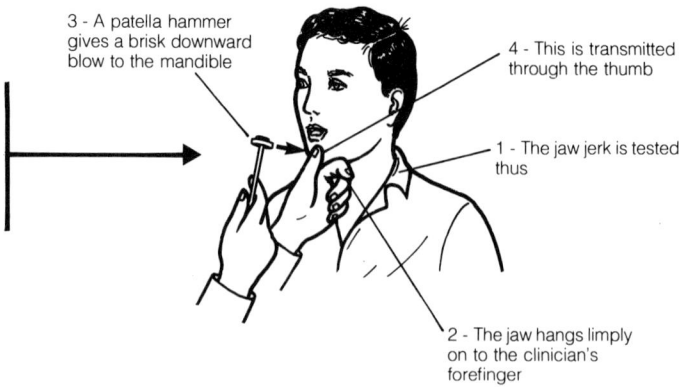

3 - A patella hammer gives a brisk downward blow to the mandible
4 - This is transmitted through the thumb
1 - The jaw jerk is tested thus
2 - The jaw hangs limply on to the clinician's forefinger

The corneal reflex depends on the Vth nerve for the sensory input, but the VIIth nerve provides the motor pathway. The reflex is elicited with a wisp of cotton-wool, brought in from the patient's side to lightly and quickly touch the cornea. In normal people such a contact should elicit an immediate bilateral blinking. A diminished corneal reflex may be the earliest sign of damage to Va, for example intra-cranial compression of V by an acoustic neuroma, a neurofibroma of Vth nerve, a herpes zoster infection, (which commonly afflicts Va). Inflammation of the air cells of the petrous apex (usually spreading from a suppurative mastoiditis), may involve and damage the semi-lunate ganglion, (**Gradenigo's syndrome**).

Within the brainstem the several and long trigeminal nuclei are particularly prone to damage (e.g. vascular, trauma, demyelinating disease, syringobulbia, syphilis etc,).

Trigeminal Neuralgia (Tic Douloureux)
This is predominantly a condition of the elderly and is slightly more common in females. The neuralgia comprises very brief, shooting paroxysms of intense pain in the distribution of V. Not infrequently, there are "trigger areas" on the skin, which if touched, will provoke a spasm — thus some patients are unable to wash or shave parts of their face for fear of eliciting a paroysm of pain.

There is no sensory loss. The condition may remit for periods but usually returns and later on becomes more persistent. Rarely, the condition occurs as part of multiple sclerosis or as a lesion affecting the trigeminal nerve (e.g. acoustic neuroma); usually there is no known underlying cause.

Carbamazepine (100-200mg tds) is the drug of first choice and phenytoin may be added usefully in some patients. A Vth nerve section or alcoholic injection of the ganglion or sensory divisions are a last recourse to be performed by experts.

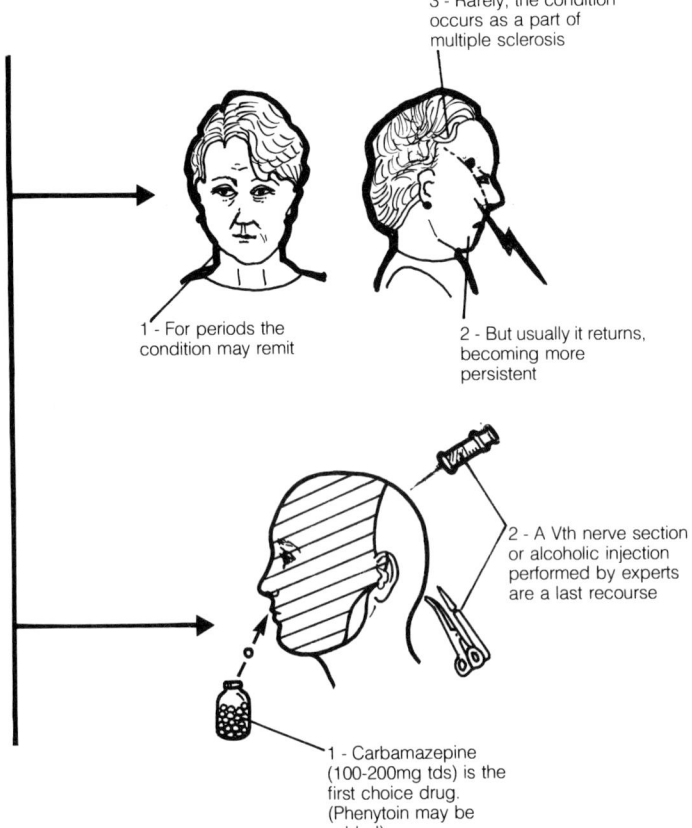

1 - For periods the condition may remit

2 - But usually it returns, becoming more persistent

3 - Rarely, the condition occurs as a part of multiple sclerosis

1 - Carbamazepine (100-200mg tds) is the first choice drug. (Phenytoin may be added)

2 - A Vth nerve section or alcoholic injection performed by experts are a last recourse

The Facial Nerve (VII)

The VIIth nerve emerges from the lateral aspect of the lower pons, crosses the posterior fossa to enter the facial canal in the petrous temporal bone. The facial canal passes laterally and then posteriorly and inferiorly to end at the stylomastoid foramen, where the VIIth nerve emerges from the skull. As the facial canal changes direction in the petrous temporal bone, the VIIth nerve expands to form the geniculate ganglion which contains the ganglion cells of the chorda tympani nerve that subserves the sense of taste from the anterior two thirds of the tongue.

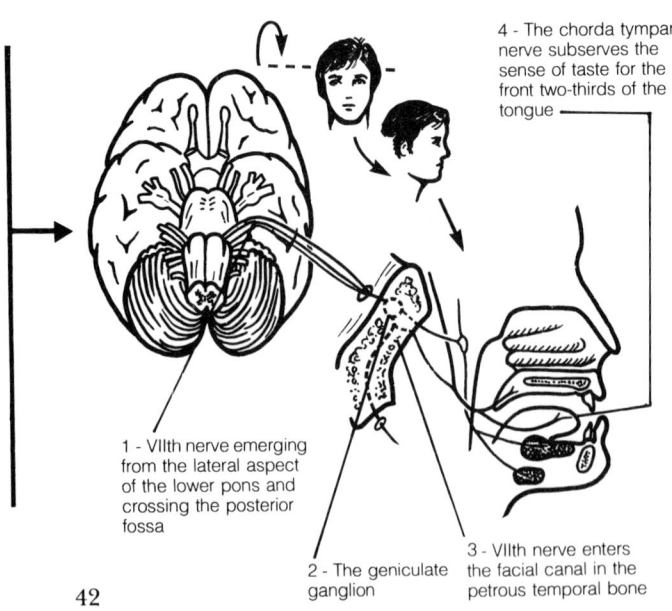

1 - VIIth nerve emerging from the lateral aspect of the lower pons and crossing the posterior fossa

2 - The geniculate ganglion

3 - VIIth nerve enters the facial canal in the petrous temporal bone

4 - The chorda tympani nerve subserves the sense of taste for the front two-thirds of the tongue

Within the facial canal the VIIth nerve gives off a branch to stapedius muscle. When the VIIth nerve is damaged at the level of the geniculate ganglion, the patient may complain of hyperacusis (due to paralysis of stapedius), and there is loss of taste from the anterior two thirds of the tongue. Parasympathetic efferent fibres leave the nerve at the geniculate ganglion via the greater superficial petrosal nerve to subserve lacrimation.

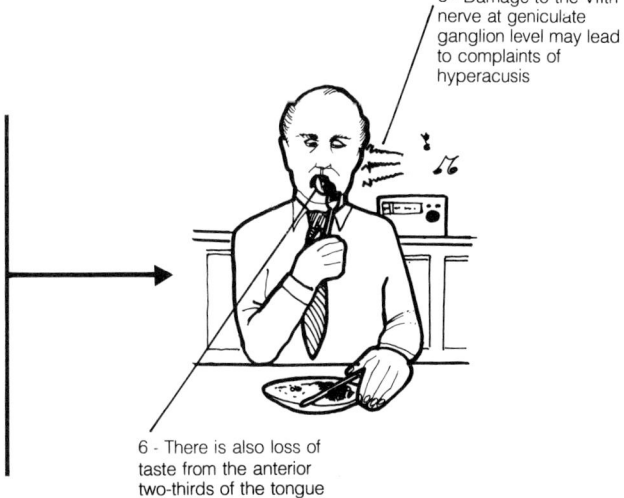

5 - Damage to the VIIth nerve at geniculate ganglion level may lead to complaints of hyperacusis

6 - There is also loss of taste from the anterior two-thirds of the tongue

After the VIIth nerve emerges from the skull, it sends motor branches to the stylohyoid muscle the posterior belly of digastric and occipito-frontalis. The VIIth nerve then passes forward into the parotid gland when it divides into several terminal motor branches which pass to supply the muscles of facial expression. **A VIIth nerve palsy** may be supected from a patient's facial expression at rest: the

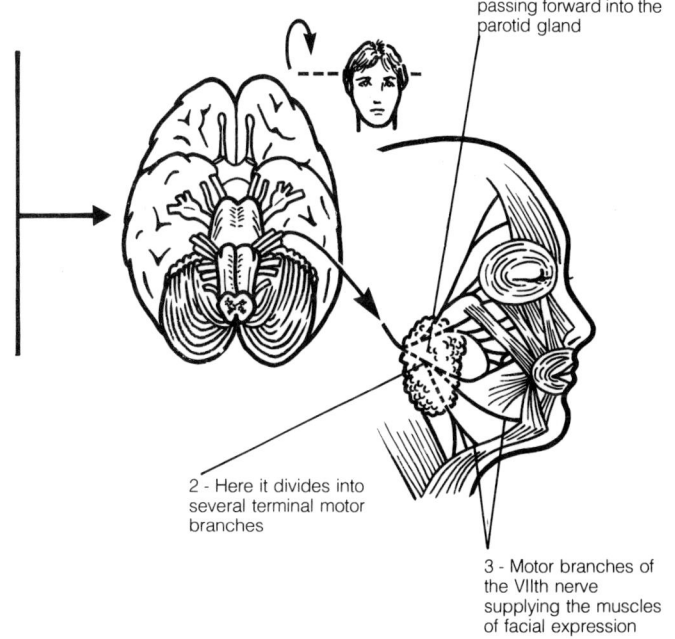

1 - The VIIth nerve passing forward into the parotid gland

2 - Here it divides into several terminal motor branches

3 - Motor branches of the VIIth nerve supplying the muscles of facial expression

Cranial Nerve Functions (continued)

nasolabial fold and furrows on the brow are smoother and the eye appears wider; the mouth is drawn slightly to the healthy side. The function of the upper branches of VII are tested clinically by asking the patient to screw up both eyes, to raise both eyebrows and then to frown; (the motor arm of the corneal reflex is subserved through the fibres to orbicularis oculi). The lower fibres of VII are clinically assessed by asking the patient to smile, purse the lips, to whistle or blow out the cheeks.

Facial paralysis is distinguishable as due to a supranuclear lesion and a VIIth nerve nuclear lesion of infranuclear type, (lower motor neurone – LMN lesion). The main difference is that a supranuclear lesion tends to spare the upper facial muscles due to bilateral innervation to those parts of the VIIth nucleus that control upper facial muscles; in nuclear or infranuclear paralysis all the facial muscles are equally affected and often perceptibly wasted. Supranuclear and brainstem nuclear lesions are often due to vascular lesions or tumours.

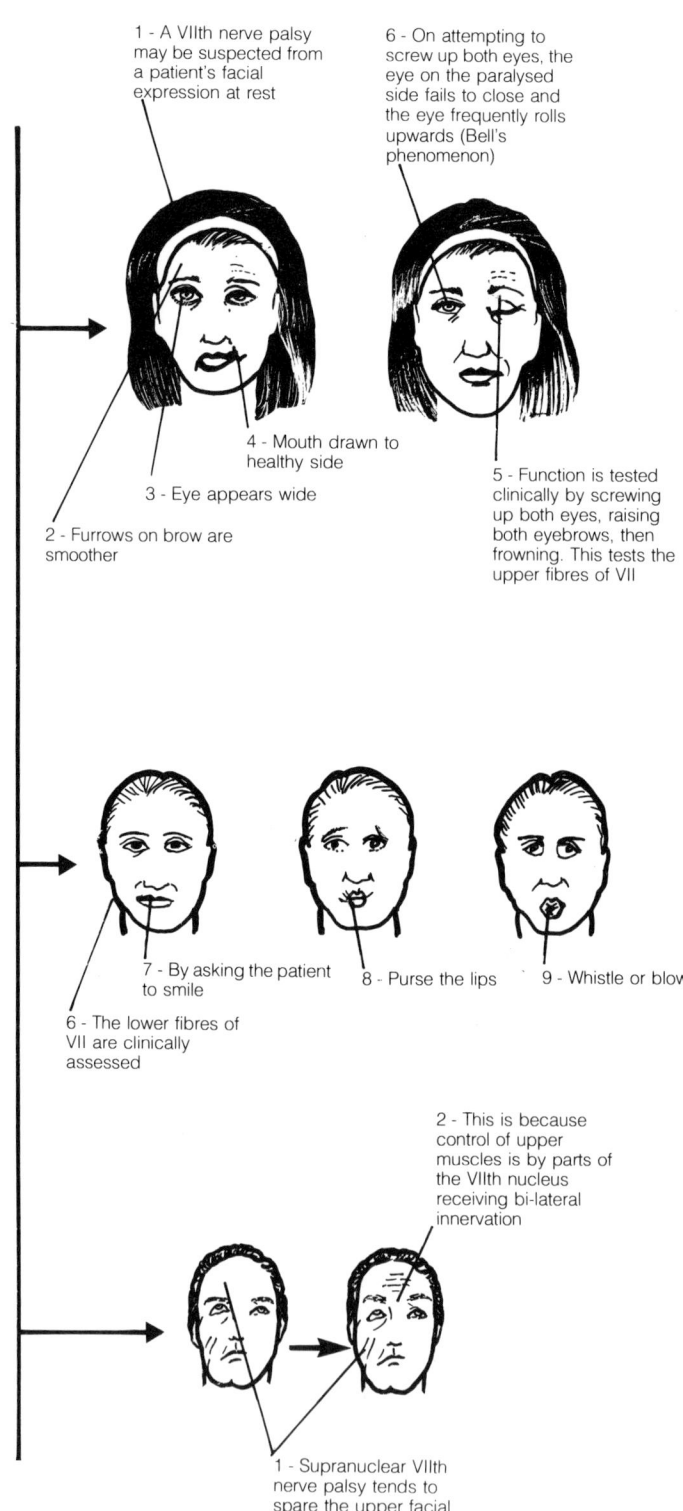

1 - A VIIth nerve palsy may be suspected from a patient's facial expression at rest

6 - On attempting to screw up both eyes, the eye on the paralysed side fails to close and the eye frequently rolls upwards (Bell's phenomenon)

2 - Furrows on brow are smoother

3 - Eye appears wide

4 - Mouth drawn to healthy side

5 - Function is tested clinically by screwing up both eyes, raising both eyebrows, then frowning. This tests the upper fibres of VII

6 - The lower fibres of VII are clinically assessed

7 - By asking the patient to smile

8 - Purse the lips

9 - Whistle or blow

1 - Supranuclear VIIth nerve palsy tends to spare the upper facial muscles

2 - This is because control of upper muscles is by parts of the VIIth nucleus receiving bi-lateral innervation

Cranial Nerve Functions (continued)

Millard-Gubler syndrome is due to a lesion of the VIIth nerve nucleus and adjacent pyramidal tract, (which is rostral to the decussation). Such a lesion results in an ipsilateral LMN Vth paresis and a crossed hemiplegia. Infranuclear lesions may be due to tumours, both intracranial (eg. acoustic neurome) or extracranial (eg. parotid tumours), or to spreading suppuration from a mastoiditis.

1 - LMN Vth nerve paresis

4 - Spreading suppuration from mastoiditis

3 - Intracranial tumour (acoustic neuroma)

2 - Extracranial parotid tumour

1 - Infranuclear lesions may be due to tumours both intracranial or extracranial

Herpes zoster may affect the geniculate ganglion, and headache may precede a zoster eruption on the pinna of the ear and external auditory canal, fauces and soft palate; an LMN VIIth paresis results which is usually recoverable, (Ramsay Hunt Syndrome).

1 - Herpes zoster may affect the geniculate ganglion

2 - Headache may precede a zoster eruption on the pinna of the ear and external auditory canal, fauces and soft palate

3 - An LMN paresis results but is usually recoverable (Ramsay-Hunt Syndrome)

Cranial Nerve Functions (continued)

Bell's palsy

Bell's palsy is a unilateral VIIth nerve palsy of acute onset and unknown aetiology although attributed to non-suppurative inflammation of the VIIth nerve within the distal facial canal. It is slightly commoner in young adult males. A slight facial ache may precede a LMN VIIth nerve palsy which may rapidly progress to complete paralysis; the sense of taste may or may not be affected. The condition must be distinguished from poliomyelitis and multiple sclerosis, which may simulate it.

Acute treatment with steroids or ACTH may reduce the severity of the condition but these should not be continued indefinitely. The prognosis depends on the severity of the acute paresis. Patients with some voluntary facial movements retained at one week from the onset of symptoms will probably recover fully albeit slowly. However, those with complete paralysis often do not recover. Electrophysiological studies showing denervation may assist in prognostication in this latter group. In cases where paresis is profound, the eye must be protected, perhaps with a lateral tarsorrhaphy or protective spectacles.

Clonic Facial Spasm – This condition of unknown aetiology tends to afflict the elderly who present with frequent, shock-like twitches of the facial muscles – usually unilateral. Orbicularis oculi is commonly the first muscle affected, but the condition may progress to other muscles and the contractions increase in strength. Drugs are not helpful in most cases but it is only in very extreme cases that surgical nerve section is indicated.

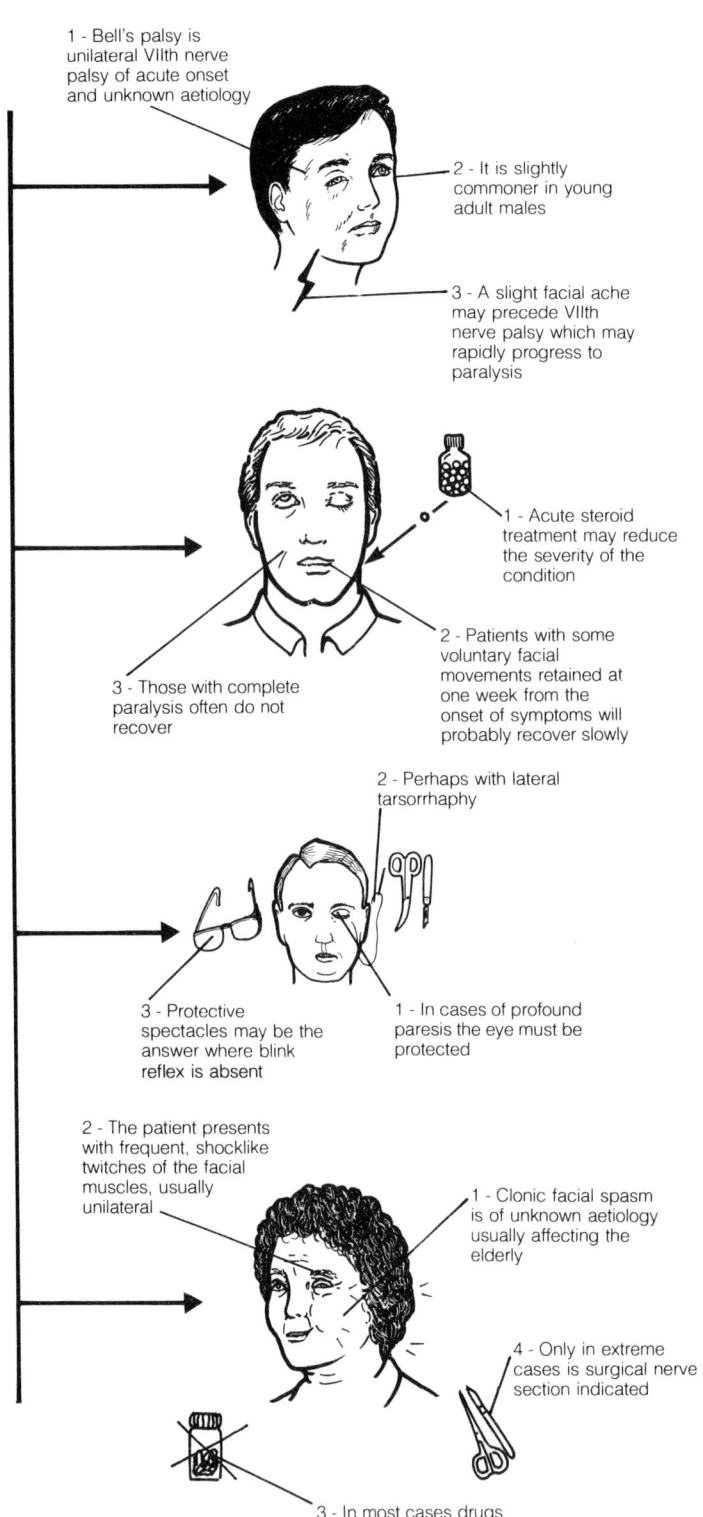

1 - Bell's palsy is unilateral VIIth nerve palsy of acute onset and unknown aetiology

2 - It is slightly commoner in young adult males

3 - A slight facial ache may precede VIIth nerve palsy which may rapidly progress to paralysis

1 - Acute steroid treatment may reduce the severity of the condition

2 - Patients with some voluntary facial movements retained at one week from the onset of symptoms will probably recover slowly

3 - Those with complete paralysis often do not recover

2 - Perhaps with lateral tarsorrhaphy

3 - Protective spectacles may be the answer where blink reflex is absent

1 - In cases of profound paresis the eye must be protected

2 - The patient presents with frequent, shocklike twitches of the facial muscles, usually unilateral

1 - Clonic facial spasm is of unknown aetiology usually affecting the elderly

4 - Only in extreme cases is surgical nerve section indicated

3 - In most cases drugs are not helpful

Cranial Nerve Functions (continued)

Vestibulocochlear Nerve (VIII) – The auditory division of VIII conveys hearing from the cochlea whilst the vestibular divisions carries fibres from the semicircular canals and otolith.

Auditory (Cochlear) Division – The cochlear fibres pass through the petrous temporal bone to the internal auditory meatus with the VIIth nerve and thence to the caudal end of the pons where the nucleus of this nerve lies.

Cortical representation of sound is bilateral. Although accurate testing of hearing can only be performed by audiometry, clinical testing may be valuable. The clinician first whispers into one ear from two feet or closer, with the other ear occluded. The tuning fork tests distinguish conduction deafness due to middle ear disease from perceptive or nerve deafness. In Rinne's test, the vibrating tuning fork is held in air next to the ear or the stem is pressed against the mastoid process (testing bone conduction). In middle ear disease, the bone conduction is unimpaired and the sound is heard louder when the stem is pressed against the mastoid.

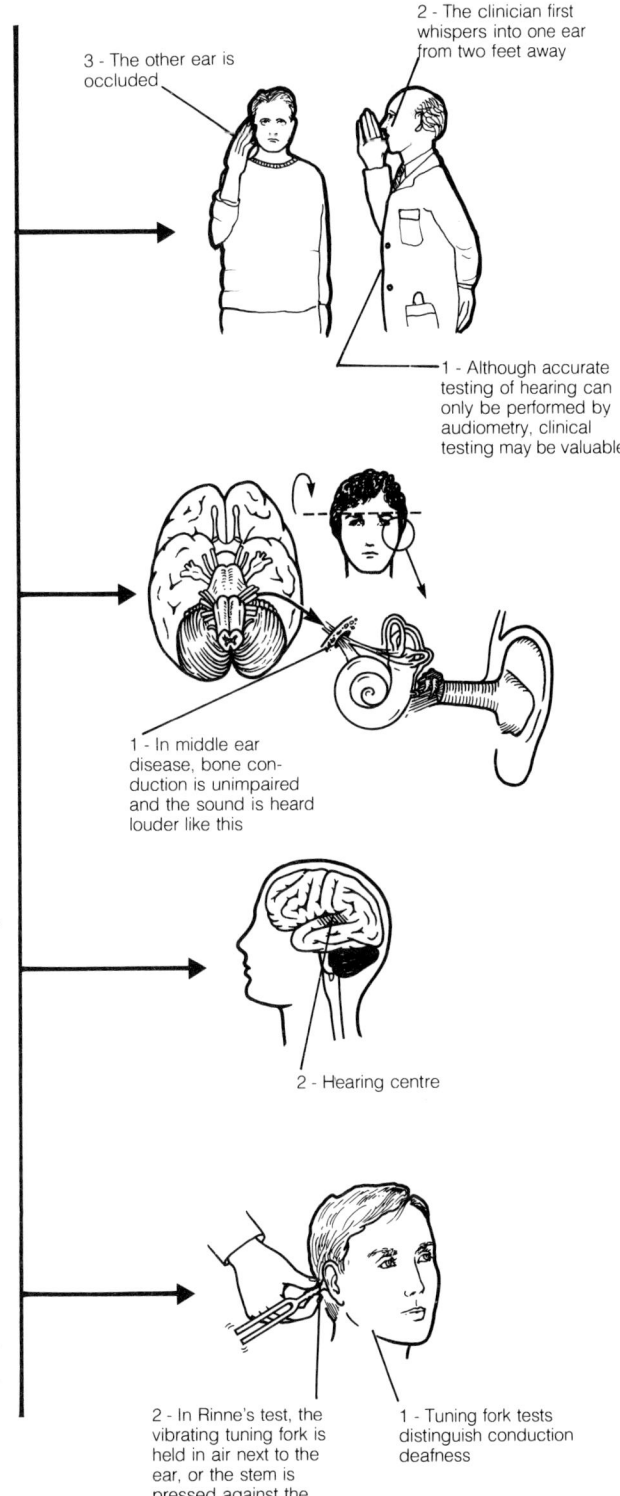

3 - The other ear is occluded

2 - The clinician first whispers into one ear from two feet away

1 - Although accurate testing of hearing can only be performed by audiometry, clinical testing may be valuable

1 - In middle ear disease, bone conduction is unimpaired and the sound is heard louder like this

2 - Hearing centre

2 - In Rinne's test, the vibrating tuning fork is held in air next to the ear, or the stem is pressed against the mastoid process

1 - Tuning fork tests distinguish conduction deafness

Cranial Nerve Functions (continued)

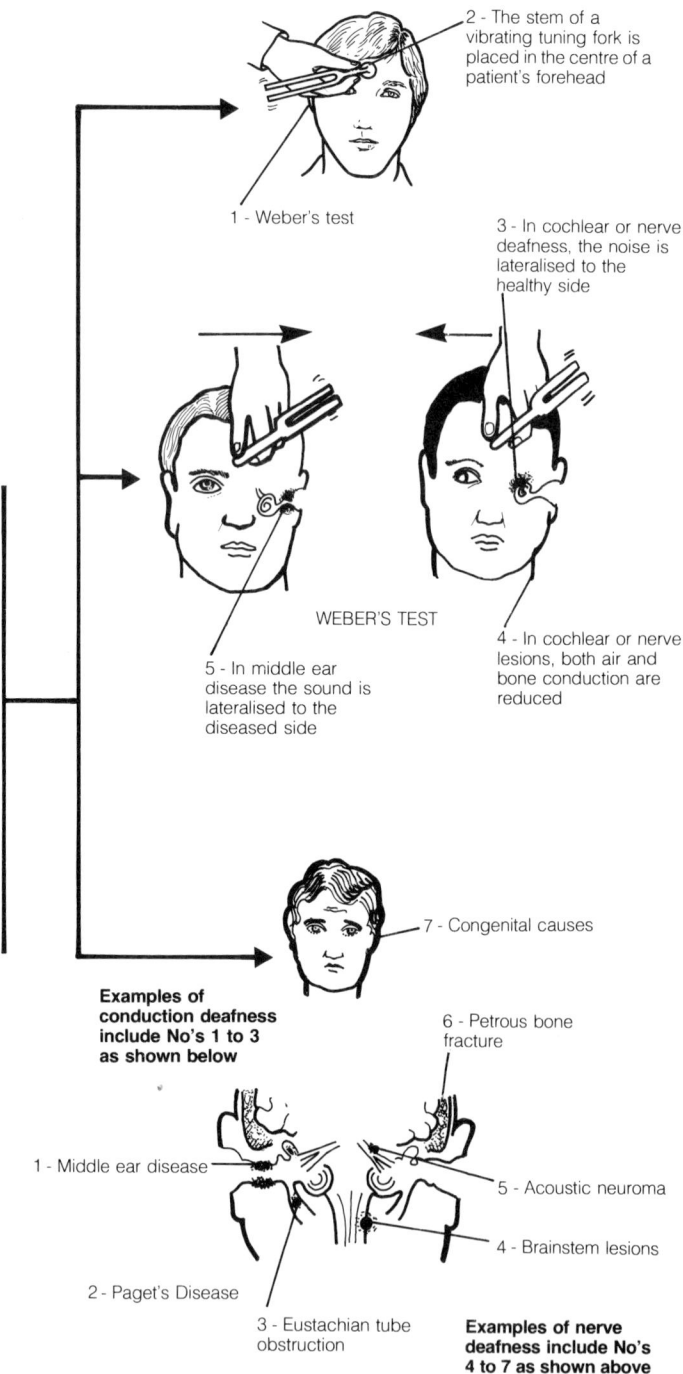

In cochlear or nerve lesions, both air and bone conduction are reduced. In Weber's test, the stem of the vibrating tuning fork is placed centrally on the patient's forehead. In middle ear disease, the sound is lateralised to the diseased side, whereas in cochlear or nerve deafness the noise is lateralised to the healthy side. Examples of conduction deafness include middle ear disease, Eustachian tube obstruction, otosclerosis, Paget's disease of bone. Examples of nerve deafness include congenital causes, fractures through the petrous bone, acoustic neuromas, brainstem lesions etc.

Cranial Nerve Functions (continued)

Vestibular Division – Within each of the semicircular canals of the labyrinth and utricle and saccule there are specialised hair-bearing cells that sense movement of the head in space and gravitational forces. These sensitive cells transmit impulses tonically via the vestibular division of VIII to enter the pons and end in the vestibular nuclei or pass via the inferior cerebellar peduncle to the cerebellar cortex. Fibres from the vestibular nuclei pass rostrally to the temporal lobes and caudally via the vestibulospinal tracts, influencing motor activity in balance and 'righting reflexes'.

Clinically, the labyrinth can be stimulated either by altering the position of the head – (eg. by rotation), or by irrigating one ear with hot or cold water, (this 'caloric test' having the advantage of only testing one labyrinth at a time).

1 - Within each of the semi-circular canals of the labyrinth, utricle and saccule are specialised hair bearing cells

2 - These sense movement of the head and gravitational forces

3 - These sensitive cells transmit impulses via the vestibular division of VIII. They are stimulated by fluid movement in the canal

4 - Vestibular division of VIII nerve

5 - They enter the pons and end in the vestibular nuclei, or pass to the cerebellar cortex

6 - Fibres pass to the temporal lobes and via the vestibulospinal tracts

At rest | Rotation of head to right | End of rotation

10 - The labyrinth is simulated on head rotation by the basic inertia of the fluid in the semi-circular canals

Cranial Nerve Functions (continued)

The caloric test is a more formal test usually performed in an ENT department. The simpler bedside test for positional nystagmus is also valuable, particularly in the assessment of 'vertigo'. The patient lies supine with the head projecting beyond the edge of the couch supported by the clinician's hands. The examiner then rotates the head to one side and extends the neck. The normal person may have one or two beats of nystagmus but not more. Where there is a peripheral vestibular lesion, nystagmus occurs after a latency of approximately ten seconds and persists for up to one minute before it disappears. With lesions of central vestibular pathways, however, immediate nystagmus occurs and persists. The nystagmus is horizontal, never vertical.

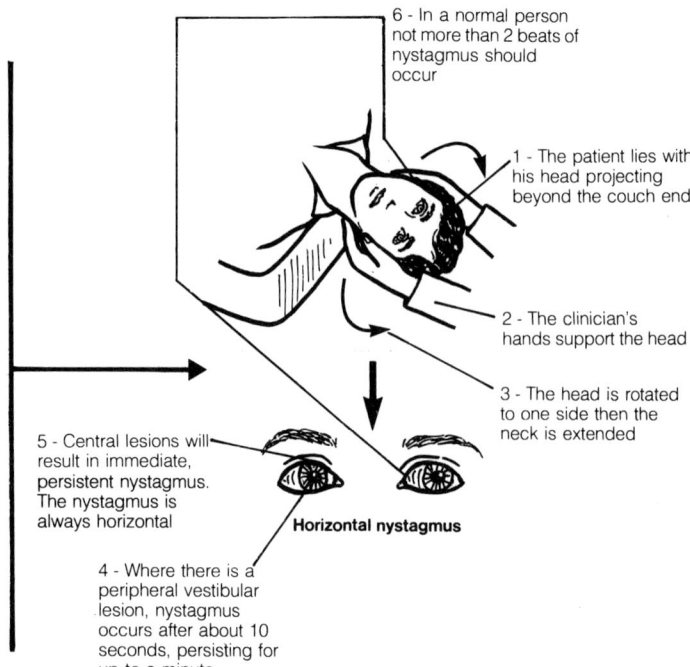

1 - The patient lies with his head projecting beyond the couch end
2 - The clinician's hands support the head
3 - The head is rotated to one side then the neck is extended
4 - Where there is a peripheral vestibular lesion, nystagmus occurs after about 10 seconds, persisting for up to a minute
5 - Central lesions will result in immediate, persistent nystagmus. The nystagmus is always horizontal
6 - In a normal person not more than 2 beats of nystagmus should occur

Horizontal nystagmus

Vertigo – Vertigo is the subjective sensation of movement of the environment and is always accompanied by a disturbance of balance. Severe vertigo may be accompanied by a reflex autonomic discharge with sweating, bradycardia, pallor – even syncope, accompanied by nausea and perhaps vomiting.

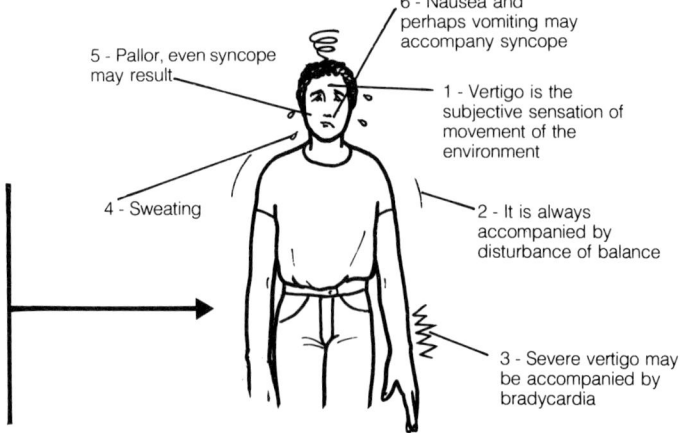

1 - Vertigo is the subjective sensation of movement of the environment
2 - It is always accompanied by disturbance of balance
3 - Severe vertigo may be accompanied by bradycardia
4 - Sweating
5 - Pallor, even syncope may result
6 - Nausea and perhaps vomiting may accompany syncope

'Peripheral' causes of vertigo include trauma to the labyrinth, labyrinthitis (often presumed acute viral), drugs (eg. streptomycin), Menière's disease, acoustic neuroma, secondary to suppurative middle ear disease or blocked Eustachian tube. Central/brainstem causes of vertigo are most commonly due to vertebrobasilar insufficiency secondary to cerebrovascular disease.

1 - Peripheral cause of vertigo as follows
2 - Acoustic neuroma
3 - Menière's disease
4 - Drugs eg. streptomycin
5 - Secondary to blocked Eustachian tube
6 - Middle ear disease

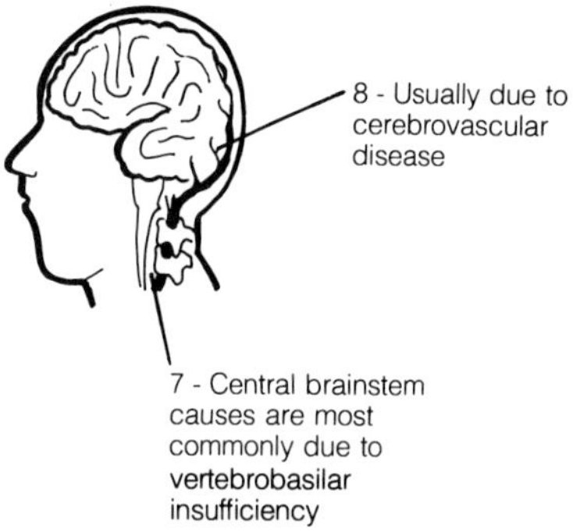

7 - Central brainstem causes are most commonly due to vertebrobasilar insufficiency
8 - Usually due to cerebrovascular disease

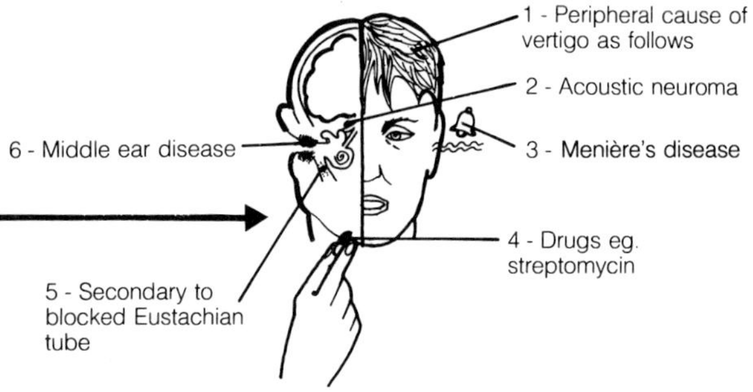

The physical examination of all these patients will always include ENT examination, tests of cochlear division function, test for positional nystagmus, caloric testing, blood pressure and auscultation for bruits in the neck and neurological examination for focal neurology.

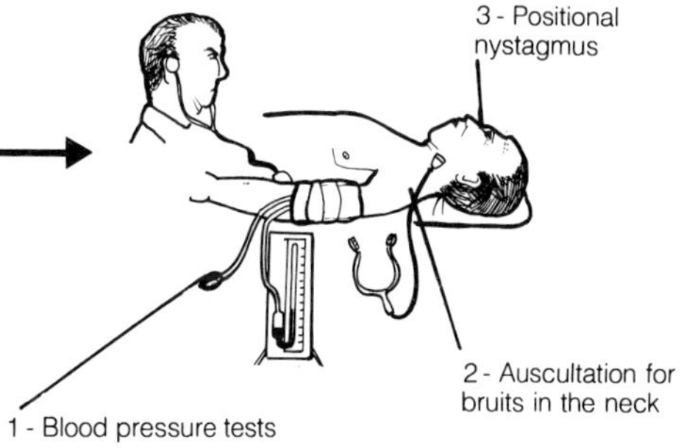

1 - Blood pressure tests
2 - Auscultation for bruits in the neck
3 - Positional nystagmus

Cranial Nerve Functions (continued)

Menière's Disease – This condition tends to afflict patients in late middle age (45-60 years) being slightly commoner in men. There is dilation of the endolymph system within the inner ear although the cause of this is unknown. The common clinical history is of unilateral or bilateral progressive deafness and tinnitus over months or even years before there is an attack of vertigo of varying severity; the attack may last for minutes or hours and the patient finds that he is least uncomfortable lying in a dark room. The attacks of vertigo recur irregularly in time and vary in severity. However, as time goes by, deafness progresses and the severity of vertigo may lessen. The coincidence of disturbed hearing, (almost invariably with some tinnitus), and disturbed vestibular function make it clear that the lesion is in the internal ear or VIIIth nerve, and caloric testing is abnormal in approximately 90% of cases of Menière's disease.

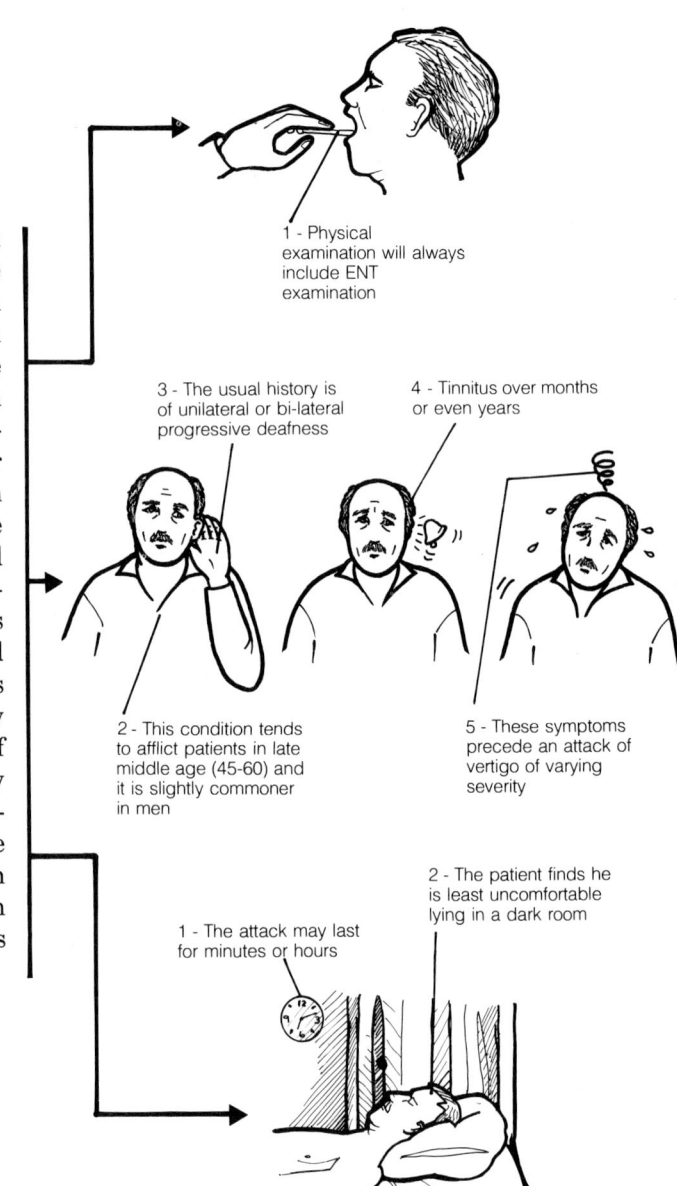

Cranial Nerve Functions (continued)

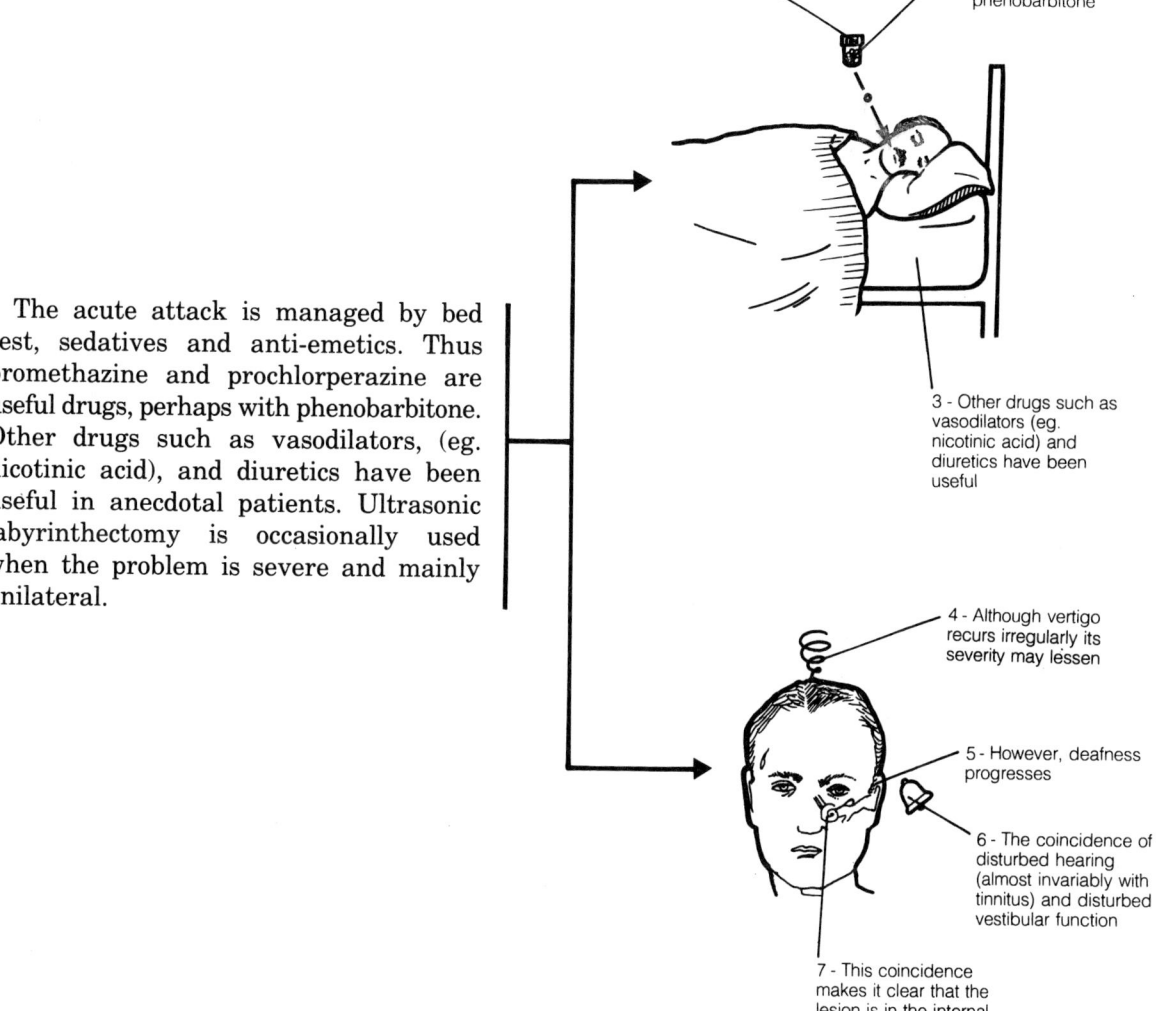

1 - An acute attack is managed by bed rest, sedatives and antiemetics

2 - Promethazine and prochlorperazine are useful and perhaps phenobarbitone

3 - Other drugs such as vasodilators (eg. nicotinic acid) and diuretics have been useful

4 - Although vertigo recurs irregularly its severity may lessen

5 - However, deafness progresses

6 - The coincidence of disturbed hearing (almost invariably with tinnitus) and disturbed vestibular function

7 - This coincidence makes it clear that the lesion is in the internal ear or VIIIth nerve

The acute attack is managed by bed rest, sedatives and anti-emetics. Thus promethazine and prochlorperazine are useful drugs, perhaps with phenobarbitone. Other drugs such as vasodilators, (eg. nicotinic acid), and diuretics have been useful in anecdotal patients. Ultrasonic labyrinthectomy is occasionally used when the problem is severe and mainly unilateral.

Cranial Nerve Functions (continued)

The Glossopharyngeal Nerve (IX) and Vagus Nerve (X) – Both these nerves leave the medulla oblongata, to cross the posterior cranial fossa and emerge from the skull through the jugular foramen. The IXth nerve conveys sensation, (including taste), from the posterior one-third of the tongue, the tonsil, oropharynx, soft palate, Eustachian tube and middle ear. The motor supply of IX is to the pharyngeal muscles concerned with swallowing and also autonomic efferent supply to the parotid gland. Motor fibres from X also supply the voluntary muscles of the pharynx and palate as well as the larynx, and the vagus nerve also has important autonomic motor fibres to the heart, bronchi and stomach. Sensory visceral fibres pass in X from the heart and great vessels, respiratory tract and gastrointestinal tract.

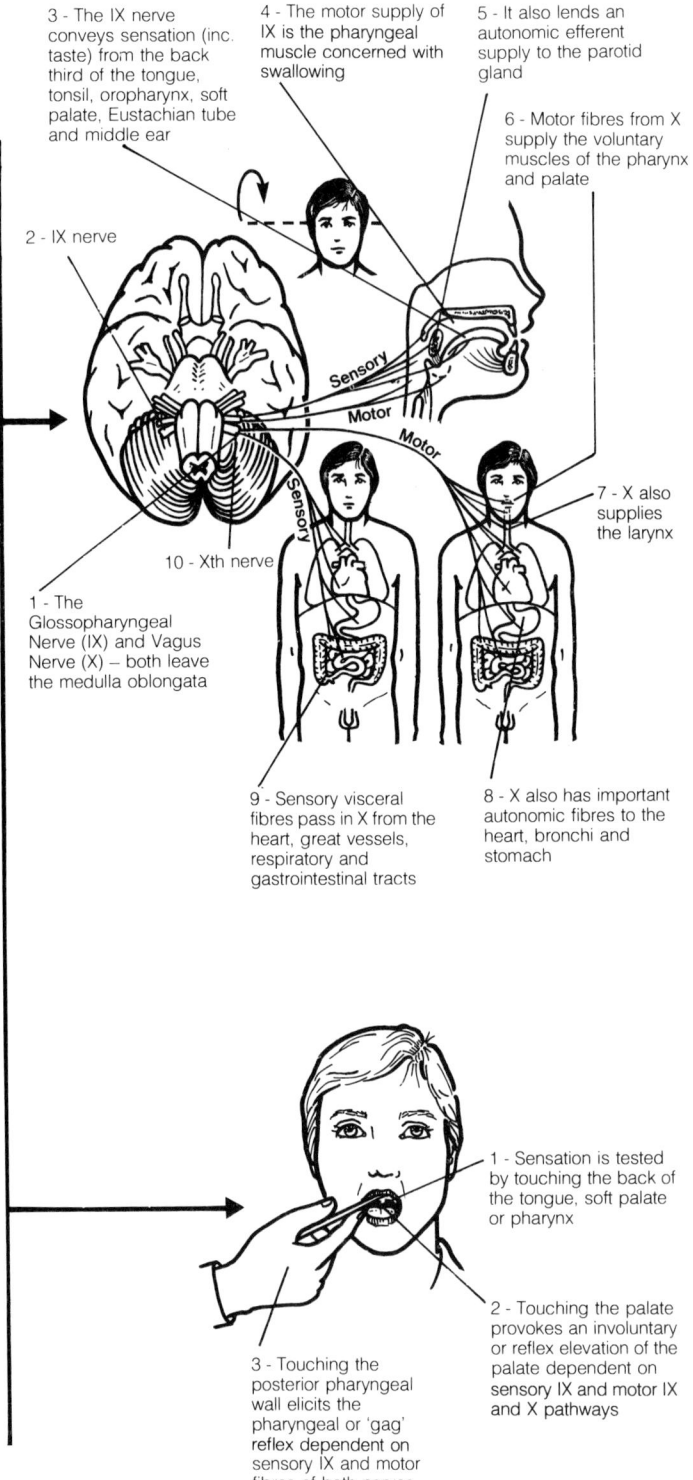

Sensation is tested by touching the back of the tongue, soft palate or pharynx; touching the palate provokes an involuntary or reflex elevation of the palate dependent on sensory IX and motor X pathways, (the palatal reflex). Touching the posterior pharyngeal wall elicits the pharyngeal or 'gag' reflex dependent on sensory IX and motor IX and X fibres.

Cranial Nerve Functions (continued)

Motor functions of IX and X are tested when the patient utters/phonates: 'Ah'. The palate should be drawn up symmetrically with the uvula remaining in the midline. If there is a peripheral lesion of one Xth nerve the palate is drawn over to the normal side; if both Xth nerves are paralysed, the palate fails to move at all and the patient may complain of regurgitation of food into the nasal cavity on swallowing. The voice of such a patient has a characteristic nasal resonance.

Unilateral pharyngeal muscle paralysis causes few problems but bilateral paralysis leads to profound dysphagia. Upper motor neurone (UMN) lesions must be bilateral to significantly influence the motor functions of IX and X.

1 - Motor functions of IX and X tested when the patient utters 'Ah'

2 - The palate should be drawn up symmetricaly with the uvula remaining in the midline

3 - Uvula

1 - Peripheral lesion of one Xth nerve

2 - Palate drawn over to normal side

3 - If both Xth nerves are paralysed the palate fails to move at all

4 - The patient may complain of regurgitation of food into the nasal cavity on swallowing

5 - The voice of such a patient has a characteristic nasal resonance

1 - Bilateral paralysis leads to profound dysphagia

2 - UMN Lesions must be bilateral to significantly influence the motor functions of IX and X

Cranial Nerve Functions (continued)

All the laryngeal muscles (except cricothyroid) are innervated by the recurrent laryngeal branch of X, and paralysis of X leads to altered voice and impaired cough; if bilateral paralysis occurs, phonation is not possible and the cough is described as 'bovine' as there is no pressure gradient across the vocal cords to produce the explosive character of a normal cough. Indirect laryngoscopy confirms the vocal cord palsy.

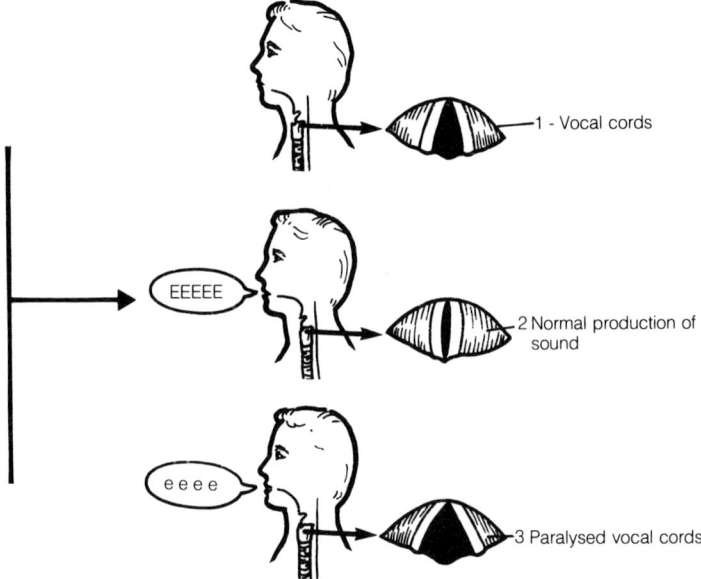

1 - Vocal cords
2 - Normal production of sound
3 - Paralysed vocal cords

The Accessory Nerve (XI) – The accessory nerve shares its motor nucleus (nucleus ambiguus) in the medulla oblongata with the vagus nerve. After emerging from the medulla, XI passes across the posterior fossa where it may be damaged by pressure (usually together with IX, X and XII) by a tumour. After emerging from the skull through the jugular foramen, XI supplies motor fibres to sternomastoid and the upper part of trapezius.

The function of XI is tested by asking the patient to shrug his shoulders (trapezius) against resistance, and to turn his chin to the contra-lateral side (sternomastoid) against resistance. Unilateral XIth nerve lesions lead to wasting and weakness of the muscles; bilateral XIth nerve lesions lead to weakness of the main flexors and extensors of the neck.

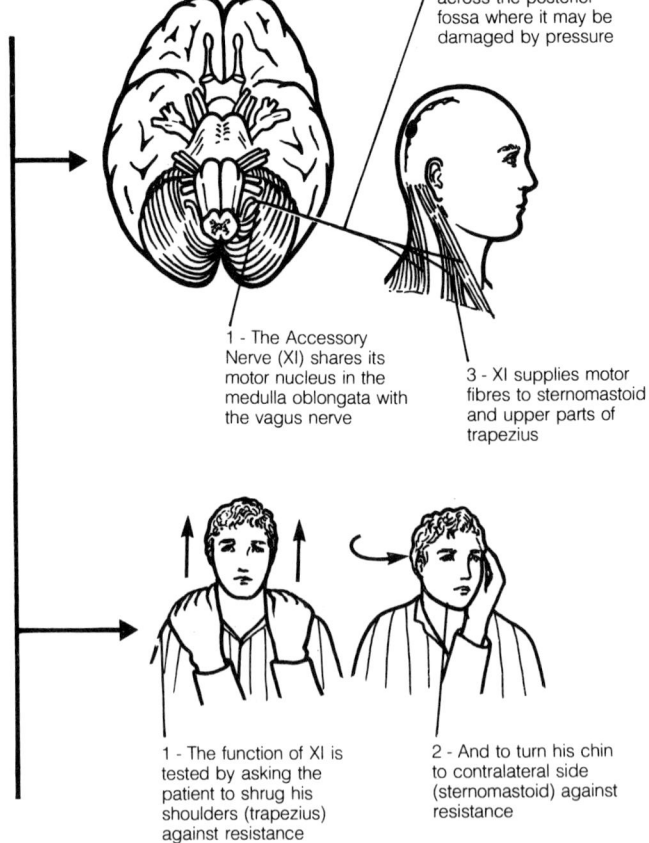

1 - The Accessory Nerve (XI) shares its motor nucleus in the medulla oblongata with the vagus nerve

2 - After emerging from the medulla, XI passes across the posterior fossa where it may be damaged by pressure

3 - XI supplies motor fibres to sternomastoid and upper parts of trapezius

1 - The function of XI is tested by asking the patient to shrug his shoulders (trapezius) against resistance

2 - And to turn his chin to contralateral side (sternomastoid) against resistance

It should be noted, however, that weak and wasted sternomastoid muscles are a prominent feature in dystrophia myotonica and that motor neurone disease and myasthenia gravis may also both afflict the muscles of 'head position'.

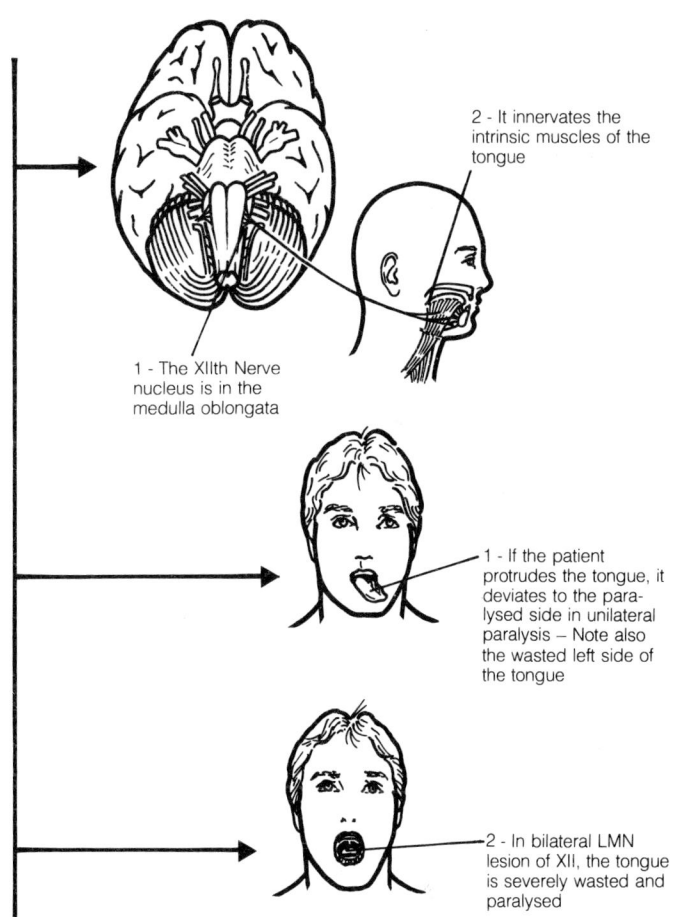

3 - It should however be noted that weak and wasted sternomastoid muscles are a prominent feature of dystrophia myotonica

2 - Bilateral XIth nerve lesions lead to weakness of the main neck flexors and extensors

1 - Unilateral nerve lesions lead to wasting and weakness of the muscles

4 - Motor neurone disease and myasthenia gravis may both affect the muscles of head position

The Hypoglossal Nerve (XII) – The XIIth nerve nucleus is in the medulla oblongata and after emerging from the skull through the hypoglossal canal, XII passes circuitously downwards and then forwards to innervate the intrinsic muscles of the tongue.

1 - The XIIth Nerve nucleus is in the medulla oblongata

2 - It innervates the intrinsic muscles of the tongue

Examination of XII commences with inspection; in an LMN XIIth lesion, there is hemiatrophy of the tongue and fibrillating muscle fibre bundles are visible. If the patient then protrudes the tongue it will be observed that, in the presence of unilateral paralysis, the tongue deviates to the paralysed side. If there are bilateral LMN lesions of XII, then the tongue is

1 - If the patient protrudes the tongue, it deviates to the paralysed side in unilateral paralysis – Note also the wasted left side of the tongue

2 - In bilateral LMN lesion of XII, the tongue is severely wasted and paralysed

severely wasted and paralysed. In a unilateral UMN lesion of XII, the tongue is not wasted but is weak and deviates to the affected side on protrusion. In bilateral UMN lesions, (which not uncommonly occur in motor neurone disease) the tongue appears 'bunched up' and severely paretic; speech is spastic and has been likened to words being squeezed out through the mouth like toothpaste from a tube (spastic dysarthria).

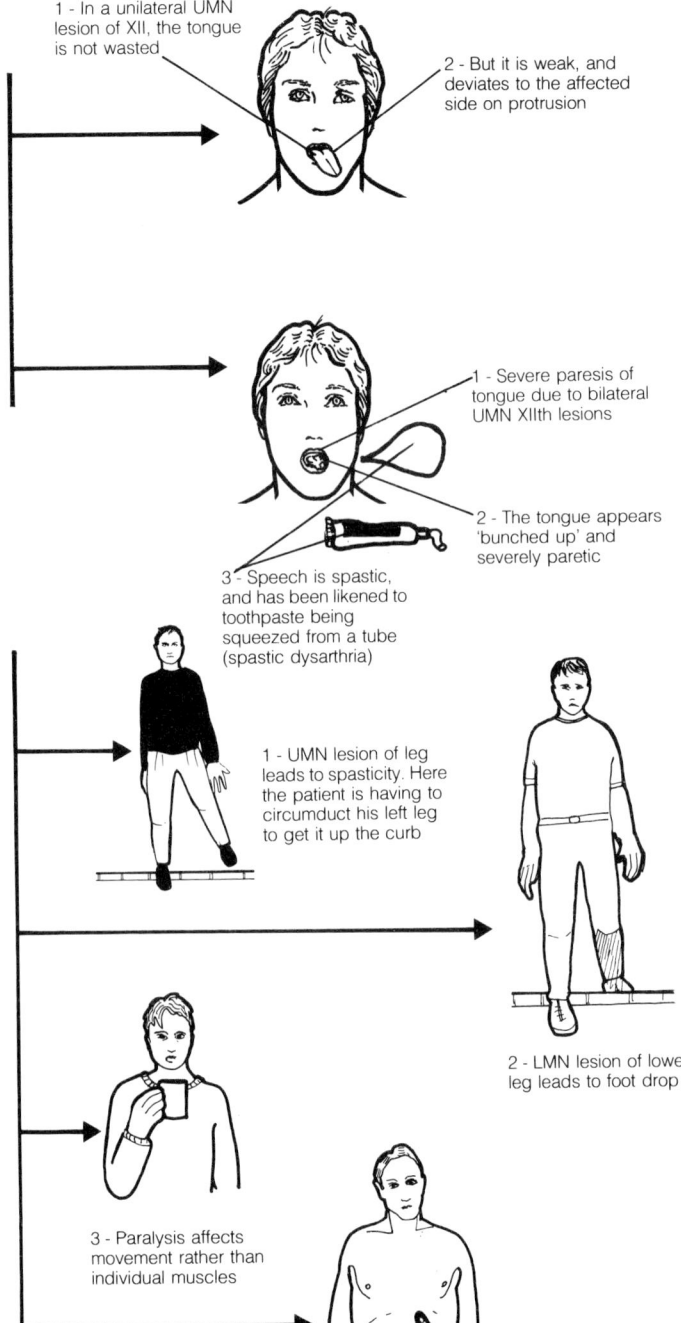

1 - In a unilateral UMN lesion of XII, the tongue is not wasted

2 - But it is weak, and deviates to the affected side on protrusion

1 - Severe paresis of tongue due to bilateral UMN XIIth lesions

2 - The tongue appears 'bunched up' and severely paretic

3 - Speech is spastic, and has been likened to toothpaste being squeezed from a tube (spastic dysarthria)

1 - UMN lesion of leg leads to spasticity. Here the patient is having to circumduct his left leg to get it up the curb

2 - LMN lesion of lower leg leads to foot drop

3 - Paralysis affects movement rather than individual muscles

4 - Superficial reflexes diminished or modified

THE PERIPHERAL MOTOR SYSTEM

UPPER MOTOR NEURONE LESION (U.M.N)	LOWER MOTOR NEURONE LESION (L.M.N)
Wasting slight (only from disuse)	Wasting marked
	Fasciculation
No trophic changes in skin	Skin blue, cold, shiny, thin
Clasp knife spasticity Clonus often present	Flaccid tone
Paralysis affects movements rather than individual muscles eg. extensors in arm flexors in leg	Individual muscles or muscle groups affected
Tendon reflexes increased	Tendon reflexes diminished or absent
Superficial reflexes diminished or modified eg. abdominal reflexes absent extensor plantar reflex (Babinski's sign)	Superficial reflexes unimpaired

The Peripheral Motor System

Apart from hysteria, the major causes of weakness can firstly be distinguished into upper motor neurone versus lower motor neurone lesions and other causes, (notably extrapyramidal or cerebellar causes and primary muscular disorders). The upper motor neurone (UMN) refers to the long corticospinal (pyramidal) tract from motor cortex to anterior horn cell whilst the lower motor neurone (LMN) refers to the peripheral nerve that springs from the anterior horn cell; (LMN lesions include poliomyelitis or motor neurone disease at anterior horn cell level or root or polyneuropathy distally).

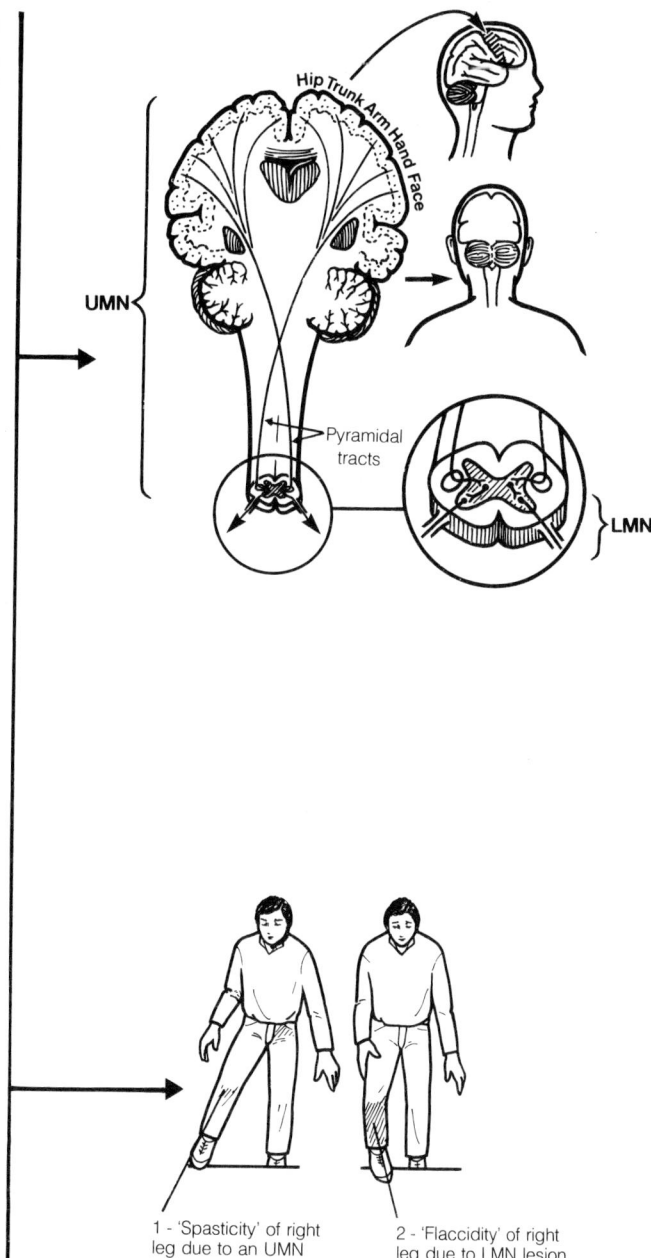

It is very important to be able to clinically distinguish paralysis or weakness due to an UMN versus a LMN lesion and these differences are tabulated on the page opposite. From this table, it will be seen that 'spasticity' of limbs is seen with UMN lesions and 'flaccidity' with LMN lesions. A man with an UMN lesion affecting his legs 'drags' his stiff leg whilst walking and has to swing his leg out and around to mount the curb when crossing a road; a patient with LNM lesion has a flapping foot or foot drop.

1 - 'Spasticity' of right leg due to an UMN lesion

2 - 'Flaccidity' of right leg due to LMN lesion

The Peripheral Motor System

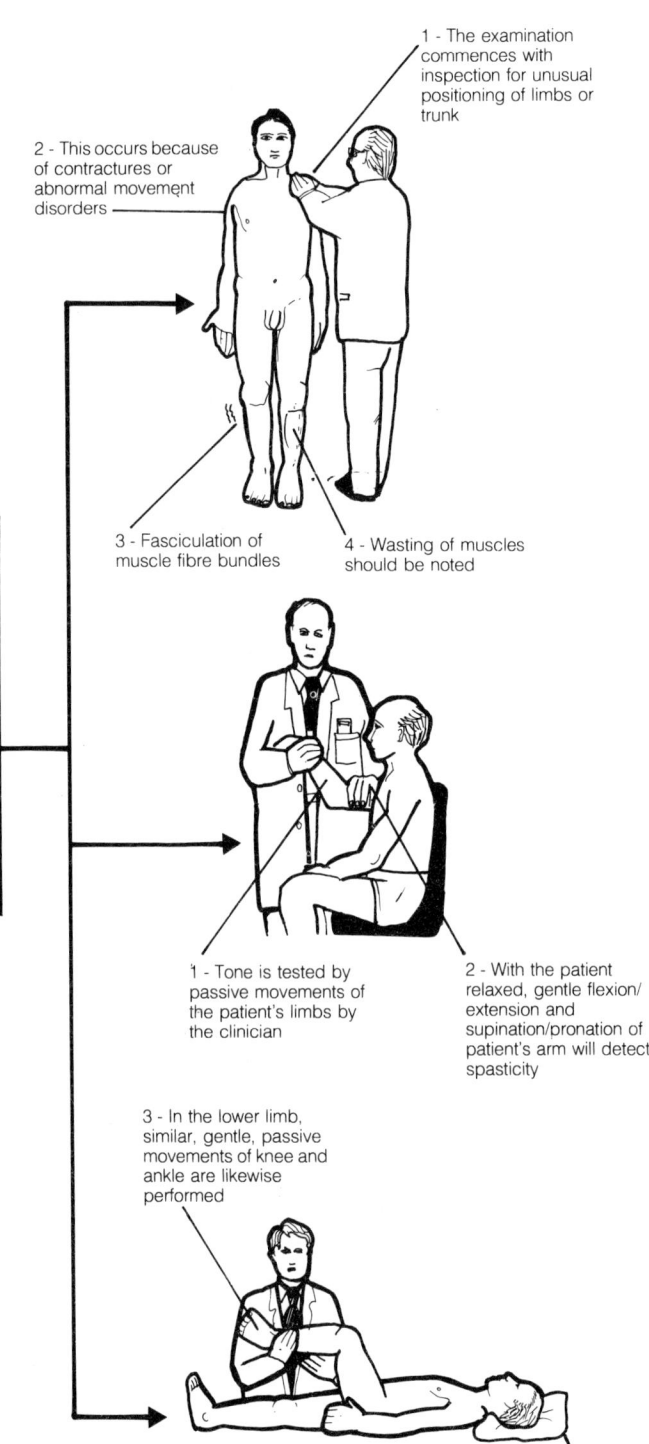

Examination of the Motor System

The examination commences with inspection for unusual positioning of limbs or trunk due to contractures or abnormal movement disorders (see later), for wasting of muscles or fasciculation of muscle fibre bundles. Tone is tested by passive movements of the patient's limbs by the clinician. With the patient relaxed, gentle flexion/extension and supination/pronation of the patient's arm will detect spasticity (hypertonicity) and in the lower limb similar gentle passive movements of knee and ankle are performed likewise.

With severely spastic limbs, a sudden passive movement against the spastic contracture leads to alternating flexor/extensor contractions (clonus) – characteristic of UMN lesions and best demonstrated as patellar and ankle clonus. Next, power is tested; in general, the clinician should request the patient to contract the muscle being tested and then the clinician attempts to overcome that action, (eg. the patient bends the elbow and then the clinician tries to overcome biceps contraction – root C5, 6 and musculocutaneous nerve).

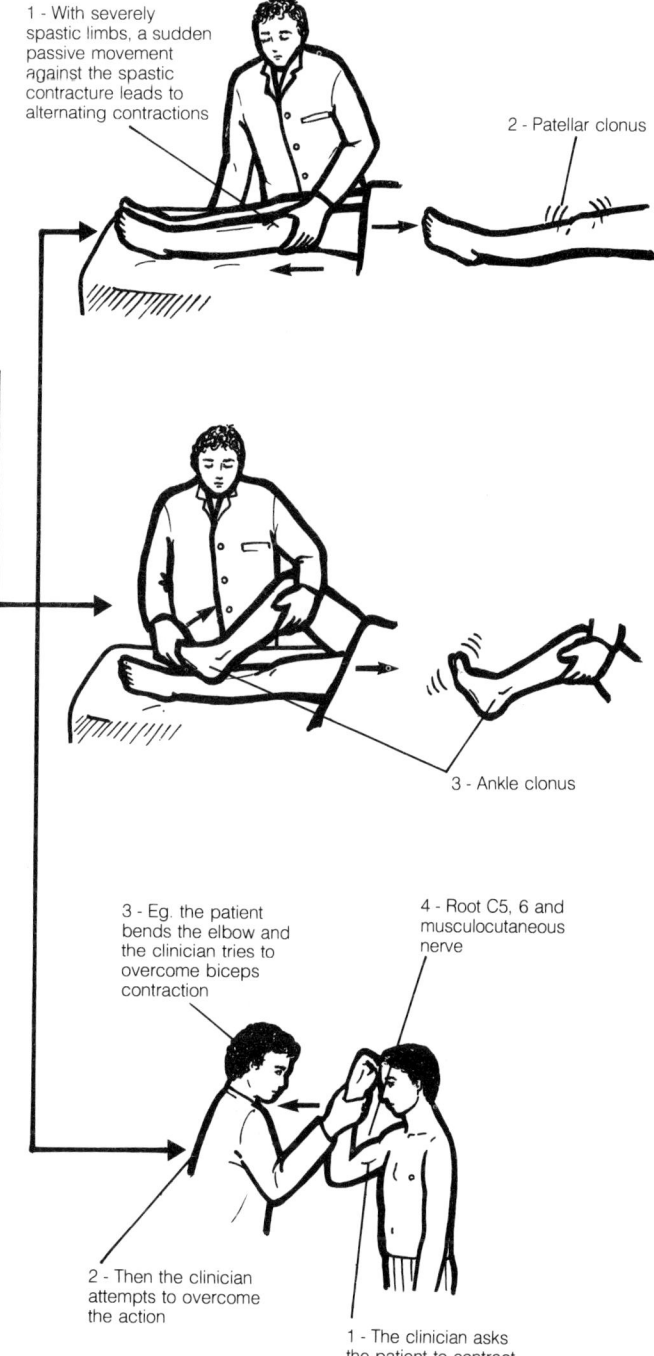

1 - With severely spastic limbs, a sudden passive movement against the spastic contracture leads to alternating contractions

2 - Patellar clonus

3 - Ankle clonus

3 - Eg. the patient bends the elbow and the clinician tries to overcome biceps contraction

4 - Root C5, 6 and musculocutaneous nerve

2 - Then the clinician attempts to overcome the action

1 - The clinician asks the patient to contract the muscle being tested

The Peripheral Motor System

When the clinician has assessed tone and power, coordination is tested, but it must be remembered that coordination also depends on proprioception, (joint position sense) and this has not yet been assessed. If the patient can hold his outstretched arms at the same level against varying pressures with his eyes closed and can stand to attention with his eyes closed without toppling over (**Romberg's test**), then joint position sense is probably not severely impaired and any clumsiness probably not therefore due to 'sensory ataxia'. Cerebellar ataxia may cause profound difficulty in coordination and the finger-nose test (where the patient puts one forefinger on his nose and then on some object at arm's length (eg. clinician's finger) before repeating this sequence over and over again) is a good way of demonstrating this.

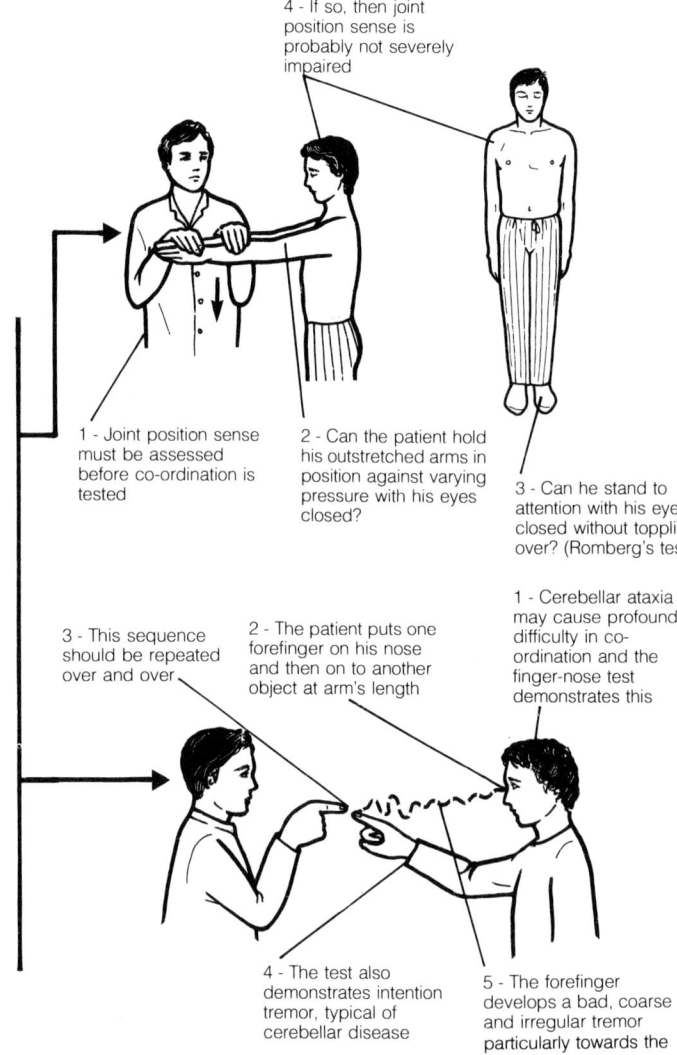

4 - If so, then joint position sense is probably not severely impaired

1 - Joint position sense must be assessed before co-ordination is tested

2 - Can the patient hold his outstretched arms in position against varying pressure with his eyes closed?

3 - Can he stand to attention with his eyes closed without toppling over? (Romberg's test)

3 - This sequence should be repeated over and over

2 - The patient puts one forefinger on his nose and then on to another object at arm's length

1 - Cerebellar ataxia may cause profound difficulty in co-ordination and the finger-nose test demonstrates this

4 - The test also demonstrates intention tremor, typical of cerebellar disease

5 - The forefinger develops a bad, coarse and irregular tremor particularly towards the end of its course

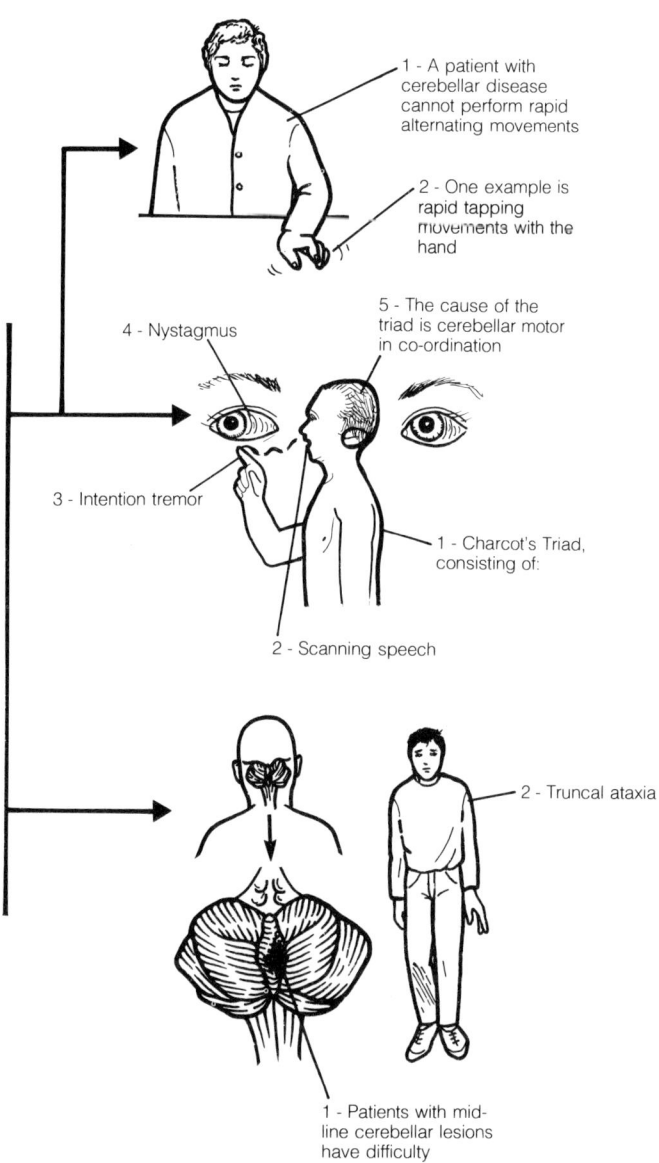

Furthermore, this test also demonstrates 'intention tremor', (so typical of cerebellar disease), where the forefinger develops a bad, coarse and irregular tremor just before it locates the clinician's finger or the patient's nose. A patient with cerebellar disease cannot perform rapid alternating movements (dysdiadokinesis) such as tapping lightly with his hand. Lastly, there is a famous clinical triad of signs (**Charcot's triad**) caused by cerebellar motor incoordination. These are: scanning speech, nystagmus and intention tremor. Patients with lesions eg. tumour in the cerebellar hemispheres demonstrate these signs, but patients with mid-line cerebellar lesions have more difficulty with maintaining their balance (truncal ataxia).

There are a group of hereditary cerebellar ataxias which may have their clinical onset at different times in life and are due to the death of neurones of cerebellar and spino-cerebellar tracts. In **Friedreich's ataxia** there is degeneration of the spino-cerebellar and pyramidal motor tracts and of the posterior columns of the cord.

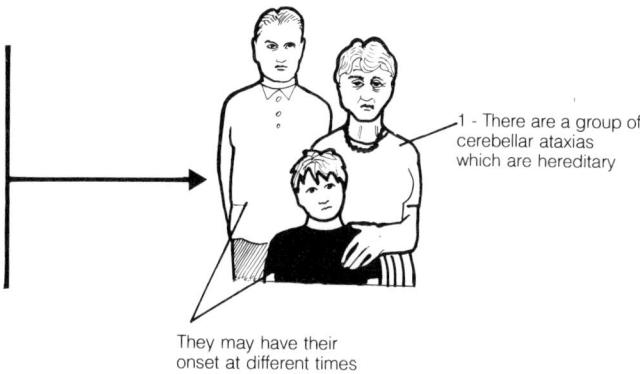

The Peripheral Motor System

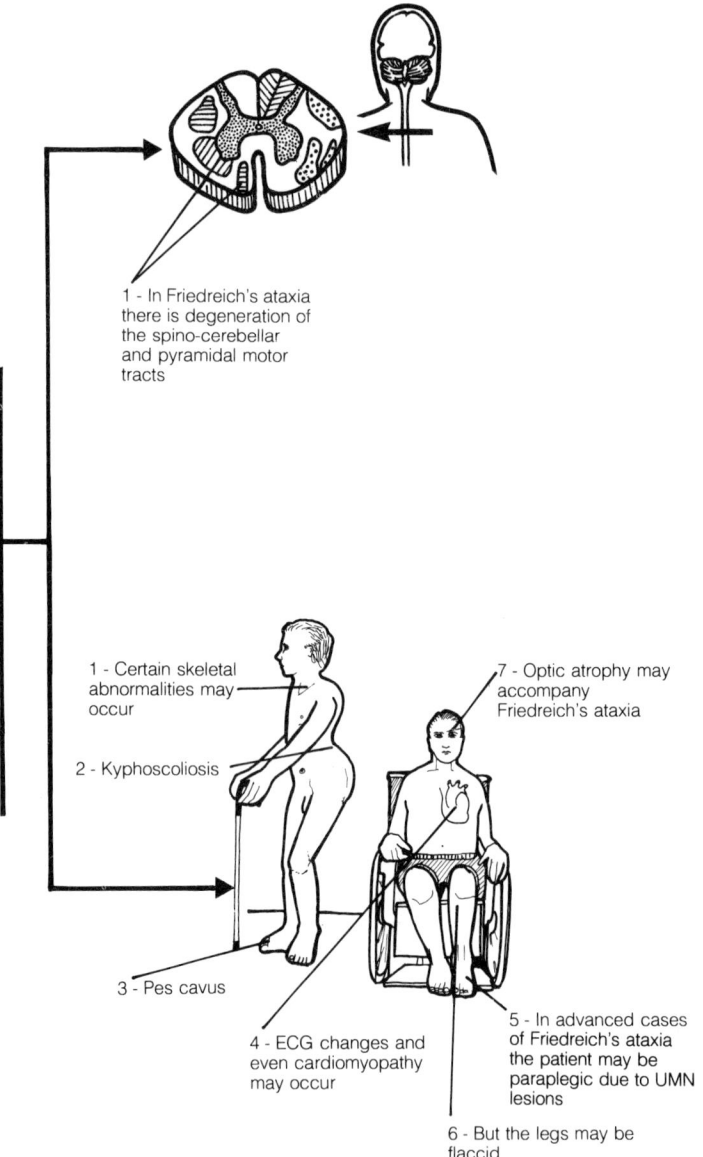

1 - In Friedreich's ataxia there is degeneration of the spino-cerebellar and pyramidal motor tracts

1 - Certain skeletal abnormalities may occur

2 - Kyphoscoliosis

3 - Pes cavus

4 - ECG changes and even cardiomyopathy may occur

5 - In advanced cases of Friedreich's ataxia the patient may be paraplegic due to UMN lesions

6 - But the legs may be flaccid

7 - Optic atrophy may accompany Friedreich's ataxia

In addition, certain skeletal abnormalities (kyphoscoliosis and pes cavus), ECG changes (even cardiomyopathy) and optic atrophy may occur. Here the cerebellar incoordination may be masked by other neurological signs – for example, in advanced cases of Friedreich's ataxia the patient may be paraplegic due to pyramidal (UMN) lesions but the legs may be flaccid, (due to degeneration of proprioceptive pathways – muscle tone depending on sensory input). This last situation is a rare example where the leg tone is flaccid but the plantar responses are upgoing (see below).

The Peripheral Motor System

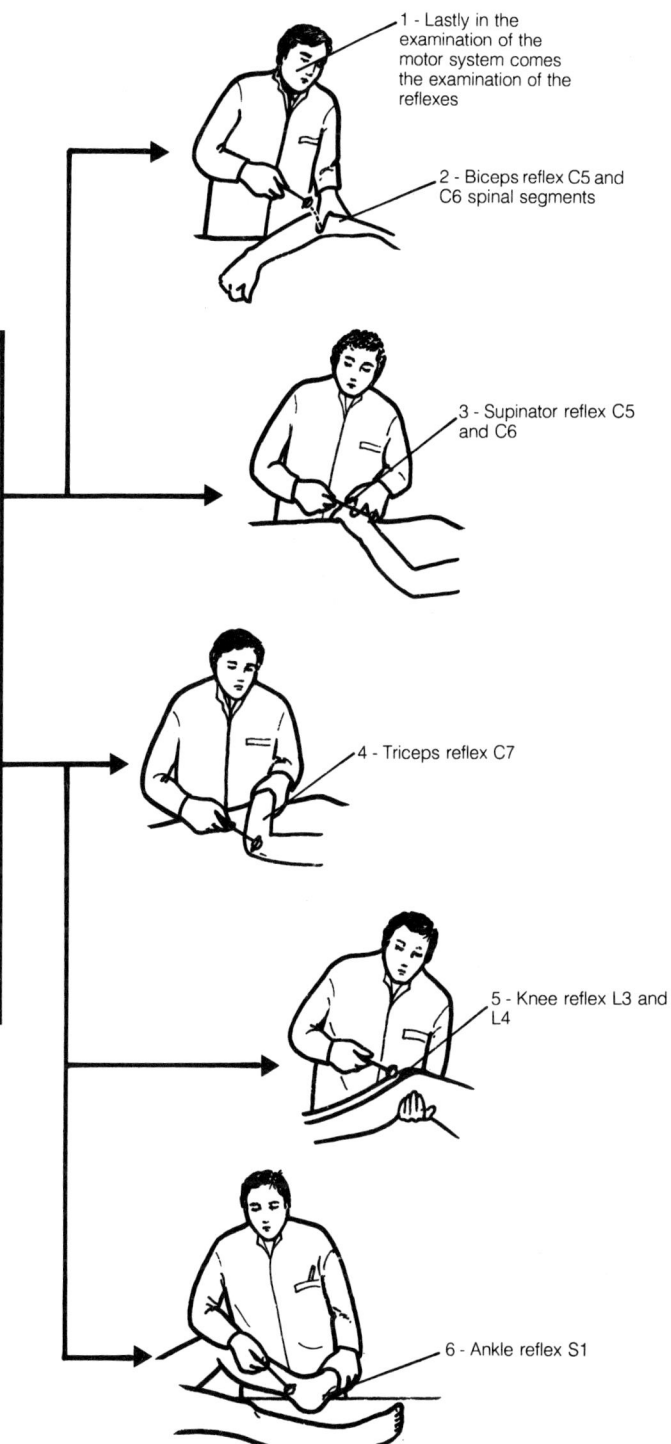

1 - Lastly in the examination of the motor system comes the examination of the reflexes

2 - Biceps reflex C5 and C6 spinal segments

3 - Supinator reflex C5 and C6

4 - Triceps reflex C7

5 - Knee reflex L3 and L4

6 - Ankle reflex S1

Lastly, in the examination of the motor system comes the examination of the reflexes. A deep tendon reflex is an involuntary muscular contraction immediately following a sudden stretching of the muscle tendon. The spinal segments upon which the common tendon reflexes are dependent are:-

Biceps reflex – C5, 6
Supinator reflex – C5, 6
Triceps reflex – C7
Finger reflex – C7, 8
Knee reflex – L3, 4
Ankle reflex – S1

Sometimes, the tendon reflexes seem sluggish or absent in otherwise normal people. The reflexes can be demonstrated in these normal people by reinforcement, (the contraction of muscles elsewhere in the body – eg. gritting the teeth hard).

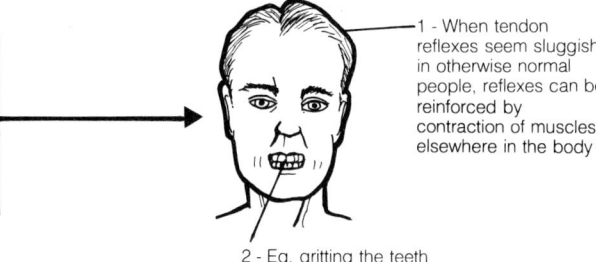

1 - When tendon reflexes seem sluggish in otherwise normal people, reflexes can be reinforced by contraction of muscles elsewhere in the body

2 - Eg. gritting the teeth hard

Superficial Reflexes

The superficial abdominal reflexes consist of brisk unilateral contraction of a segment of the abdominal wall in response to a cutaneous stimulus, (eg. drawing a cocktail stick lightly across the skin). A similar light scratch on the inner aspect of the upper thigh elicits a cremasteric contraction.

The plantar response is elicited by a light scratching sensation elicited by a key drawn forwards over the outer aspect of the sole. An upgoing plantar response (**Babinski sign**) is pathognomonic of an UMN lesion and comprises firstly dorsiflexion of the great toe and then fanning out of the other toes. In certain UMN lesions, the response may be elicited from further afield (eg. firm moving pressure over the anterior shin – **Oppenheim's reflex**), or the motor response may involve a whole reflexor contraction of the limb.

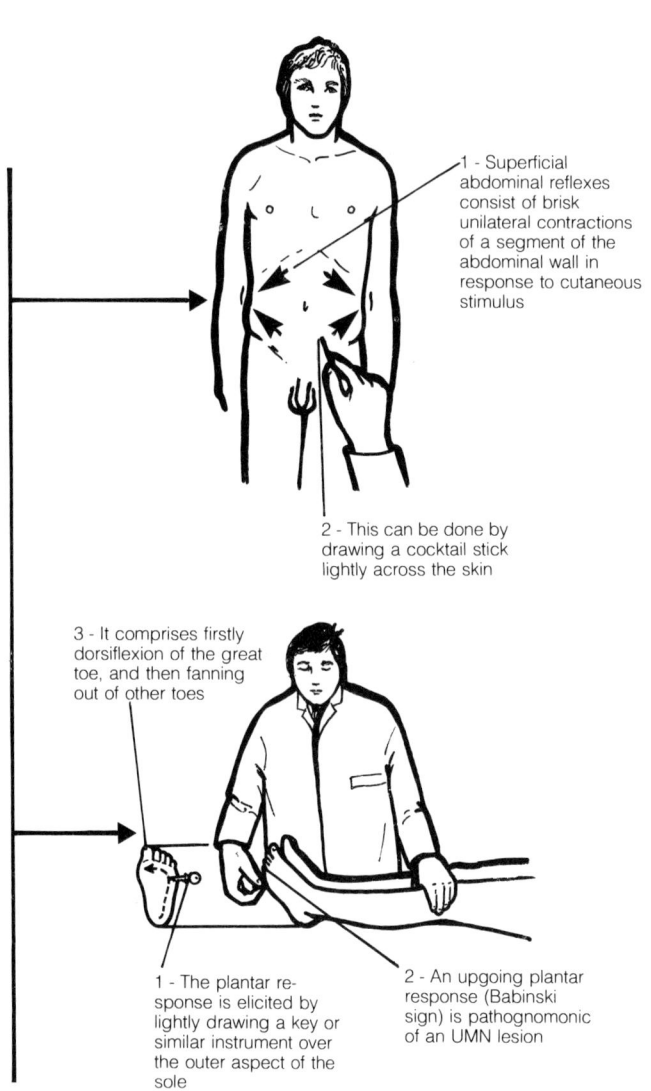

1 - Superficial abdominal reflexes consist of brisk unilateral contractions of a segment of the abdominal wall in response to cutaneous stimulus

2 - This can be done by drawing a cocktail stick lightly across the skin

3 - It comprises firstly dorsiflexion of the great toe, and then fanning out of other toes

1 - The plantar response is elicited by lightly drawing a key or similar instrument over the outer aspect of the sole

2 - An upgoing plantar response (Babinski sign) is pathognomonic of an UMN lesion

THE PERIPHERAL SENSORY SYSTEM

Sensation is conveyed via peripheral nerves to the spinal cord, entering this through the posterior roots. Fibres conveying pain and temperature cross to the contralateral side of the cord within a few segments of entering the cord to ascend to the brain in the lateral spinothalamic tract. Sensations of light touch, joint position sense (proprioception) and vibration sense ascend in the ipsilateral dorsal columns (decussating to the other side in the medulla oblongata).

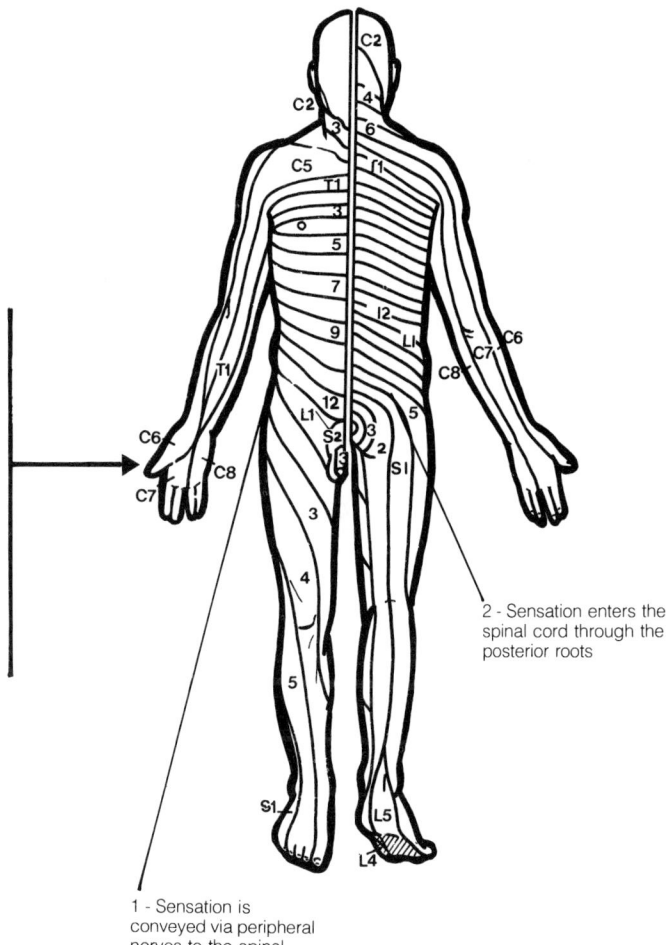

2 - Sensation enters the spinal cord through the posterior roots

1 - Sensation is conveyed via peripheral nerves to the spinal cord

The Peripheral Sensory System

5 - Sensations of light touch joint position, sense and vibration ascend in the ipsilateral dorsal columns to the medulla where they decussate and then pass on to the contralateral sensory cortex

4 - Pain and a temperature sense are carried in the lateral spinothalamic tract

Sensory testing depends on an alert, attentive, co-operative patient. First, any area of sensory loss or impairment needs to be mapped out and the distinction between selective sensory loss (eg. sparing pain and temperature sense) versus unselective anaesthesia, must be made. Thus, it is often possible to distinguish peripheral nerve, nerve root, cord and brain lesions – particularly when taken in conjunction with motor or other neurological deficit.

3 - Fibres conveying pain and temperature cross to the contralateral side of the cord

2 - Any area of sensory loss or impairment must be mapped out

3 - It is often possible to distinguish peripheral nerve, nerve root, cord or brain lesions

1 - Sensory testing depends on an alert, attentive co-operative patient

4 - Brain

5 - Cord

6 - Root

8 - Distinction must be made between selective sensory loss and unselective anaesthesia

7 - Peripheral nerve

Spinal Cord Compression

SPINAL CORD COMPRESSION

This short section on spinal cord compression comes immediately after the clinical examination of the CNS because the physical signs of this important, urgent and often treatable condition must be known by all practitioners.

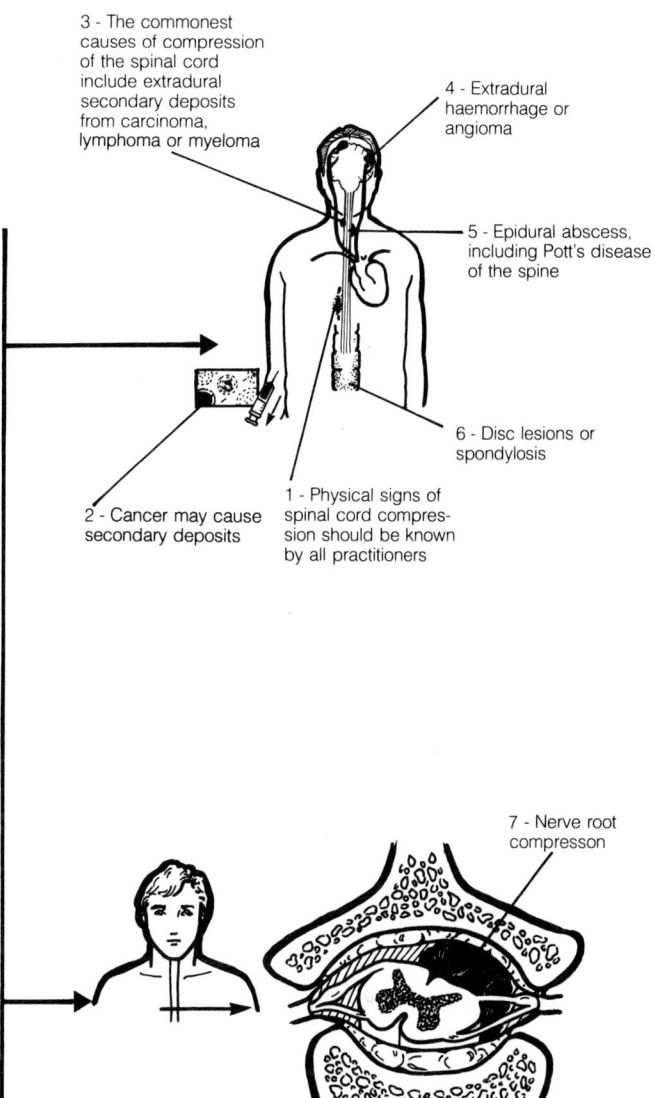

1 - Physical signs of spinal cord compression should be known by all practitioners

2 - Cancer may cause secondary deposits

3 - The commonest causes of compression of the spinal cord include extradural secondary deposits from carcinoma, lymphoma or myeloma

4 - Extradural haemorrhage or angioma

5 - Epidural abscess, including Pott's disease of the spine

6 - Disc lesions or spondylosis

7 - Nerve root compresson

The commonest causes of compression of the spinal cord include extradural secondary deposits from carcinoma or leukaemia or myeloma, epidural abscess (including Pott's disease of spine), an extradural haemorrhage or angioma, disc lesions or spondylosis, and meningiomas.

Spinal Cord Compression

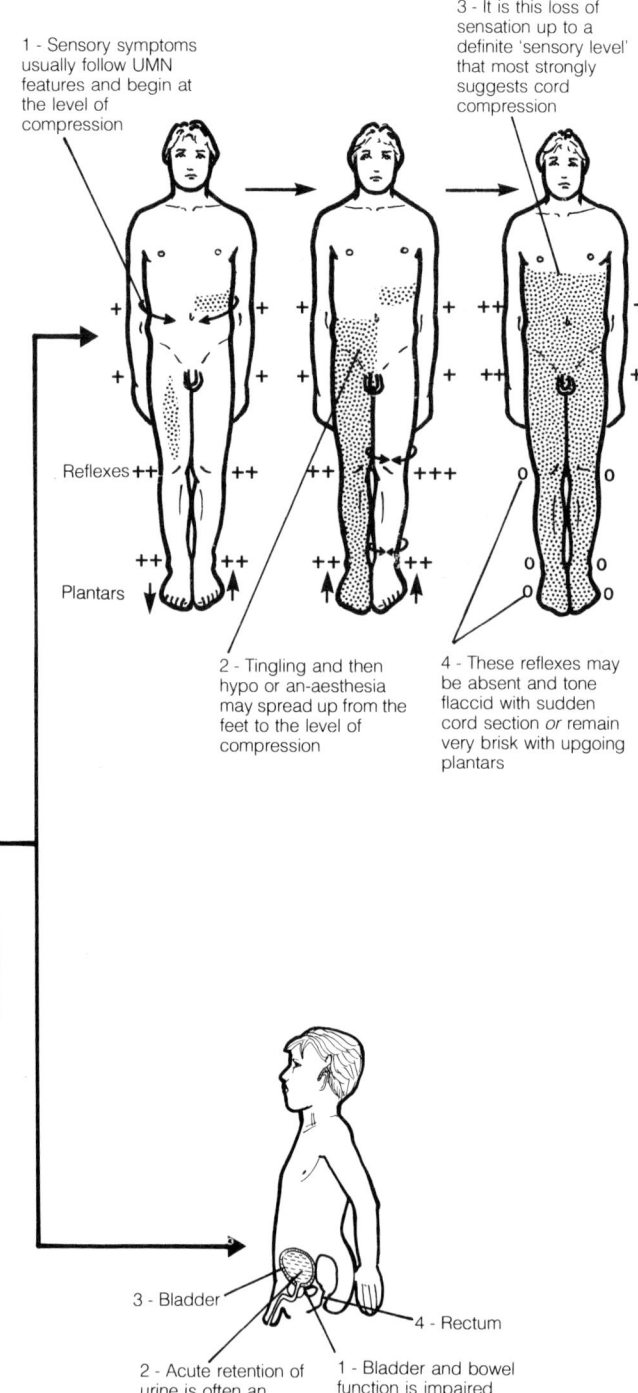

1 - Sensory symptoms usually follow UMN features and begin at the level of compression

2 - Tingling and then hypo or an-aesthesia may spread up from the feet to the level of compression

3 - It is this loss of sensation up to a definite 'sensory level' that most strongly suggests cord compression

4 - These reflexes may be absent and tone flaccid with sudden cord section *or* remain very brisk with upgoing plantars

The **signs of cord compression** will include UMN signs caudal to the lesion, (and usually these are fairly symmetrical), thus usually a spastic paraparesis occurs. Sensory symptoms usually follow UMN features and may begin with root symptoms at the level of compression; tingling and then hypo- or anaesthesia may spread upwards from the feet to the level of compression. It is this loss of sensation up to a definite **'sensory level'** that most strongly suggests spinal cord compression. Bladder and bowel function is impaired, and acute retention of urine is often an important early feature.

3 - Bladder

4 - Rectum

2 - Acute retention of urine is often an important early feature

1 - Bladder and bowel function is impaired

Spinal Cord Compression

Having **diagnosed** cord compression, plain X-rays of the whole vertebral column precede urgent neurosurgical referral and a myelogram. For malignant disease, neurosurgical decompression and radiotherapy are the appropriate first therapies prior to review of systemic management. The degree of recovery is inversely related to severity of the neurological deficit. For radiosensitive tumours (e.g Myeloma), radiotherapy alone may be indicated.

1 - Having diagnosed cord compression, plain X-rays of the whole vertebral column are needed

2 - These precede urgent neurosurgical referral and a myelogram

1 - For malignant disease, neurosurgical decompression with radiotherapy are appropriate first therapies

2 - Neurosurgical decompression

3 - Radiotherapy

4 - Then systemic management is reviewed

5 - Degree of recovery is inversely related to the severity of the neurological deficit

Occasionally, compression of the spinal cord from one side may lead to impairment of light touch, proprioception and vibration sense from the ipsilateral dermatomes caudal to the compression and impaired temperature and pain sensation from contralateral dermatomes caudal to the lesion (**Brown Séquard lesion**).

1 - Compression of the spinal cord on one side

2 - Impairment of light touch, proprioception and vibration sense from the ipsilateral dermatomes caudal to the compression

3 - Impaired temperature and pain sensation from contralateral dermatomes caudal to the lesion

4 - This comprises a Brown Séquard lesion

Spinal Cord Compression

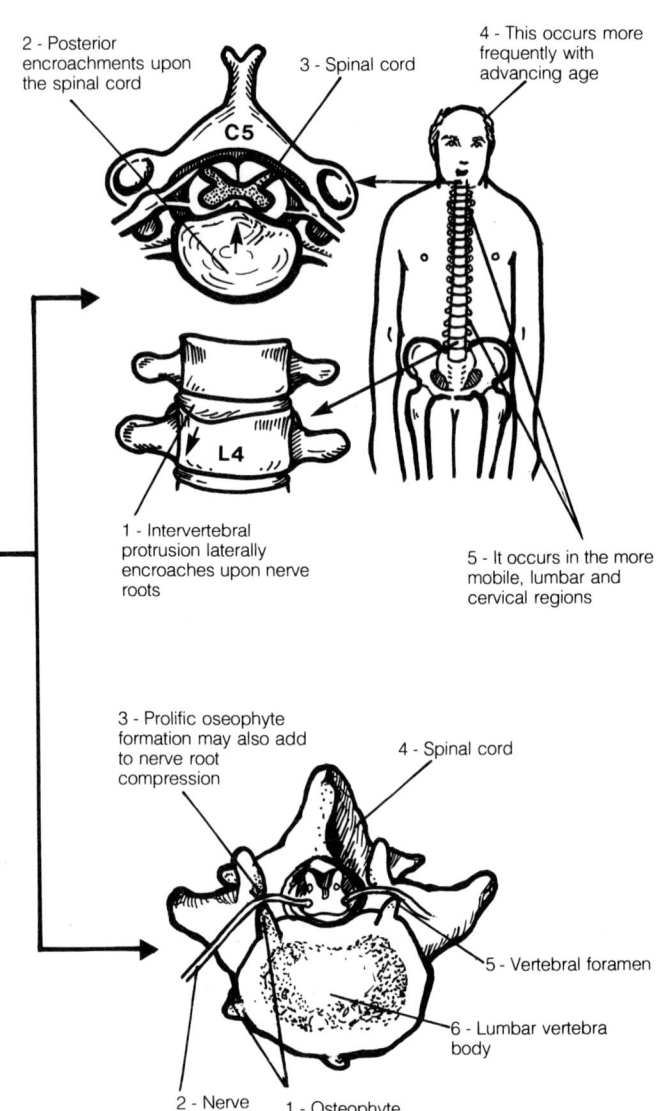

Intervertebral Disc Prolapse and Spondylosis

Intervertebral disc degeneration and protrusion laterally, (to encroach upon segmental nerve roots), or posteriorly (to encroach and compress the spinal cord) occur more frequently with advancing age and in the more mobile regions of the spine – particularly cervical and lumbar regions. Secondary osteoarthritic changes with prolific osteophyte formation may also add to the compression of nerve roots.

Spinal Cord Compression

In the cervical spine the C6/7 disc is most frequently involved and the C7 nerve root is compressed leading to pain in the myotomal distribution of the nerve root, wasting and weakness of triceps, extensor digitorum and extensor carpi ulnaris together with a reduced triceps jerk (ie. LMN signs).

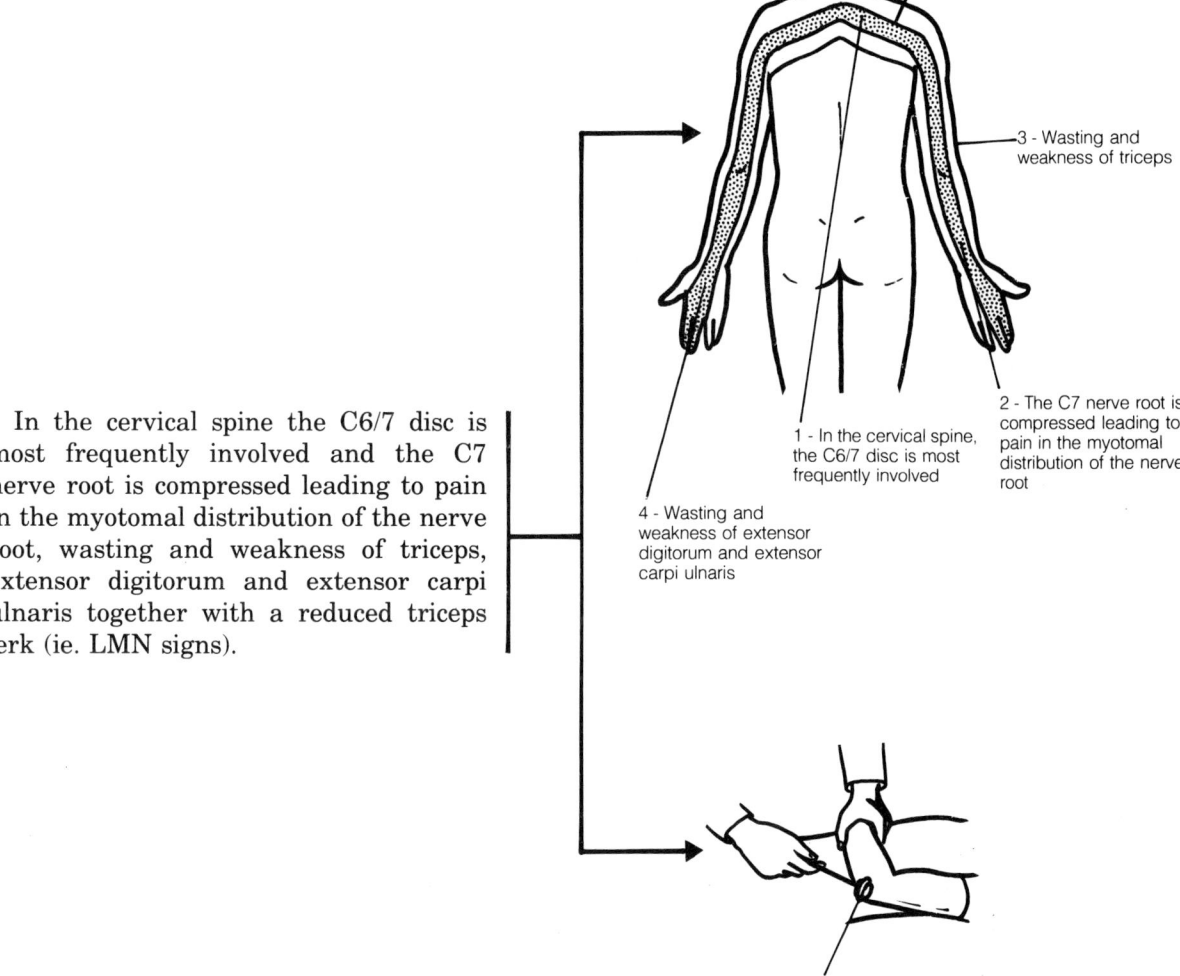

1 - In the cervical spine, the C6/7 disc is most frequently involved

2 - The C7 nerve root is compressed leading to pain in the myotomal distribution of the nerve root

3 - Wasting and weakness of triceps

4 - Wasting and weakness of extensor digitorum and extensor carpi ulnaris

5 - Reduced triceps jerk (LMN sign)

Spinal Cord Compression

A careful search for UMN signs in the legs must be performed such that concurrent cord compression is not missed, (although in the acute lateral root compression syndrome this is unusual). Plain X-rays of the cervical spine show disc space narrowing with or without osteophytes and perhaps minor subluxation; in the absence of long tract signs, (UMN signs in the legs or bladder dysfunction), myelography is not indicated. **Treatment** is by rest and gentle traction and immobilisation of the cervical spine, provided by a light but stiff collar. Decompressive surgery is rarely required unless cord compression occurs.

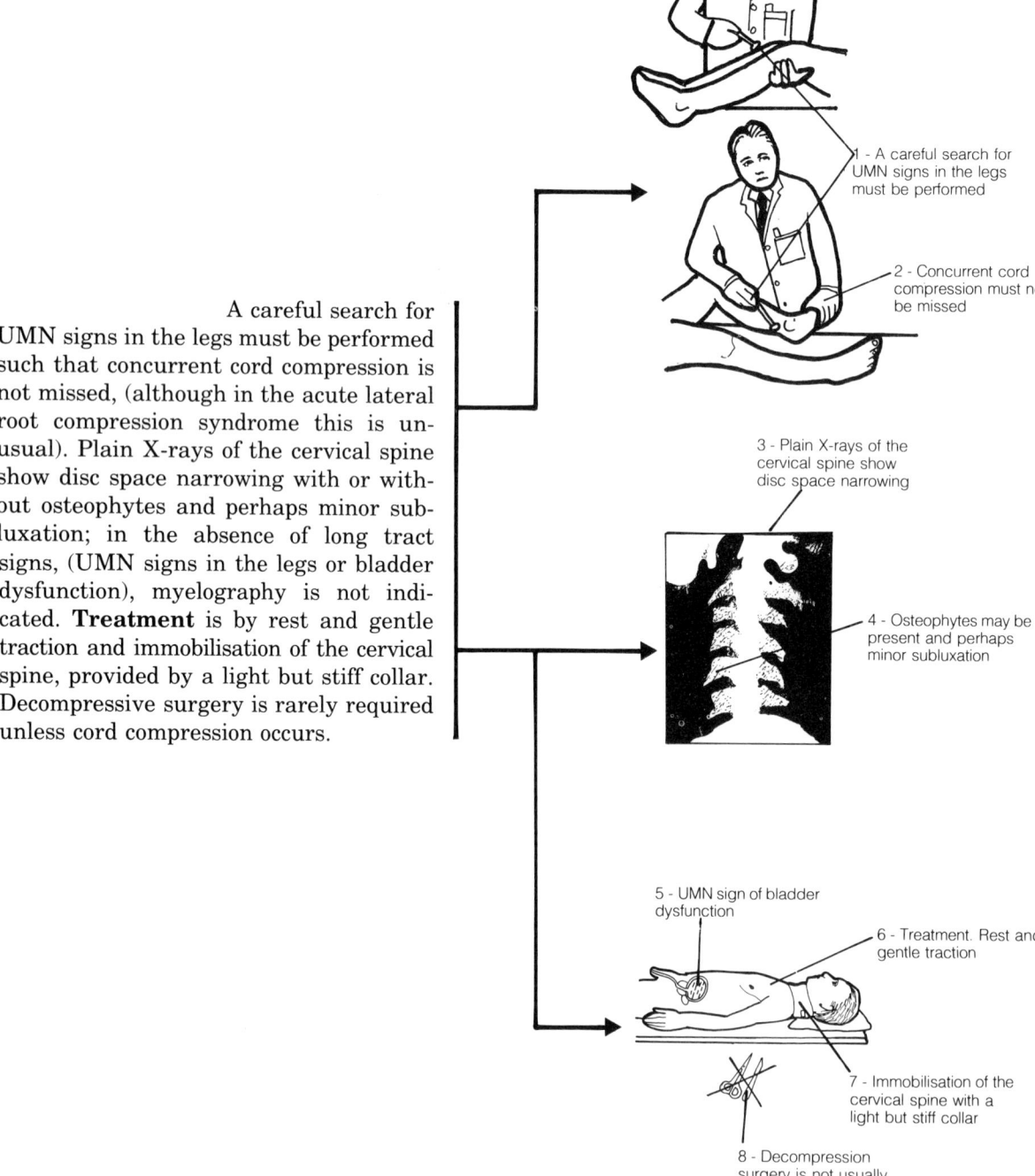

1 - A careful search for UMN signs in the legs must be performed

2 - Concurrent cord compression must not be missed

3 - Plain X-rays of the cervical spine show disc space narrowing

4 - Osteophytes may be present and perhaps minor subluxation

5 - UMN sign of bladder dysfunction

6 - Treatment. Rest and gentle traction

7 - Immobilisation of the cervical spine with a light but stiff collar

8 - Decompression surgery is not usually required

Osteophytes due to cervical spondylosis may also encroach upon the vertebral artery as it passes upwards to the brain. Occasionally, 'drop attacks' – precipitated by neck movements – are due to this vertebral artery compression.

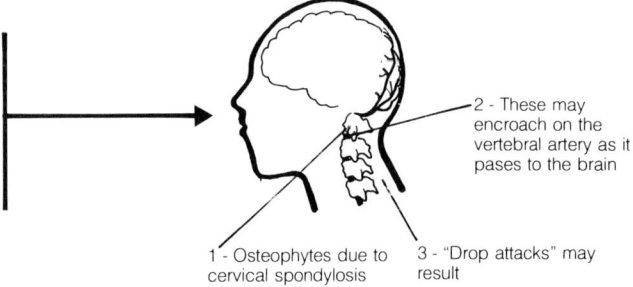

LUMBAGO

Lumbago refers to pain in the lumbar spine, (worse on bending down) and sciatica to pain radiating down the back of the leg in the distribution of the sciatic nerve, (exacerbated by sneezing and coughing). The commonest cause of these symptoms is intervertebral disc prolapse, but there is always a differential diagnosis which includes infiltration of the lumbar spine by malignancy, (often from a

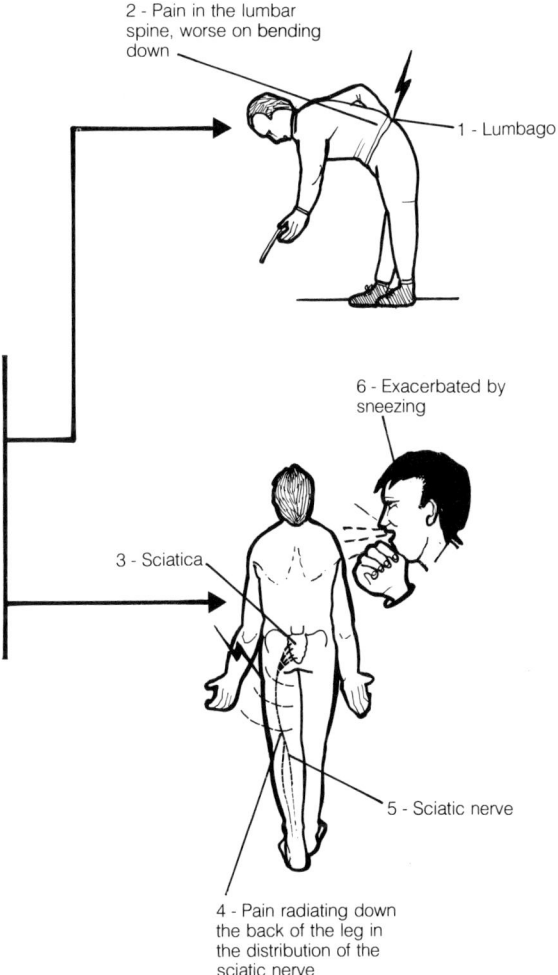

Lumbago

pelvic neoplasm, making it mandatory for the clinician to perform a full pelvic examination during the work-up of lumbago/sciatica), and intraspinal tumour, (which may require myelographic investigation). Plain X-rays of the lumbar spine (frontal and lateral views) and pelvis are mandatory in all cases.

The commonest lumbar discs to be affected are L4-L5 and L5-S1 compressing roots L5 and S1 respectively, due to the oblique course of these roots. A midline prolapse at this level may compress the cauda equina, (with 'saddle anaesthesia', sphincter disturbance and other variable neurology). A midline prolapse requires investigation by myelography and neurosurgical decompression.

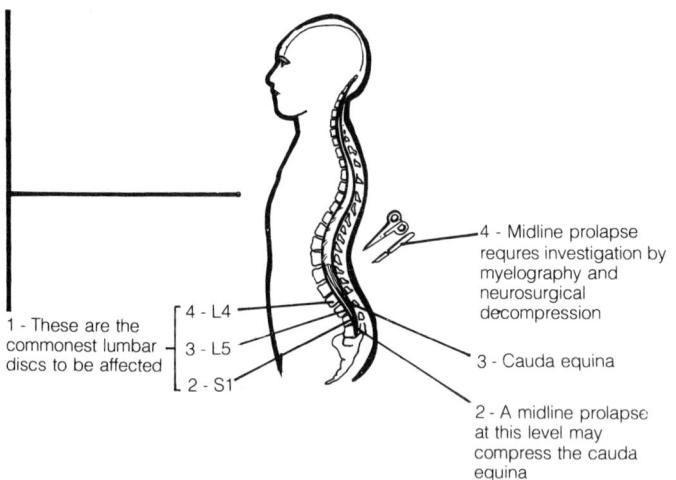

Once again, the neurological signs of root compression can be deduced from knowledge of anatomy; thus an S1 root lesion leads to weak plantar flexion of the foot, a diminished ankle jerk (LMN signs for S1), and variable sensory loss over the outer border of the foot. A useful sign of pressure on these nerve roots is the pain and limitation of passive hip flexion with the knee extended, caused by reflex spasm in the hamstring muscles, (straight leg raising test or Lasègue's sign). The angle to which the straight leg can be raised is recorded.

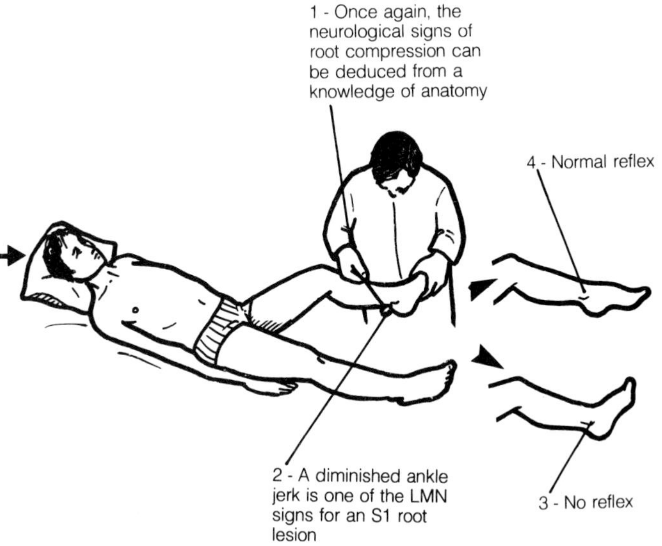

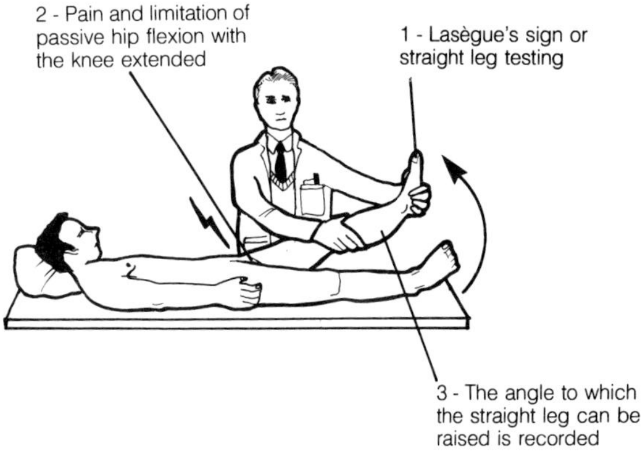

Treatment comprises supine bed rest on a firm (and preferably hard), mattress or board with no rotation or flexion of the spine; this should be maintained for 2-4 weeks before gentle, gradual mobilisation with back-strengthening exercises is implemented, probably with provision of a lumbar corset.

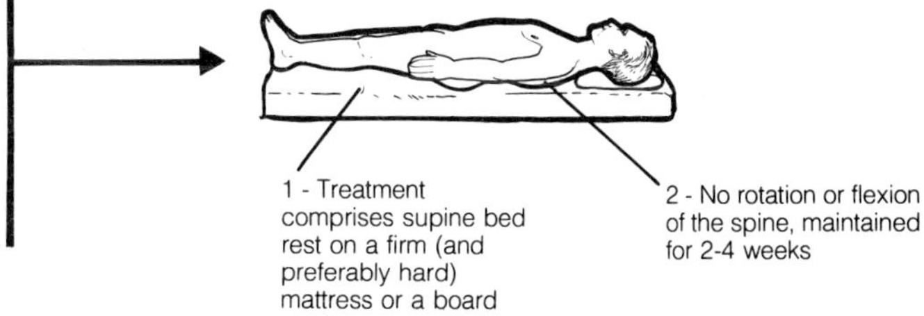

Lumbago

Some Examples Of Root Innervation Of Muscles

C5	Deltoid (shoulder abduction)
C5-6	Biceps (flexion at elbow)
C6	Brachioradialis, extensor carpi radialis (main wrist extensor)
C7	Triceps, extensor digitorum, latissimus dorsi
C8	Finger flexors
T1	Intrinsic muscles of the hand
L1-2	Iliopsoas (hip flexion)
L2-3	Adductors of the hip
L3-4	Quadriceps (knee extension and jerk)
L4	Tibialis anterior (main dorsiflexor of ankle)
L4-5	Tibialis posterior (invertor at ankle) Gluteus medius and minimus (internal rotators at hip)
L5-S1	Peronei (evertors at ankle), extensors of toes
L5-S2	Hamstrings, Gluteus maximus (hip extension)
S1	Gastrocnemius and soleus (plantar flexion and ankle jerk)

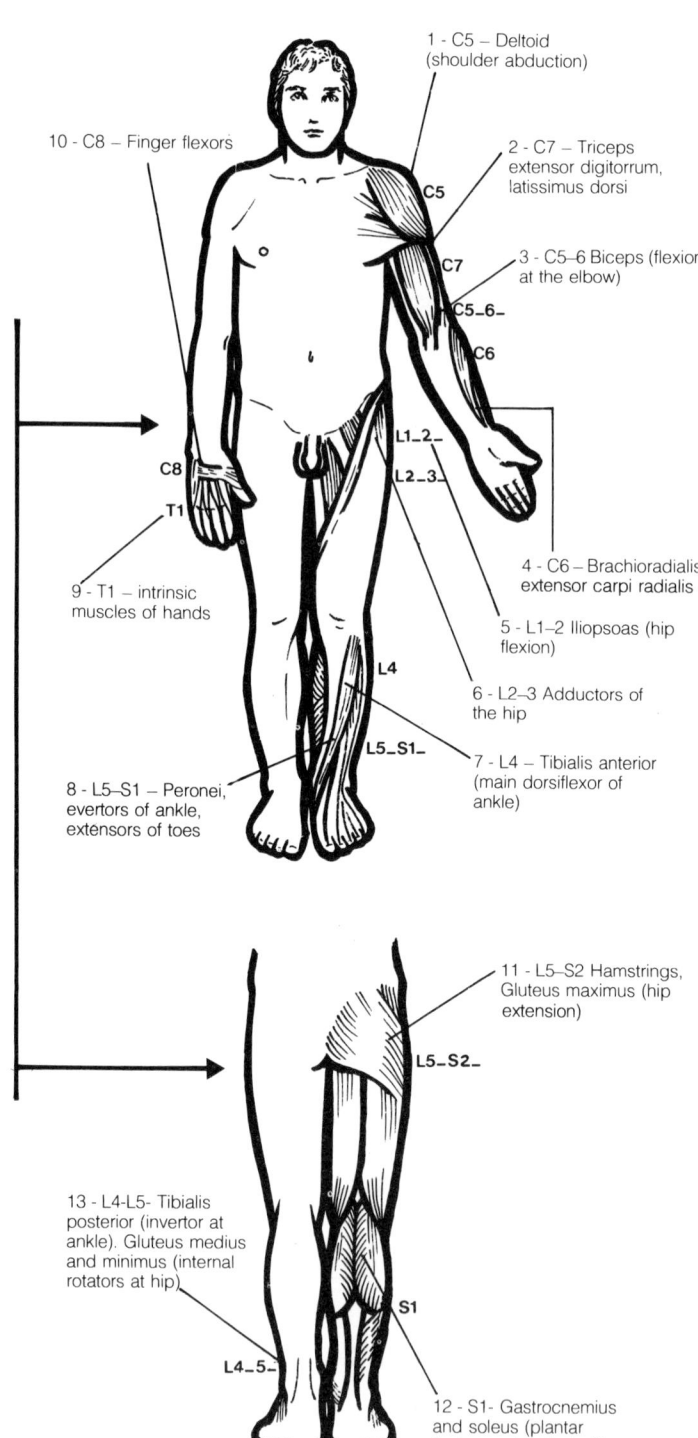

1 - C5 – Deltoid (shoulder abduction)
2 - C7 – Triceps extensor digitorrum, latissimus dorsi
3 - C5–6 Biceps (flexion at the elbow)
4 - C6 – Brachioradialis, extensor carpi radialis
5 - L1–2 Iliopsoas (hip flexion)
6 - L2–3 Adductors of the hip
7 - L4 – Tibialis anterior (main dorsiflexor of ankle)
8 - L5–S1 – Peronei, evertors of ankle, extensors of toes
9 - T1 – intrinsic muscles of hands
10 - C8 – Finger flexors
11 - L5–S2 Hamstrings, Gluteus maximus (hip extension)
12 - S1- Gastrocnemius and soleus (plantar flexion and ankle jerk)
13 - L4-L5- Tibialis posterior (invertor at ankle). Gluteus medius and minimus (internal rotators at hip)

THE CEREBROSPINAL FLUID (CSF)

The CSF is formed by the choroid plexus in the ventricles and flows throughout the ventricular system to pass via the cerebral aqueduct into the IVth ventricle and thence, (via the foramina of Magendie and Luschka), into the subarachnoid space. The CSF then bathes the whole surface of the brain and spinal cord. CSF is absorbed into the intracranial venous sinuses via arachnoid villi.

The lumbar puncture is used to sample the CSF and the secret of this simple technique is to position the patient in the left lateral position with his knees and hips flexed (to open up the lumbar intervertebral spaces) and to ensure that the plane of the iliac crests is vertical. The level of the iliac crests is approximately L3-L4 disc space and the clinician locally anaesthetises the skin and subcutis before inserting the lumbar puncture needle at this space, keeping strictly to the midline. A lumbar puncture is contraindicated when the intracranial pressure is raised (suggested by papilloedema) or when a space-occupying lesion in the posterior fossa is suspected; a drop in the lumbar CSF pressure in such patients may allow a cerebellar pressure cone to develop in the foramen magnum. When the lumbar puncture needle has penetrated the subarachnoid space, the pressure is tested and the fluid sampled (5-7ml) for cytological, biochemical, bacteriological, and virological studies. The normal CSF pressure is 60-200mm CSF.

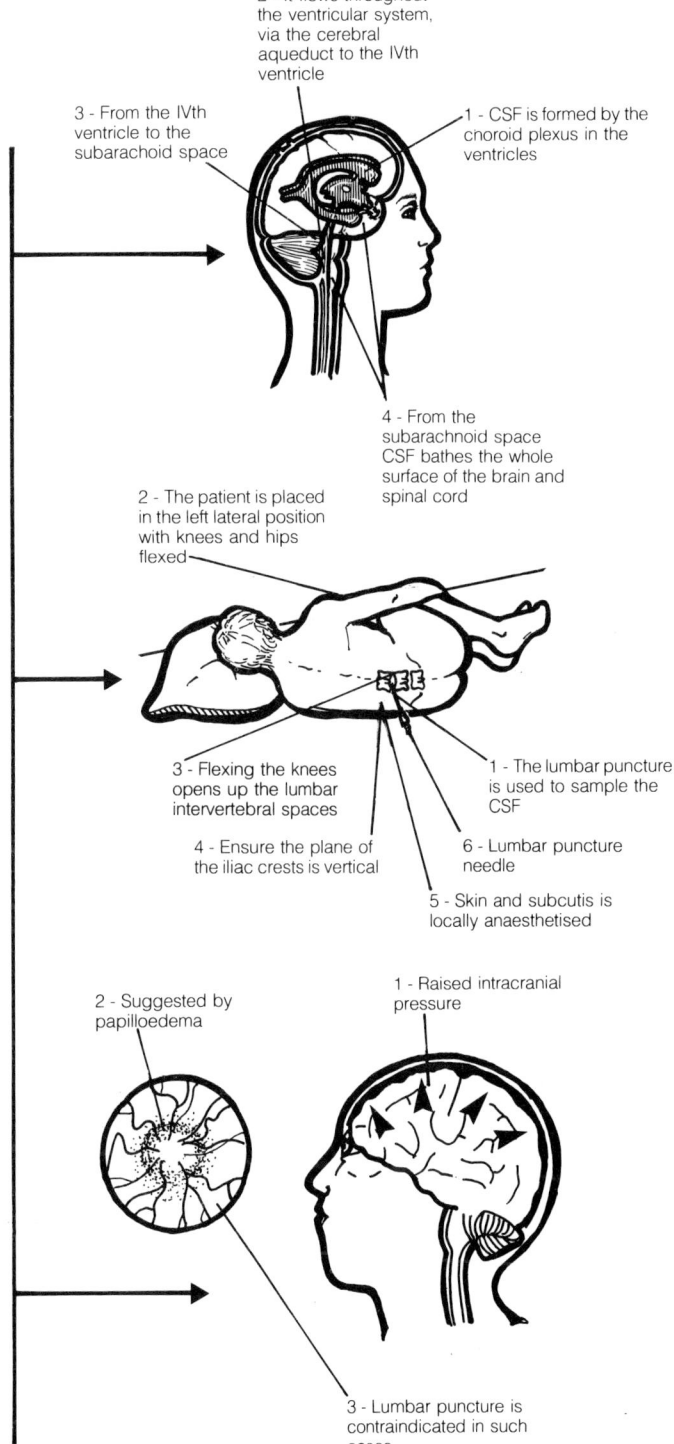

The Cerebrospinal Fluid (CSF)

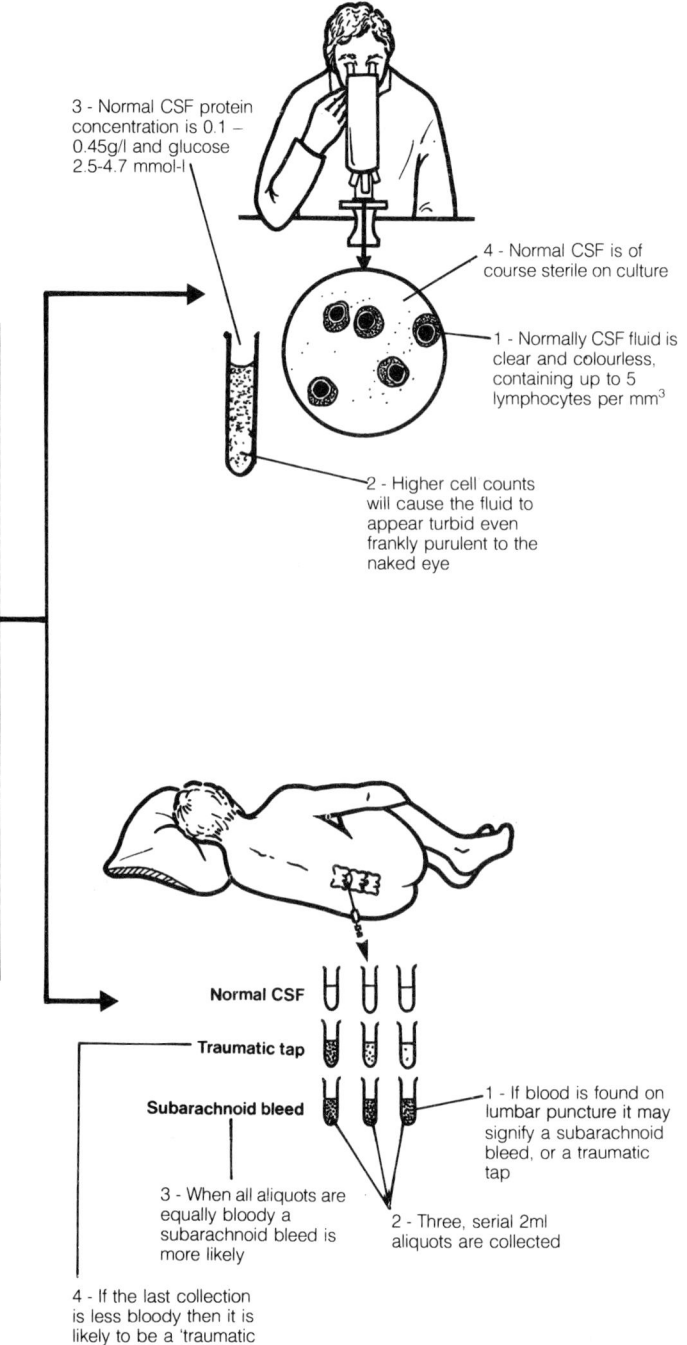

The normal CSF fluid is clear and colourless containing up to 5 lymphocytes per mm^3. High cell counts will cause the fluid to appear turbid or even frankly purulent to the naked eye. The normal CSF protein concentration is 0.1 - 0.45g/l and glucose 2.5 - 4.7mmol/l; normal CSF is of course sterile on culture. If blood is found in the CSF on lumbar puncture it may signify a subarachnoid bleed or a traumatic tap. If the CSF flow is collected in three, serial 2ml aliquots and the last collection appears less bloody, then it is likely to be a 'traumatic tap'. When all the aliquots are equally bloody, a subarachnoid bleed is more likely. For some weeks after a subarachnoid bleed, the CSF will retain a yellow tinge – xanthochromia. A bloody tap can confuse the clinician in his attempt to diagnose meningitis.

The Cerebrospinal Fluid (CSF)

In the patient with a normal peripheral blood count, a CSF cell count with a red cell: white cells ratio of less than 10:1 suggests meningitis.

If the CSF protein is raised, then other tests may be appropriate. Lange's colloidal gold reaction detects an increase in gamma globulin that is so typical of neurosyphilis, but also occurs in other pathologies. Protein electrophoresis and IgG quantitation are the modern and refined tests.

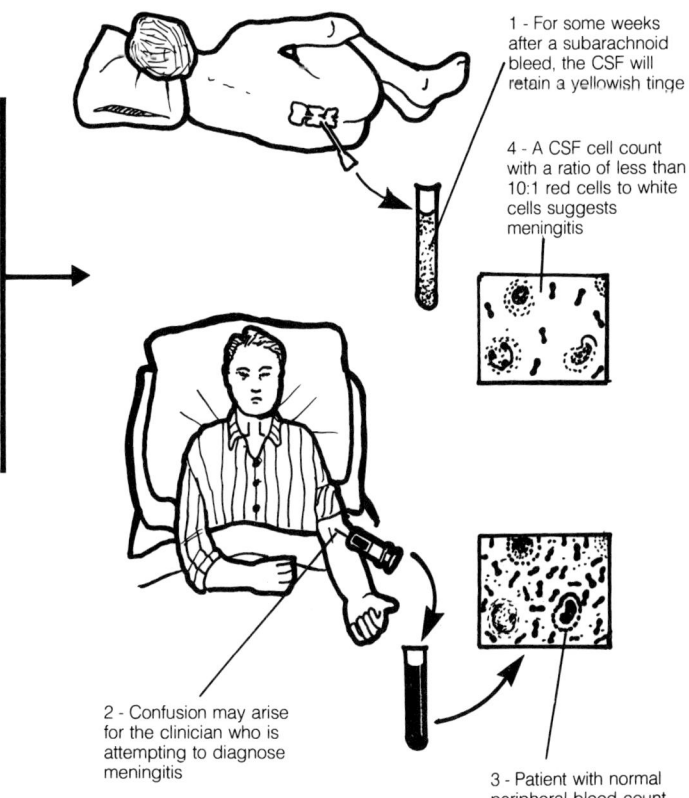

1 - For some weeks after a subarachnoid bleed, the CSF will retain a yellowish tinge

4 - A CSF cell count with a ratio of less than 10:1 red cells to white cells suggests meningitis

2 - Confusion may arise for the clinician who is attempting to diagnose meningitis

3 - Patient with normal peripheral blood count

Meningitis

Meningitis refers to inflammation of the pia and arachnoid membranes. This may be caused by infection (bacterial, viral, fungal, others), chemicals, malignant cells, sarcoidosis or even a subarachnoid bleed may cause meningeal irritation with the physical signs of meningitis.

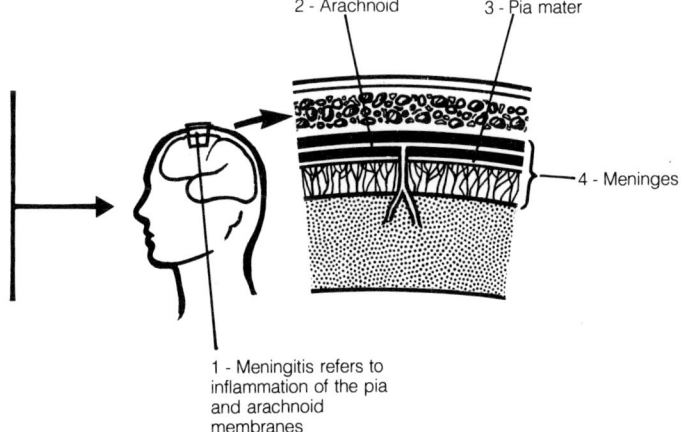

2 - Arachnoid 3 - Pia mater

4 - Meninges

1 - Meningitis refers to inflammation of the pia and arachnoid membranes

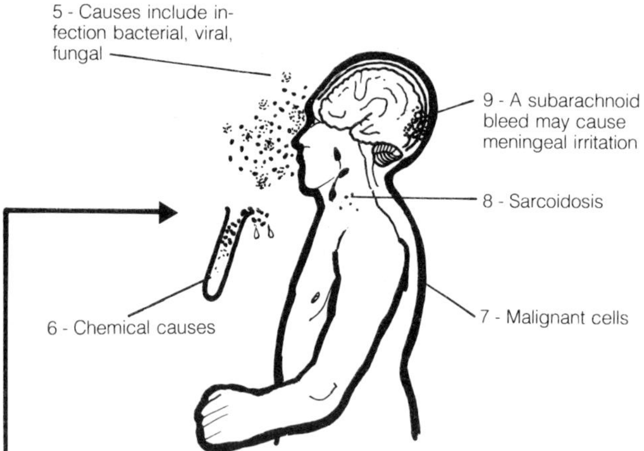

The Cerebrospinal Fluid (CSF)

5 - Causes include infection bacterial, viral, fungal

9 - A subarachnoid bleed may cause meningeal irritation

8 - Sarcoidosis

6 - Chemical causes

7 - Malignant cells

The clinical picture is of a patient with headache, fever, dizziness, nausea, vomiting and photophobia who lapses into light stupor and then coma. The **physical signs** include neck stiffness (due to a reflex spasm of the paravertebral muscles) and a positive Kernig's sign. Kernig's sign is elicited with the patient's knee and hip flexed; the clinician then

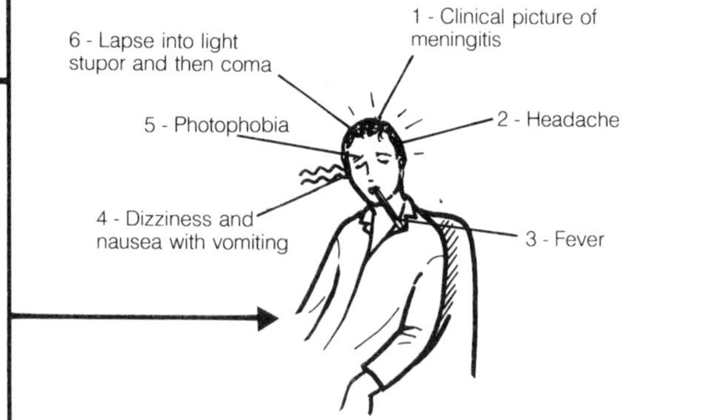

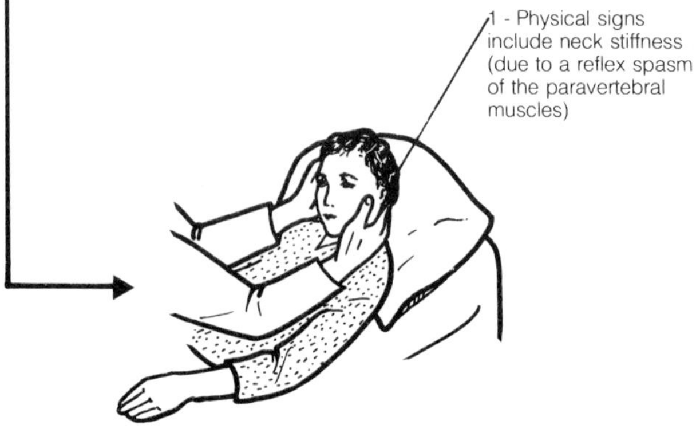

1 - Clinical picture of meningitis

2 - Headache

3 - Fever

4 - Dizziness and nausea with vomiting

5 - Photophobia

6 - Lapse into light stupor and then coma

1 - Physical signs include neck stiffness (due to a reflex spasm of the paravertebral muscles)

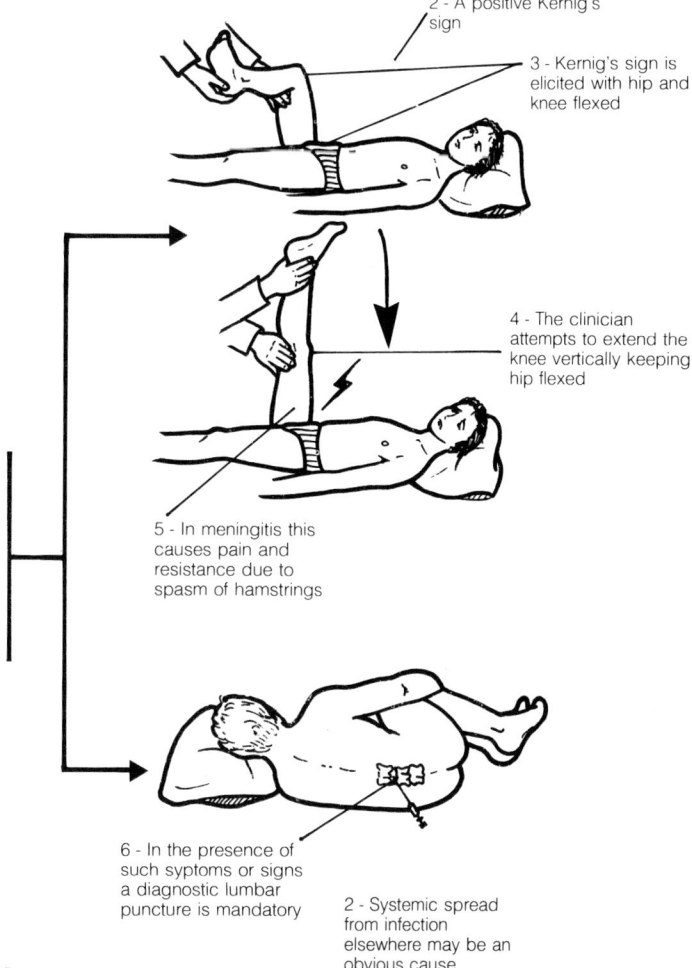

attempts to extend the knee, keeping the hip flexed. This causes pain and resistance in meningitis due to spasm of the hamstrings (positive Kernig's sign). In the presence of such symptoms or signs, a diagnostic lumbar puncture is mandatory.

Acute Pyogenic Meningitis

Although it is often obvious how a pyogenic infection may reach the CSF, (eg. local spread from a middle ear infection or sinusitis, or systemic spread from an infected focus elsewhere – septicaemia, septic embolism), in many cases the derivation of the organism is unknown. Many organisms are capable of causing meningitis but *N. meningitidis* (meningococcus), *Streptococcus pneumoniae* and *Haemophilus influenzae* are the most common pathogens. In the immunosuppressed patient, the list of potential pathogens is considerably longer with yeasts and fungi being prominent amongst the opportunist pathogens.

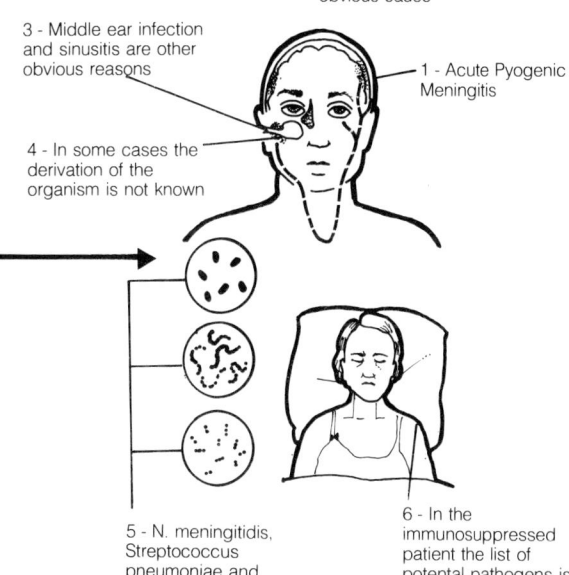

The Cerebrospinal Fluid (CSF)

The **clinical onset** may be acute with headaches, vomiting and drowsiness. Examination may demonstrate stupor, photophobia, neck stiffness and a positive Kernig's sign.

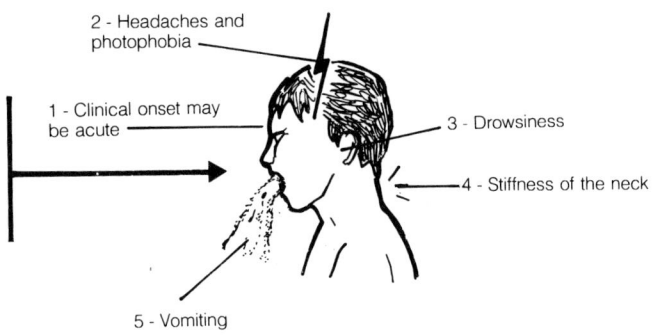

1 - Clinical onset may be acute
2 - Headaches and photophobia
3 - Drowsiness
4 - Stiffness of the neck
5 - Vomiting

Lumbar puncture (LP) will give turbid, cloudy or frankly purulent fluid due to the vast excess of polymorphs, and Gram stain may demonstrate the bacterium microscopically; the CSF protein and pressure are raised. Even before the causative organism is identified, a tap of purulent CSF is an indication for immediate initiation of therapy with an intrathecal dose of benzyl penicillin 10,000 units, (diluted prior to injection).

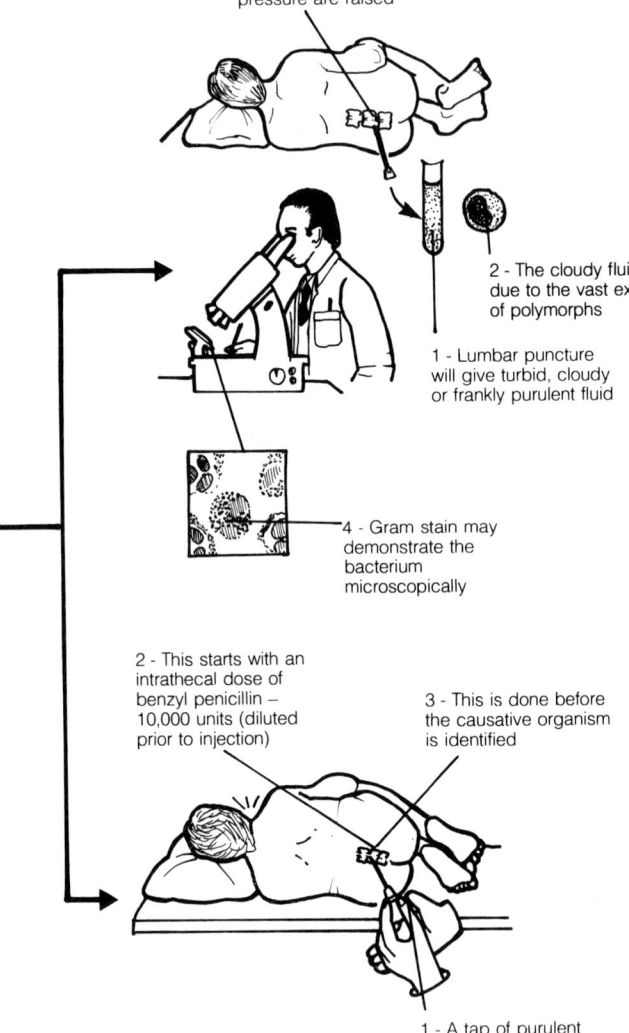

1 - Lumbar puncture will give turbid, cloudy or frankly purulent fluid
2 - The cloudy fluid is due to the vast excess of polymorphs
3 - CSF protein and pressure are raised
4 - Gram stain may demonstrate the bacterium microscopically

1 - A tap of purulent CSF is an indication for immediate initiation of therapy
2 - This starts with an intrathecal dose of benzyl penicillin – 10,000 units (diluted prior to injection)
3 - This is done before the causative organism is identified

The Cerebrospinal Fluid (CSF)

Until the bacteriological result is known, systemic combination antibiotics are given:- benzyl penicillin 4 mega-units, four hourly intravenously and sulphadiazine 6g orally stat and 2g four hourly; in comatose patients this must be given parenterally.

In severe cases of acute pyogenic meningitis, it may be thought necessary to add Chloramphenicol (20mg/Kg i.m. 6 hourly, up to 4g per day maximum).

When the bacteriological results are known, the antibiotic regime is modified appropriately. Pneumococcus is penicillin sensitive. In meningococcal infection, chloramphicol is not needed. In *H. influenzae* meningitis, (usually young children), chloramphenicol remains the drug of first choice and that rare side effect of severe blood dyscrasia is far outweighted by its potential for cure.

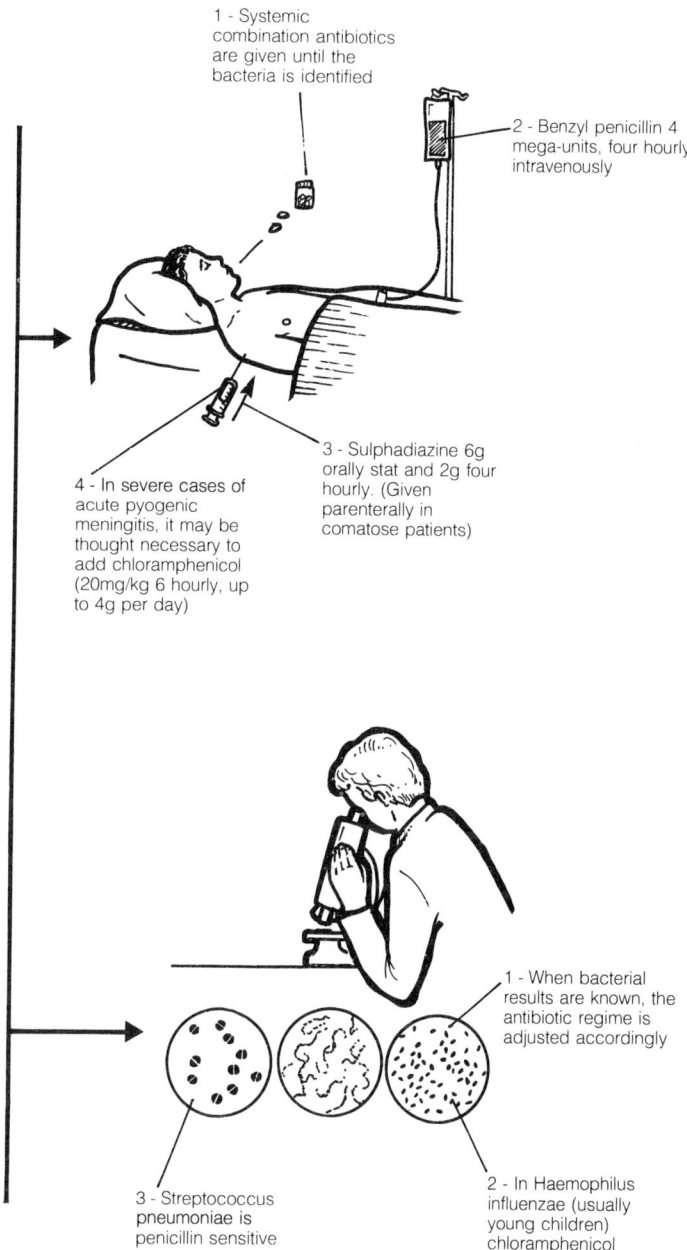

1 - Systemic combination antibiotics are given until the bacteria is identified

2 - Benzyl penicillin 4 mega-units, four hourly intravenously

3 - Sulphadiazine 6g orally stat and 2g four hourly. (Given parenterally in comatose patients)

4 - In severe cases of acute pyogenic meningitis, it may be thought necessary to add chloramphenicol (20mg/kg 6 hourly, up to 4g per day)

1 - When bacterial results are known, the antibiotic regime is adjusted accordingly

2 - In Haemophilus influenzae (usually young children) chloramphenicol remains the drug of first choice

3 - Streptococcus pneumoniae is penicillin sensitive

The Cerebrospinal Fluid (CSF)

Meningococcal meningitis may be attended by purpura – usually more marked in the skin of the buttocks and legs. Very occasionally in meningococcal meningitis, a fulminating septicaemia occurs with haemorrhagic destruction of the adrenals, (causing an acute **Addisonian crisis**) and leading to circulatory collapse and death unless rapid resuscitation including intravenous steroids and antibiotics is given (Waterhouse-Friderichsen syndrome).

1 - Meningococcal meningitis may be attended by purpura – usually more marked in the skin of the legs and buttocks

6 - Waterhouse-Friderichsen syndrome

2 - A fulminating septicaemia very occasionally occurs in meningococcal meningitis

3 - This involves haemorrhagic destruction of the adrenals (causing an acute Addisonian crisis)

5 - In the absence of treatment circulatory collapse will occur

4 - Intravenous steroids and antibiotics must be administered

Tuberculous Meningitis – T.B. meningitis is due to spread from a focus of tuberculous infection elsewhere in the body, although this other focus may not be known to the patient or clinician. The clinical onset may be insidious over a

1 - TB meningitis is due to spread from a focus of tuberculous infection elsewhere in the body

2 - This other focus may not be known to the patient or clinician

couple of weeks with vague ill health and lassitude preceding apathy, confusion and stupor; headaches, vomiting and neck stiffness may all be late and cranial nerve palsies are a late feature also. There is usually a fever often intermittent and low grade.

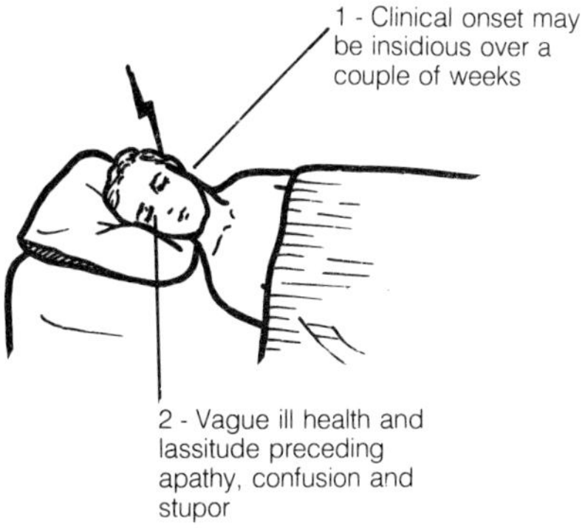

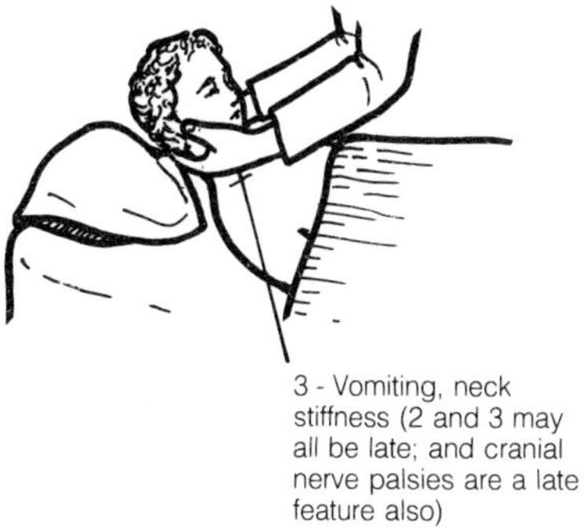

1 - Clinical onset may be insidious over a couple of weeks

2 - Vague ill health and lassitude preceding apathy, confusion and stupor

3 - Vomiting, neck stiffness (2 and 3 may all be late; and cranial nerve palsies are a late feature also)

If present, choroidal tubercles are strongly suggestive of the diagnosis. Lumbar puncture is an essential diagnostic test: the pressure is raised, the fluid usually clear but forming a cobweb clot on standing, a lymphocytosis is present and the CSF protein is raised whilst the CSF glucose is low. Ziehl-Nielsen staining of the centrifuged pellet may directly demonstrate AAFB, but culture takes several weeks.

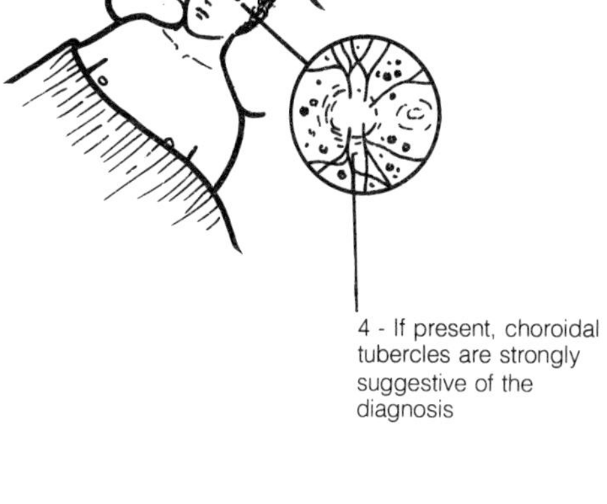

4 - If present, choroidal tubercles are strongly suggestive of the diagnosis

The Cerebrospinal Fluid (CSF)

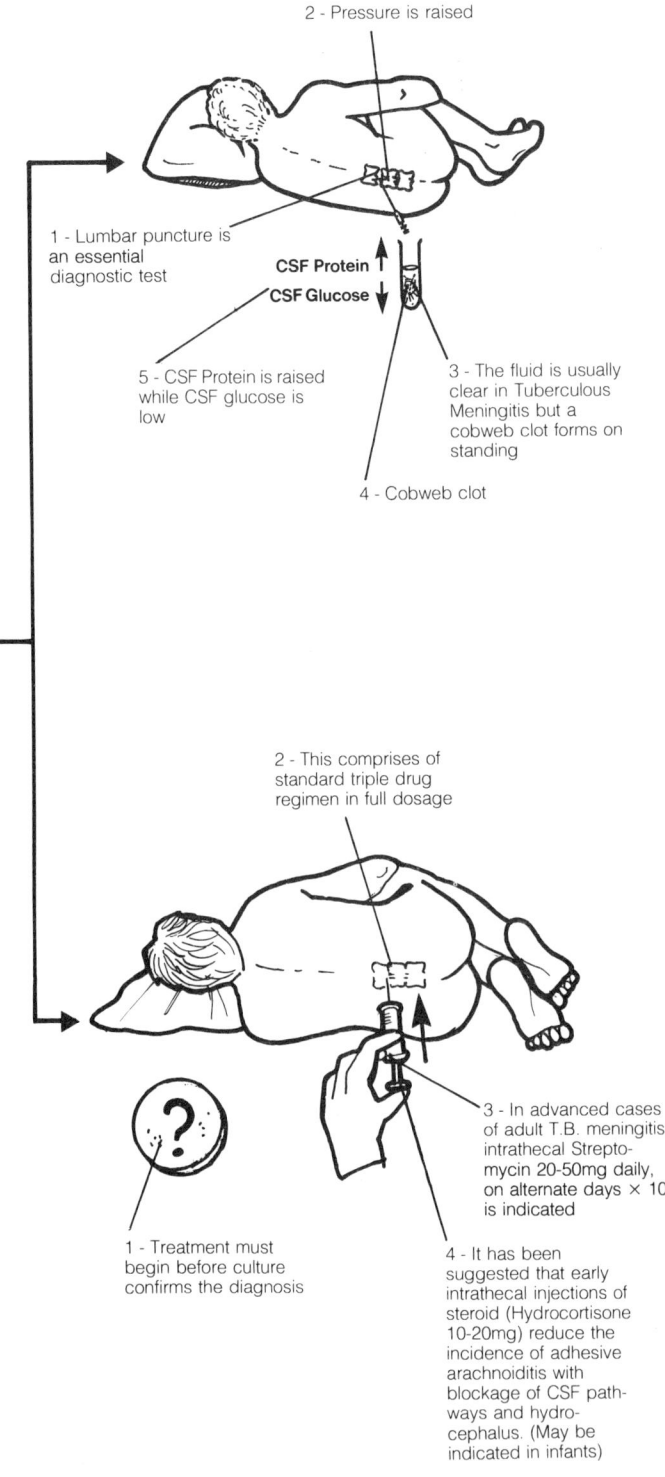

Treatment must begin before the culture confirms the diagnosis. This comprises the standard triple drug regimen in full dosage. In advanced cases of adult T.B. meningitis, intrathecal streptomycin 20-50mg daily on alternate days × 10 is indicated. It has been suggested that early intrathecal injections of steroid, (hydrocortisone 10-20mg), reduce the incidence of adhesive arachnoiditis with blockage of CSF pathways and hydrocephalus. This may be indicated in infants.

The Cerebrospinal Fluid (CSF)

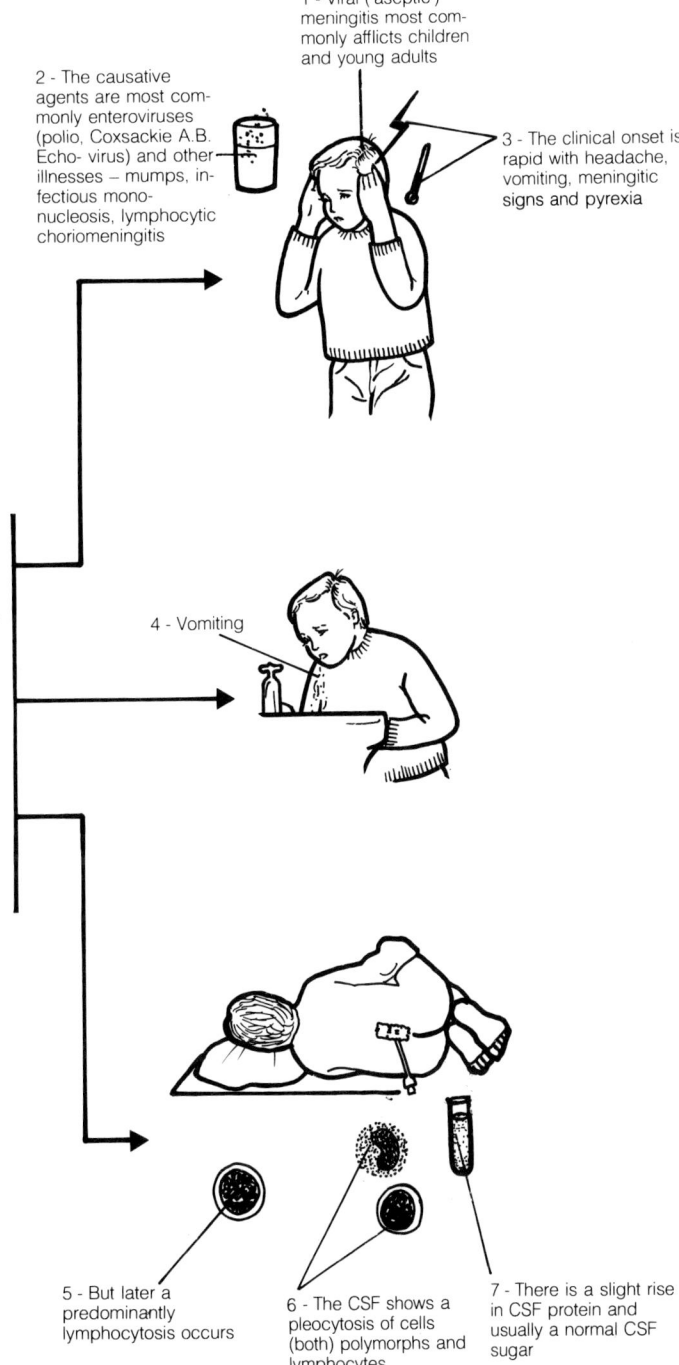

Viral Meningitis – Viral ('aseptic') meningitis most commonly afflicts children and young adults. The causative agents are most commonly: enteroviruses (polio, Coxsackie A, B, Echo-virus), mumps, infectious mononucleosis, lymphocytic choriomeningitis. The clinical onset is rapid with headache, vomiting, meningitic signs and pyrexia. The CSF shows a pleocytosis of cells (both polymorphs and lymphocytes) but later a predominantly lymphocytosis occurs. There is a slight rise in CSF protein and usually a normal CSF sugar. Specific viral tests based on serology may be diagnostic. There is no specific therapy but fortunately these acute viral menigitides are usually self-limiting and the prognosis is good.

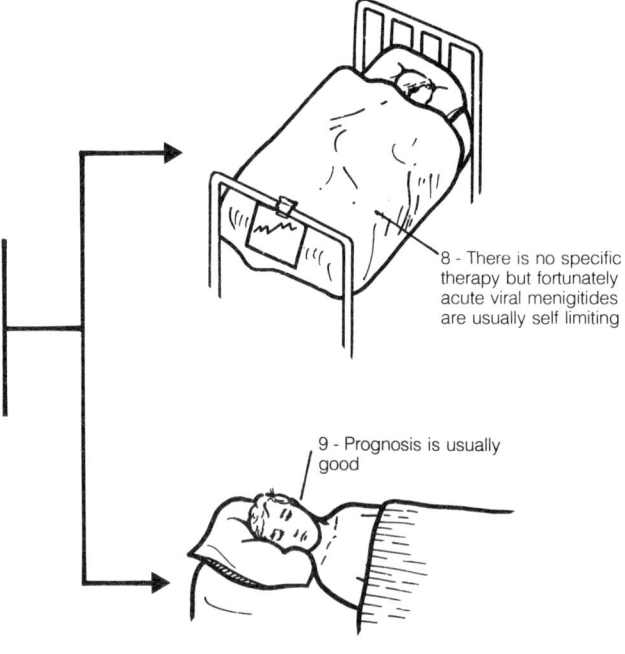

8 - There is no specific therapy but fortunately acute viral menigitides are usually self limiting

9 - Prognosis is usually good

Viral Encephalitis

Most causes of viral meningitis may also cause a meningo-encephalitis – (ie. the inflammation spreads to the brain substance). Herpes simplex may cause an acute fatal necrotising encephalitis usually starting in one temporal lobe and spreading predominantly to other sites in the limbic system including the other temporal region. Encephalitis tends to present with early alteration in consciousness and herpes encephalitis is suspected by low density C.T. changes in the temporal regions and the diagnosis confirmed by brain biopsy. There is specific therapy for herpes encephalitis and therefore early diagnosis is important – the therapy includes acyclovir and perhaps adenine arabinoside.

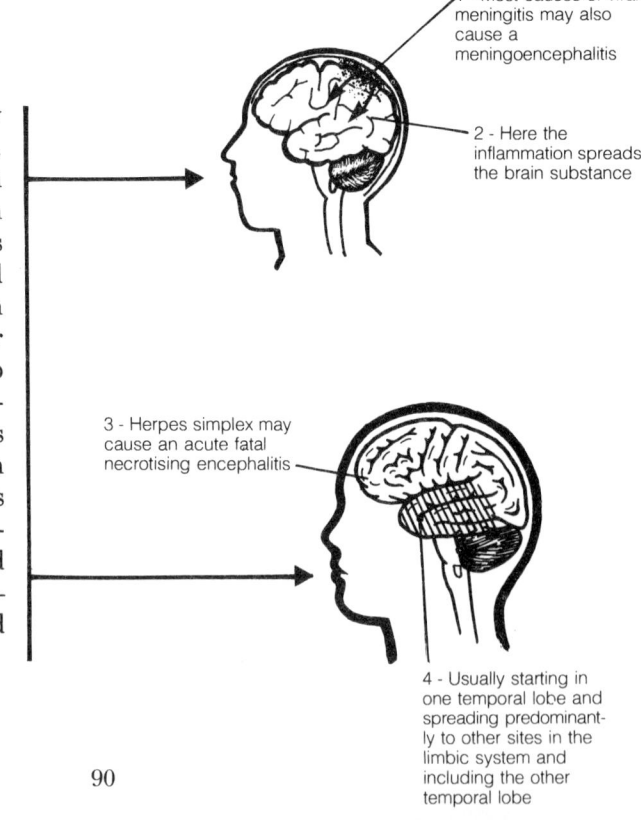

1 - Most causes of viral meningitis may also cause a meningoencephalitis

2 - Here the inflammation spreads to the brain substance

3 - Herpes simplex may cause an acute fatal necrotising encephalitis

4 - Usually starting in one temporal lobe and spreading predominantly to other sites in the limbic system and including the other temporal lobe

Dexamethasone is indicated to reduce dangerously severe oedema, although steroids are not to be recommended in other cases.

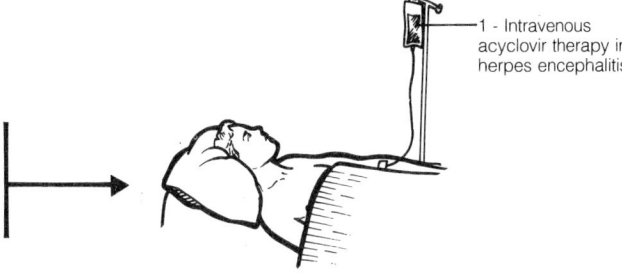

1 - Intravenous acyclovir therapy in herpes encephalitis

In tropical countries, arboviruses (arthropod borne viruses) are an important cause of encephalitis and, after its long incubation period, rabies finds its way to the brain to produce the typical spasms, hydrophobia, fits and encephalitogenic death. The **treatment** of viral encephalitis is usually symptomatic but preventative measures (eg. inoculations) may reduce the risk of infection for arboviruses and rabies.

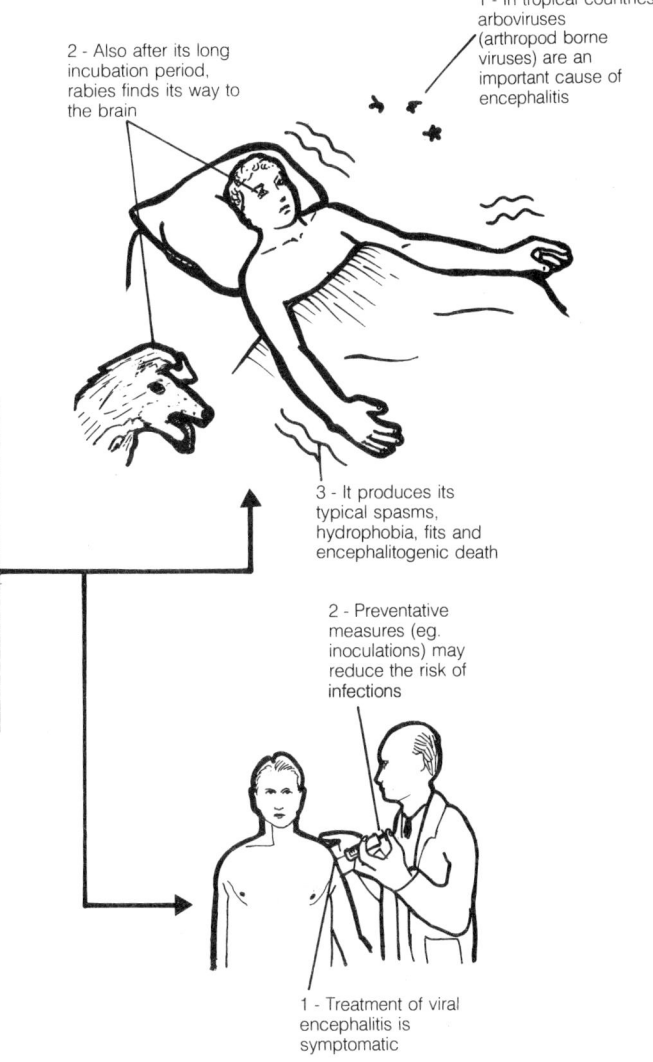

1 - In tropical countries arboviruses (arthropod borne viruses) are an important cause of encephalitis

2 - Also after its long incubation period, rabies finds its way to the brain

3 - It produces its typical spasms, hydrophobia, fits and encephalitogenic death

2 - Preventative measures (eg. inoculations) may reduce the risk of infections

1 - Treatment of viral encephalitis is symptomatic

The Cerebrospinal Fluid (CSF)

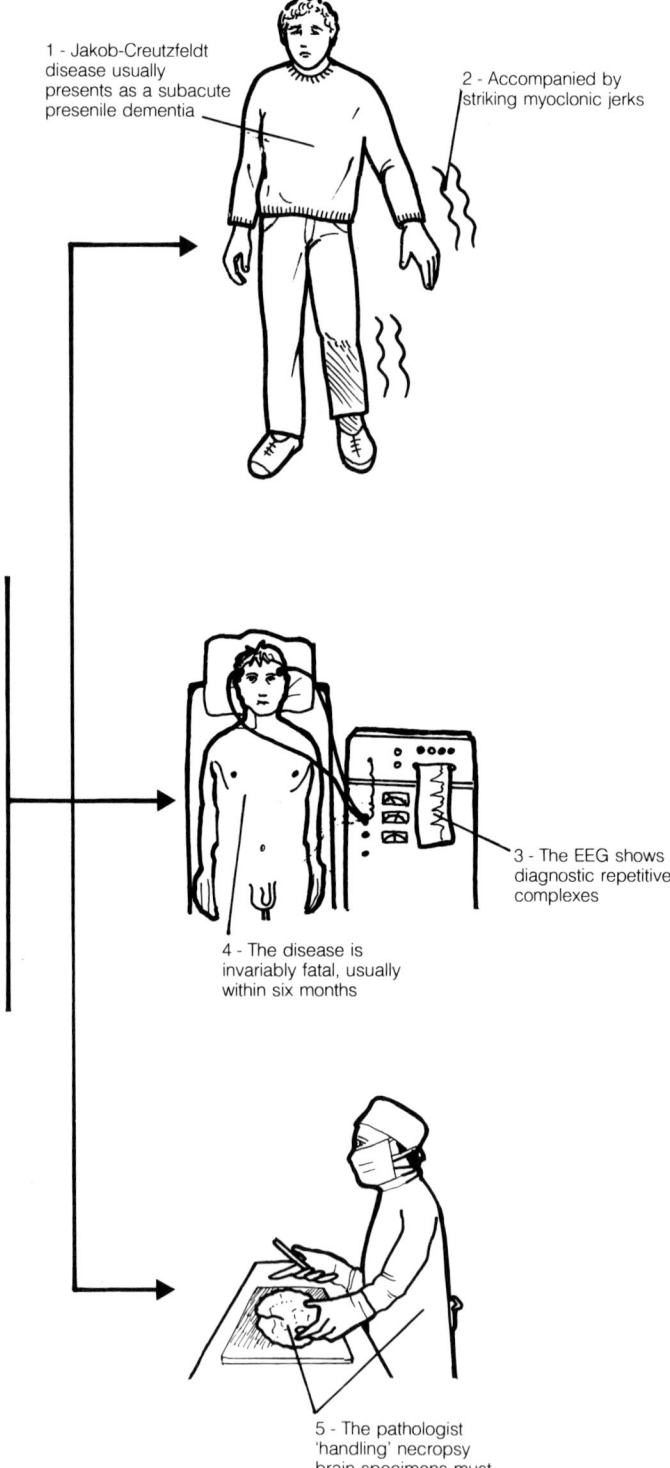

There are some viral encephalopathies with a very much slower time course, ('slow virus infections'). **Jakob-Creutzfeldt disease** usually presents as a subacute presenile dementia accompanied by striking myoclonic jerks or extrapyramidal features, motor paresis and perhaps long tract or cerebellar signs. The EEG shows diagnostic repetitive complexes. The disease is inexorably fatal usually within 6 months and the pathologist 'handling' necropsy brain specimens must consider them highly infectious.

Subacute sclerosing panencephalitis (SSPE) is another established slow virus infection here caused by measles virus. SSPE develops months or years after measles infection and intellectual dulling and myoclonic jerks herald the clinical onset. Frank dementia and fits occur as the disease progresses. The EEG is highly suggestive and the diagnosis is established by a high CSF measles antibody titre. The illness is usually fatal.

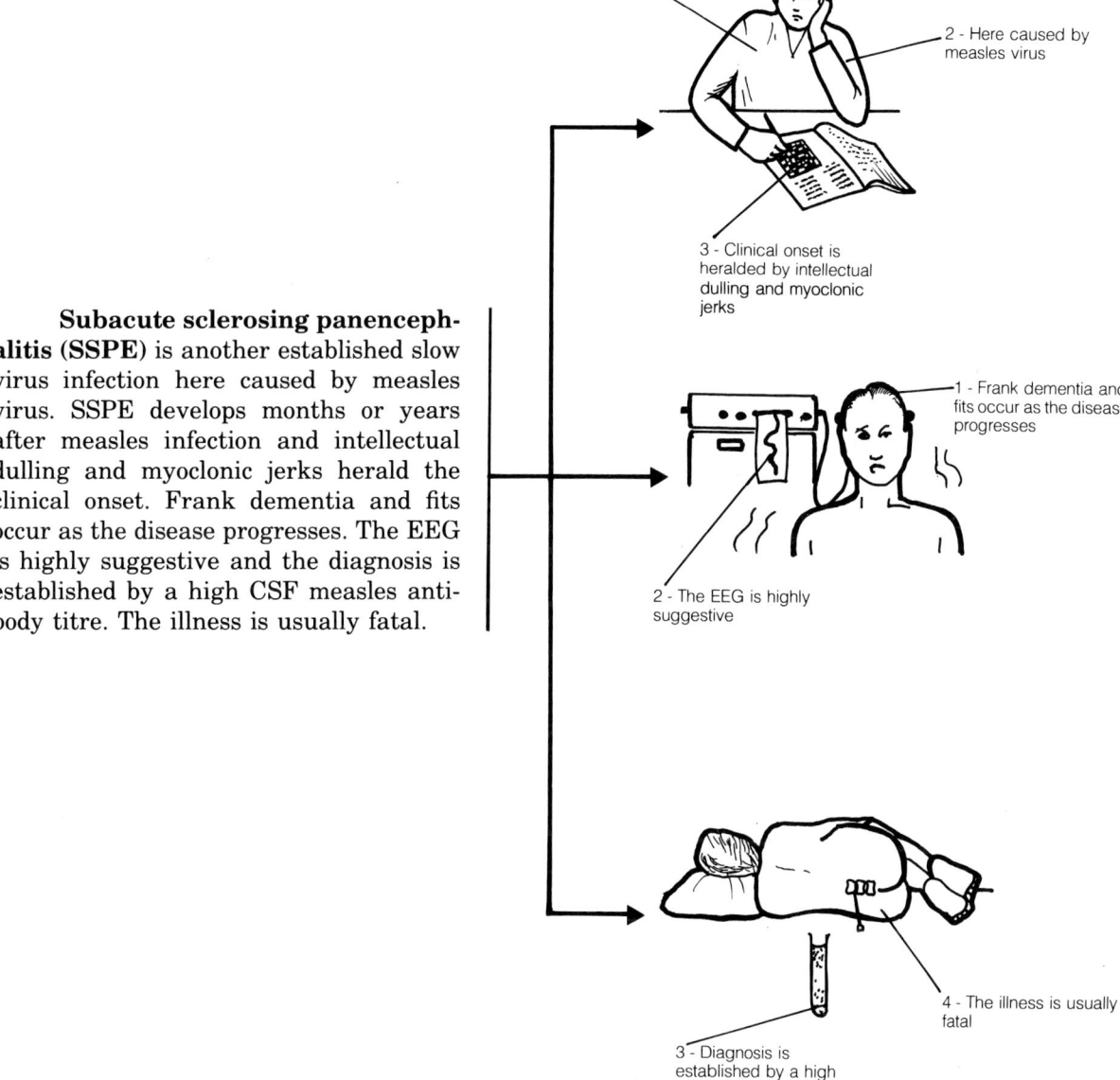

The Cerebrospinal Fluid (CSF)

In both Jakob-Creutzfeldt disease and SSPE there are the typical pathological features of spongy degeneration and gliosis in the grey matter and these features are shared by two other established slow virus infection of brain viz. kuru, (a fatal, human, cerebellar degeneration seen in New Guinea tribes practising cannibalism) and scrapie, (a similar degenerative brain condition but afflicting sheep).

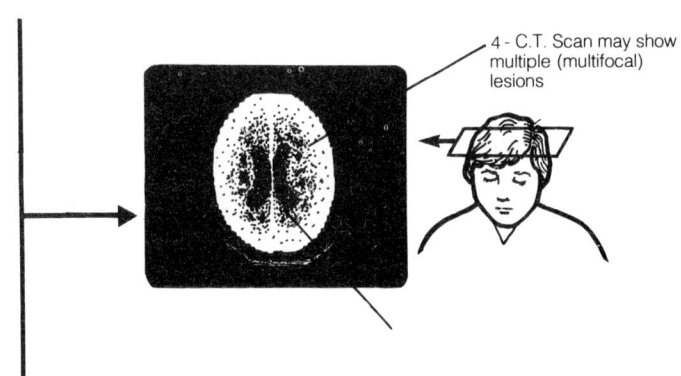

Progressive multifocal leucoencephalopathy (PML) is a rare condition most commonly seen complicating immunosuppressed patients (eg. lymphoma patients). Over the course of a few months patients become mentally disturbed and develop focal neurological signs at many CNS sites. The condition usually progresses and is fatal. Brain biopsy or post-mortem examination reveals many focal areas of demyelination and some of the distorted glial cells contain inclusion bodies, thought to be the causative papova virus.

Brain Abscess – An acute bacterial abscess in the brain usually occurs secondary to a septicaemia, (particularly in the immunosuppressed), acute infective endocarditis or lung infection. Skull fracture or suppurative middle ear disease

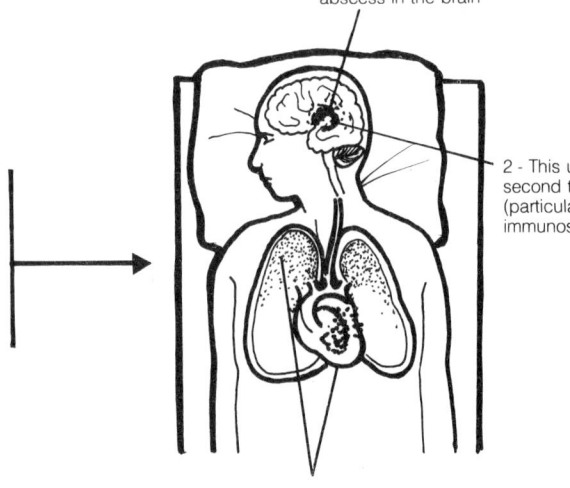

are local causes allowing a portal of entry of the pathogen to the CNS. The patient presents clinically with the signs of raised intracranial pressure with or without features of infective toxaemia, (fever, leucocytosis etc). EEG and C.T. brain scan are helpful and neurosurgical drainage is the treatment, together with antibiotics.

In the immunosuppressed, various opportunist pathogens (fungi, yeast, unusual bacteria etc) may be the cause of a cerebral abscess or meningitis.

Neurosyphilis – Although the CNS may be involved at an earlier stage of syphilis, it is usually tertiary syphilis that produces clinically important neurological syndromes. Indeed, neurosyphilis can present is such diverse ways that it is well to exclude syphilis by serological and CSF tests in any neurological disease that

1 - Skull fracture or supppurative middle ear disease are local causes

2 - This allows a portal of entry of the pathogen to the CNS

3 - These may be with the features of infective toxaemia (fever, leucocytosis etc.)

4 - Cerebral abscess appearance on a C.T. scan

1 - Although the CNS may be involved at an earlier stage, it is usually at the stage of tertiary syphilis that clinically important neurological syndromes occur

2 - Its presentation is so diverse that it is always as well to exclude syphilis by serological and CSF tests

3 - CSF test to exclude syphilis in any neurological disease proving difficult to diagnose

The Cerebrospinal Fluid (CSF)

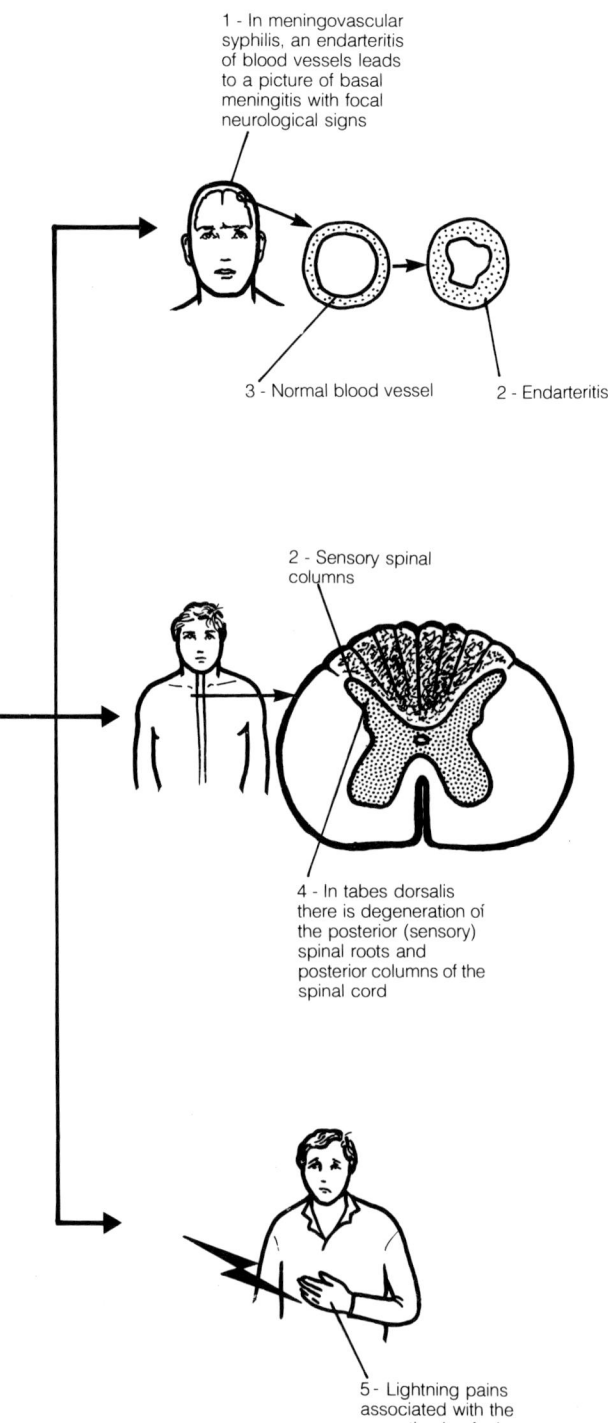

is proving difficult to diagnose. In meningovascular syphilis, an endarteritis of blood vessels leads to a picture of basal meningitis with focal neurological signs (eg. cranial nerve lesions, cord lesions – even transverse myelitis). In tabes dorsalis there is degeneration of the posterior (sensory) spinal roots and posterior columns of the spinal cord with pains (often excruciatingly severe 'lightning pains') associated with anaesthesia, sensory ataxia and the bladder and bowel sphincter disturbances. There are also secondary neuropathic skin ulcers and anatomically deranged joints (**Charcot's joints**) due to the unwitting abuse of skin and joints by the patient, whose actions are not inhibited by pain and normal sensory input. It is in this form of neurosyphilis that the **Argyll Robertson pupil** occurs.

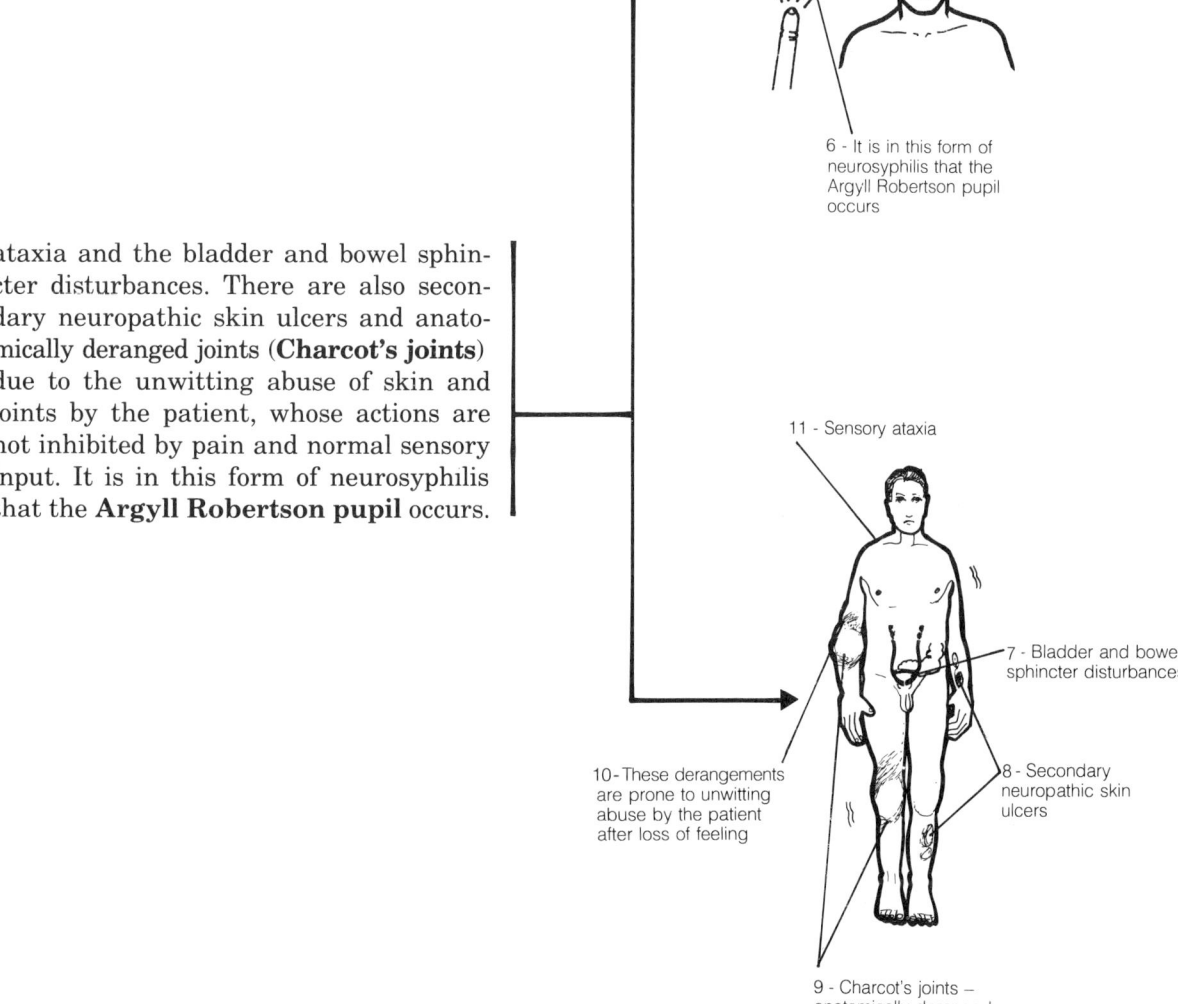

6 - It is in this form of neurosyphilis that the Argyll Robertson pupil occurs

11 - Sensory ataxia

7 - Bladder and bowel sphincter disturbances

10 - These derangements are prone to unwitting abuse by the patient after loss of feeling

8 - Secondary neuropathic skin ulcers

9 - Charcot's joints – anatomically deranged joints

The Cerebrospinal Fluid (CSF)

In the form of neurosyphilis called **General paralysis of the insane (GPI)**, a spirochaetal meningoencephalitis leads to florid changes in personality and dementia associated with peripheral motor neurological signs (eg. a spastic paraparesis, dysarthria etc) and tremor. Optic atrophy is common and in tabo-paresis there are mixed signs of both conditions including the Argyll Robertson pupil.

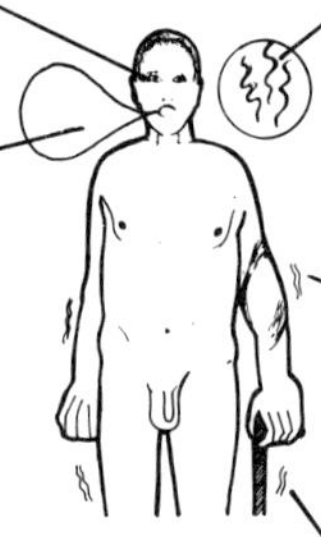

5 - Optic atrophy is common in taboparesis and the Argyll Robertson pupil

4 - Dysarthria

1 - In the form of neurosyphilis called General Paralysis of the Insane (GPI) a spirochaetal meningo-encephalitis leads to florid changes in personality and dementia

2 - Peripheral motor neurological signs also occur eg. a spastic paraparesis, dysarthria etc.)

3 - Tremor

Treatment of neurosyphilis is with high dose intramuscular penicillin (eg. procaine penicillin 600,000 u i.m. daily x 21).

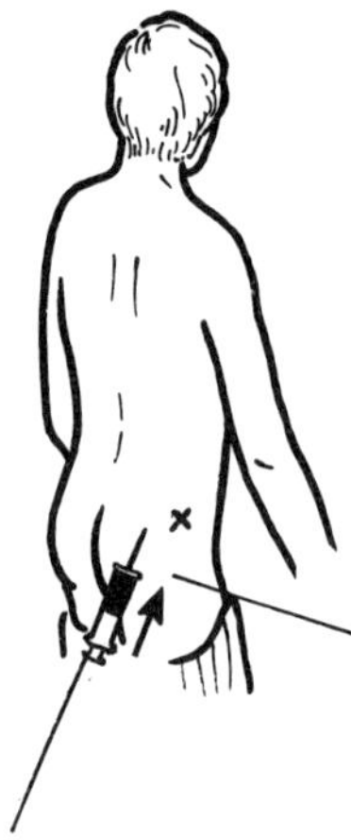

1 - Treatment of neurosyphilis is high dose intramuscular penicillin

2 - Procaine penicillin 600,000 u.i.m. daily × 21

BRAIN TUMOURS

Although cerebral metastases from primary tumours outside the CNS (notably bronchus and breast cancers), may masquerade as primary brain tumours in up to 20% of cases, nevertheless the commonest form of brain tumour in adults is the glioma (45% of total). Glial cells are the supportive cells of the CNS and comprise the astrocytes, oligodendrocytes and ependymal cells. Malignant tumours may arise from any of these three cell types but most commonly from the astrocytes. Unfortunately, the com-

1 - Cerebral metastases masquerade as primary brain tumours

4 - But the commonest form of brain tumour in adults is the glioma (45% of total)

2 - Metastases from primary tumours outside the CNS (notably bronchus and breast cancers)

3 - This happens in up to 20% of cases

GLIOMAS

ASTROCYTOMA   OLIGODENDROGLIOMA   EPENDYMOMA

5 - Glial cells are the supportive cells of the CNS as follows:

8 - Ependymal cells

6 - Astrocytes, from which the commonest malignant tumour develops

7 - Oligodendrocytes

Brain Tumours

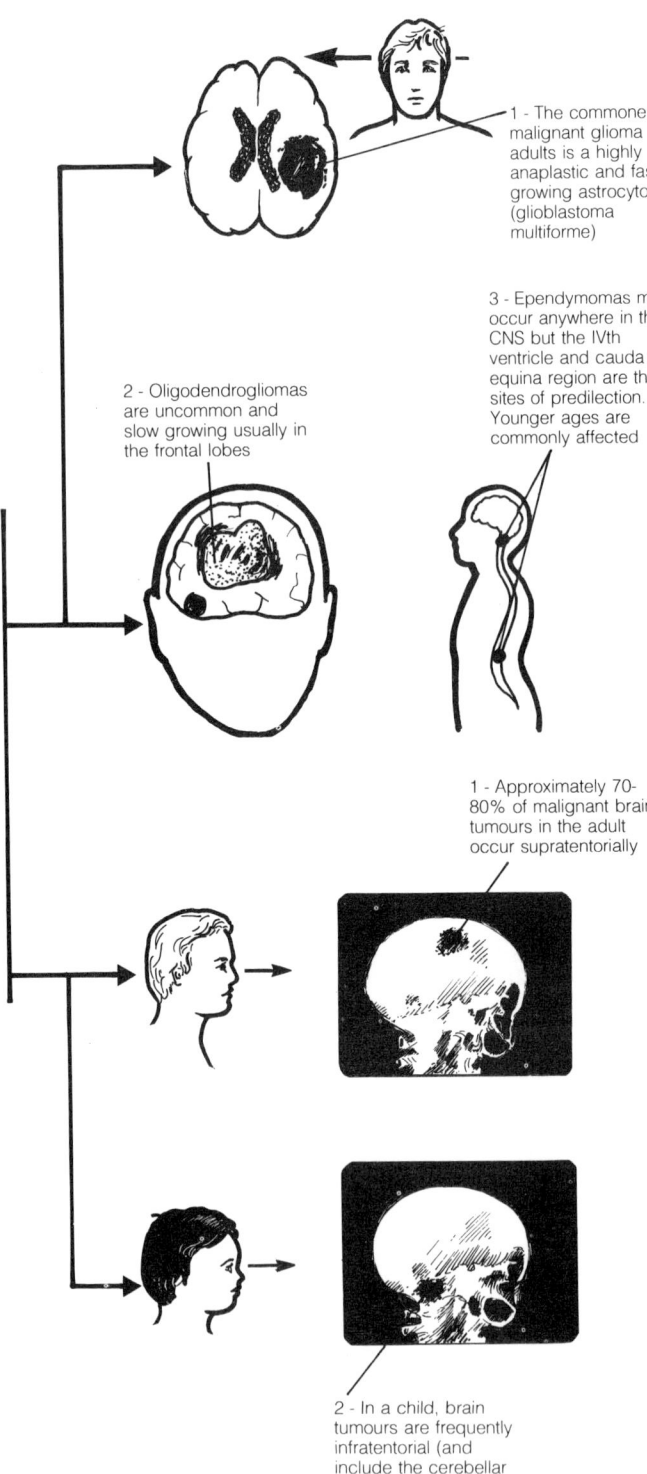

1 - The commonest malignant glioma in adults is a highly anaplastic and fast growing astrocytoma (glioblastoma multiforme)

2 - Oligodendrogliomas are uncommon and slow growing usually in the frontal lobes

3 - Ependymomas may occur anywhere in the CNS but the IVth ventricle and cauda equina region are the sites of predilection. Younger ages are commonly affected

1 - Approximately 70-80% of malignant brain tumours in the adult occur supratentorially

2 - In a child, brain tumours are frequently infratentorial (and include the cerebellar medulloblastoma)

monest malignant glioma in adults is the highly anaplastic and fast-growing astrocytoma, (called: **glioblastoma multiforme**). Oligodendrogliomas are uncommon, very slow growing, and usually occur in the frontal lobes. Ependymomas may occur anywhere in the CNS but the IVth ventricle and cauda equina region are the sites of predilection, and younger age groups are more commonly afflicted. Approximately 75-80% of malignant brain tumours in the adult occur supratentorially, and this contrasts with the child in whom brain tumours are frequently infratentorial, (and include the cerebellar medulloblastoma).

Brain Tumours

Brain tumours present clinically in one of several typical ways:- The first is adult onset epilepsy which is unusual for the idiopathic variety and always suggestive of underlying pathology; (it should be also noted that cerebrovascular disease in the elderly is also a cause of late onset epilepsy).

In particular, the occurrence of focal fits suggests an organic lesion. The second way in which tumours may present is as slowly and relentlessly progressive focal neurological signs – eg. progressively worsening hemiparesis, speech defect or hemianopia (depending on the site of the lesion); a tumour in the frontal lobe may present as a personality change or as dementia. Lastly, a tumour may present with symptoms and signs of raised intracranial pressure – headache, (typically intermittent and worse in the mornings), vomiting and later drowsiness with that cardinal physical sign: **papilloedema**.

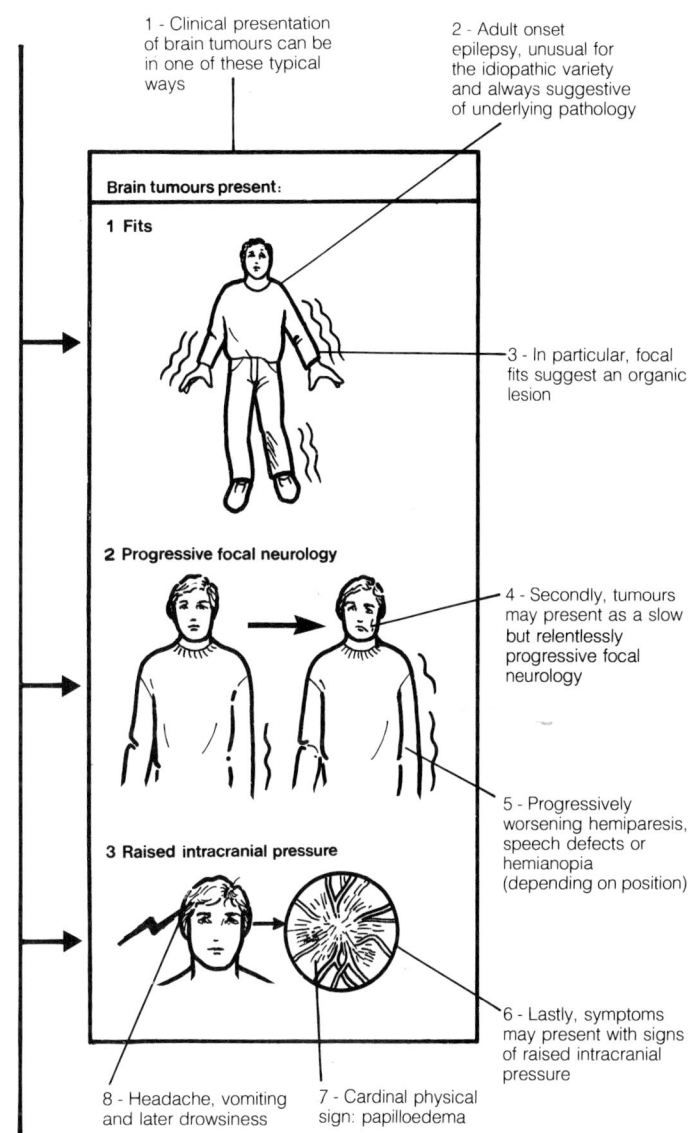

1 - Clinical presentation of brain tumours can be in one of these typical ways

2 - Adult onset epilepsy, unusual for the idiopathic variety and always suggestive of underlying pathology

3 - In particular, focal fits suggest an organic lesion

4 - Secondly, tumours may present as a slow but relentlessly progressive focal neurology

5 - Progressively worsening hemiparesis, speech defects or hemianopia (depending on position)

6 - Lastly, symptoms may present with signs of raised intracranial pressure

7 - Cardinal physical sign: papilloedema

8 - Headache, vomiting and later drowsiness

Brain Tumours

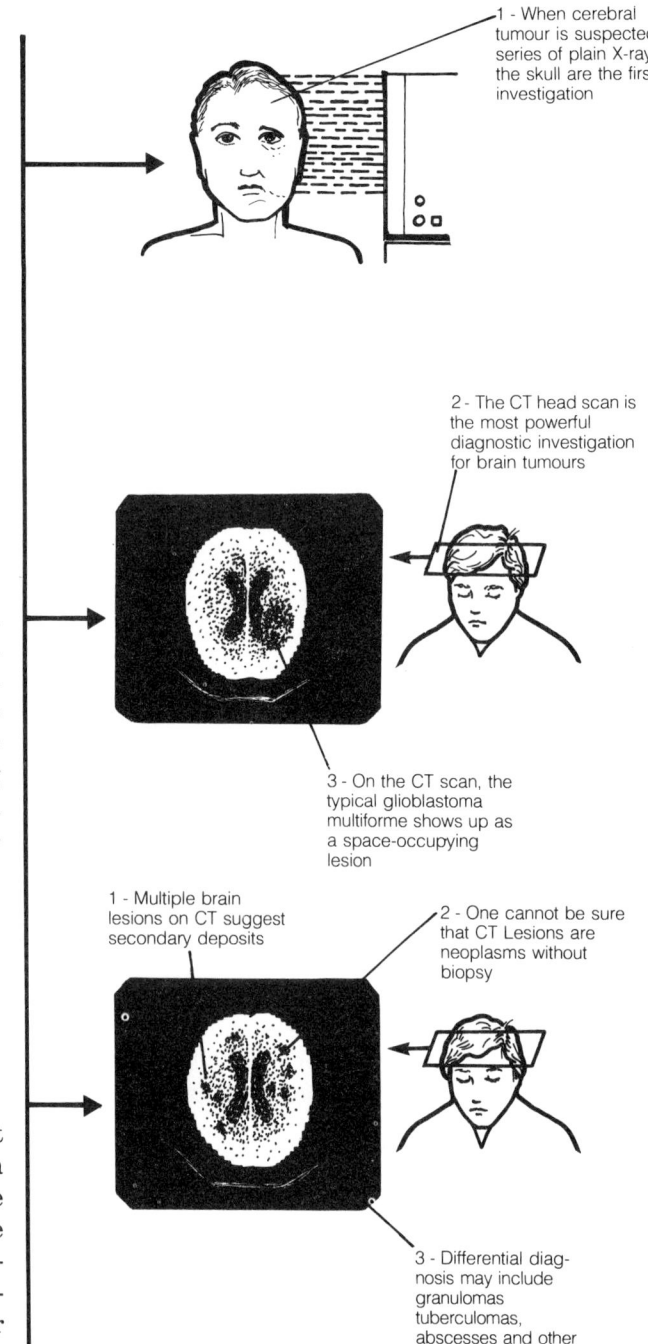

In a patient in whom one suspects a cerebral tumour, the first investigation is the plain skull X-ray series. Shifts in midline structures caused by any space occupying lesion may be deduced from displacement of a calcified pineal. Long-standing raised intracranial pressure causes erosion of the posterior clinoid process. Some tumours calcify – notably oligodendrogliomas, craniopharygiomas and some angiomas.

1 - When cerebral tumour is suspected, a series of plain X-rays of the skull are the first investigation

The C.T. head scan is the most powerful diagnostic investigation for brain tumours but arteriography is still useful in some situations. On the C.T. scan, the typical glioblastoma multiforme shows up as a space occupying lesion, enhancing peripherally with contrast but with a non-enhancing (necrotic) centre and surrounding oedema.

2 - The CT head scan is the most powerful diagnostic investigation for brain tumours

3 - On the CT scan, the typical glioblastoma multiforme shows up as a space-occupying lesion

Multiple brain lesions on C.T. suggest secondary deposits, (metastases from a systemic primary cancer). Of course, one can never be sure that C.T. lesions are neoplasms without a biopsy and the differential diagnosis may include granulomas, tuberculomas, abscesses and other infections.

1 - Multiple brain lesions on CT suggest secondary deposits

2 - One cannot be sure that CT Lesions are neoplasms without biopsy

3 - Differential diagnosis may include granulomas tuberculomas, abscesses and other infections

Neurosurgical biopsy and **decompression**, (rarely a radical excision), is indicated unless the tumour is situated in a particularly critical area of the brain, (eg. brainstem, primary motor cortex, deep thalamus etc.). This procedure provides a histological diagnosis upon which prognosis depends. In patients who are in a reasonable general medical condition, mega voltage radiotherapy to a high dose equivalent is indicated. The St. Bartholomew's Hospital data accord with those of the large American study groups, that the median survival duration of such glioma patients may be doubled by this treatment, although it is also true that the vast majority of glioma patients will still die of their disease. **Glioblastoma multiforme** is particularly lethal, with half the patients dead by one year despite radiotherapy. By contrast, in the best treatment centres, cure rates approaching 50% are obtainable for medulloblastoma following radiotherapy. The nitroso urea cytotoxic drugs may add marginally to the survival and may be indicated in some tumours.

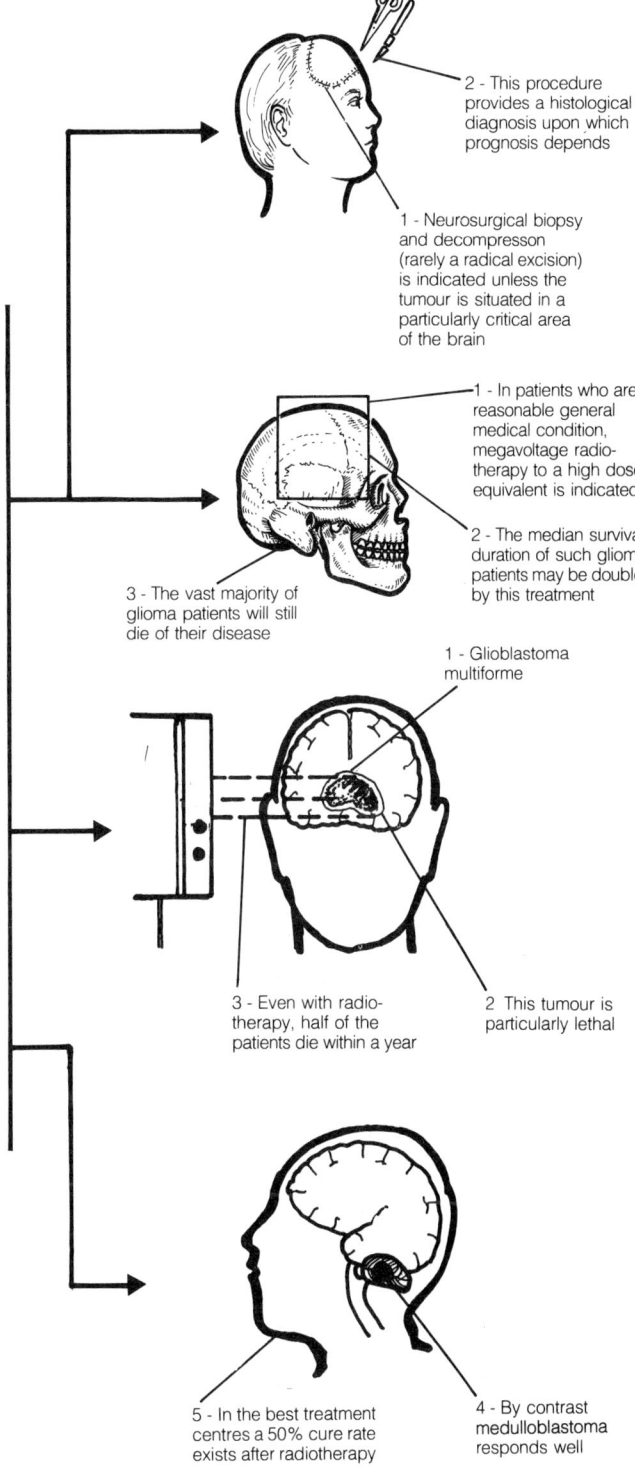

Brain Tumours

Radiotherapy is also indicated for cerebral metastases from systemic cancer in patients in reasonable medical condition. This radiotherapy will often lead to remarkable and long periods of remission.

Dexamethasone (4mg qds reducing to 2mg qds), is a useful drug in that, by reducing the cerebral oedema that surrounds all malignant brain tumours, it can greatly improve a patient's neurological status even though is has no specific effect on the tumour. Patients on high dose Dexamethasone become iatrogenically cushingoid; the tendency of dexamethasone to cause peptic ulceration can be overcome largely by the administration of cimetidine.

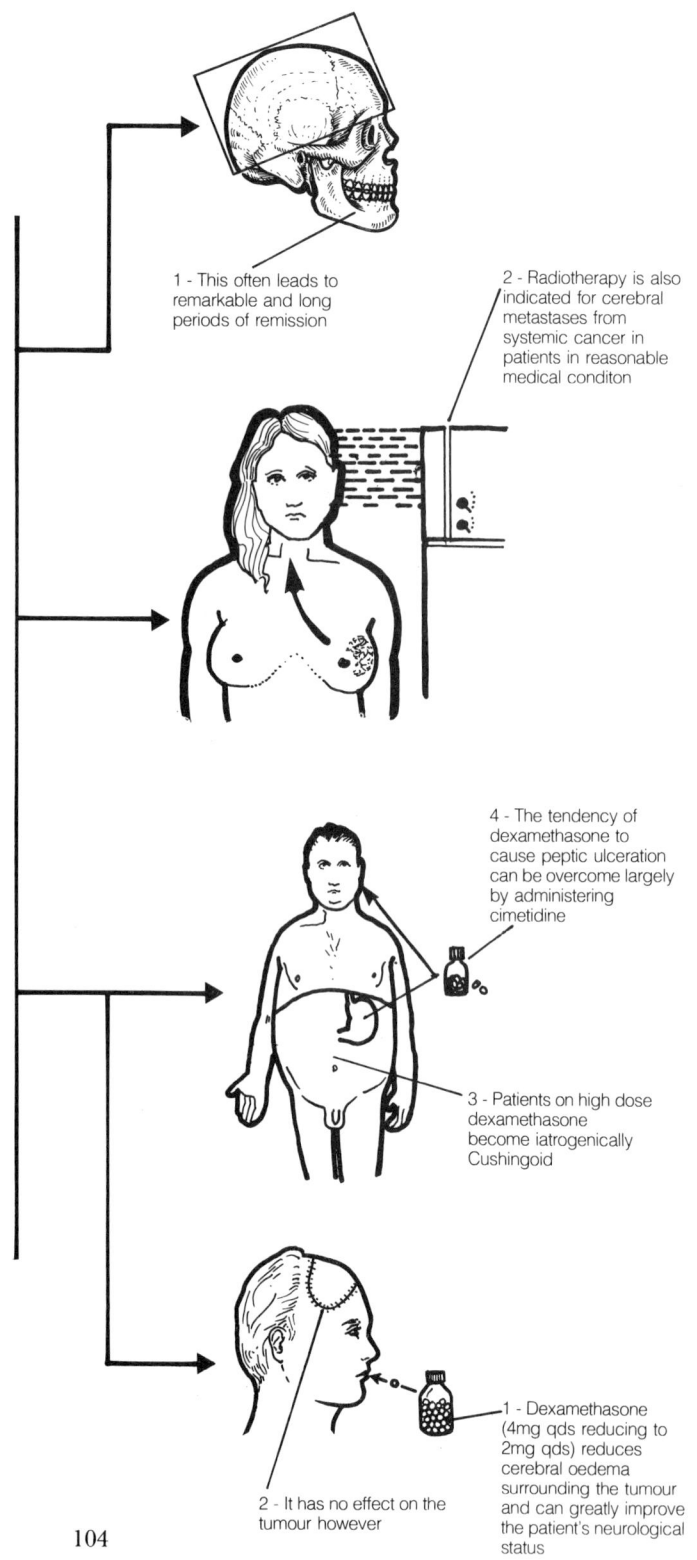

1 - This often leads to remarkable and long periods of remission

2 - Radiotherapy is also indicated for cerebral metastases from systemic cancer in patients in reasonable medical conditon

4 - The tendency of dexamethasone to cause peptic ulceration can be overcome largely by administering cimetidine

3 - Patients on high dose dexamethasone become iatrogenically Cushingoid

2 - It has no effect on the tumour however

1 - Dexamethasone (4mg qds reducing to 2mg qds) reduces cerebral oedema surrounding the tumour and can greatly improve the patient's neurological status

Meningiomas are usually benign tumours deriving from the arachnoid fibroblast; they comprise 15% of all intracranial tumours. They present clinically because of compression of the brain or cranial nerves. Meningiomas enhance dramatically on C.T. scan and have a characteristic angiographic appearance. Meningiomas are usually well-encapsulated growths and curable by surgery; unless there are certain aggressive histological features, radiotherapy is not indicated.

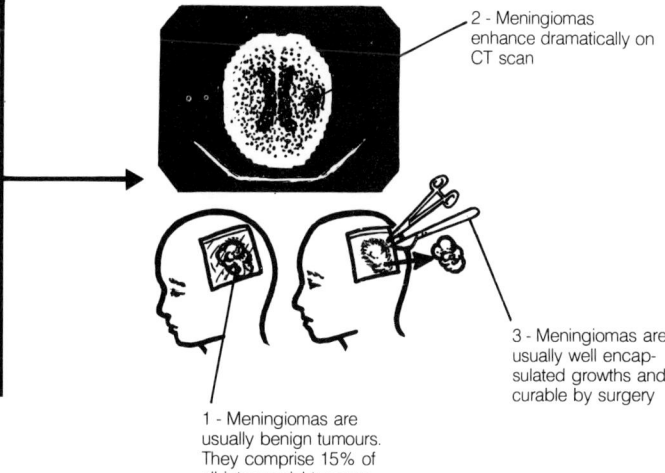

1 - Meningiomas are usually benign tumours. They comprise 15% of all intracranial tumours

2 - Meningiomas enhance dramatically on CT scan

3 - Meningiomas are usually well encapsulated growths and curable by surgery

Pituitary tumours comprise perhaps 8% of all intracranial tumours and present either due to expanding pressure on the crossing optic nerve fibres in the optic chiasm – causing the classic bitemporal hemianopia, or they present due to the endocrine secretions of the neoplastic cells – (acromegaly, Cushing's, secondary amenorrhoea); rarely, rapid swelling of a

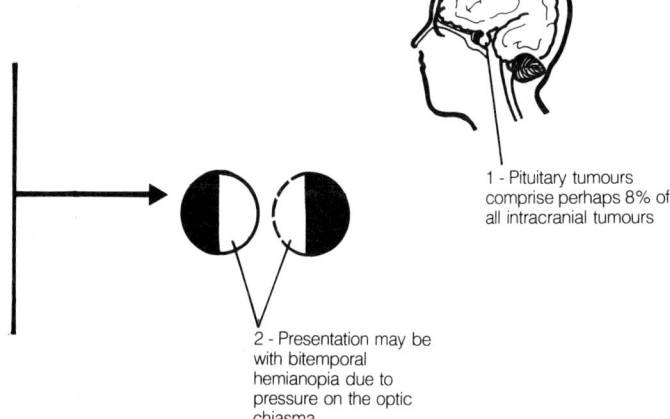

1 - Pituitary tumours comprise perhaps 8% of all intracranial tumours

2 - Presentation may be with bitemporal hemianopia due to pressure on the optic chiasma

Brain Tumours

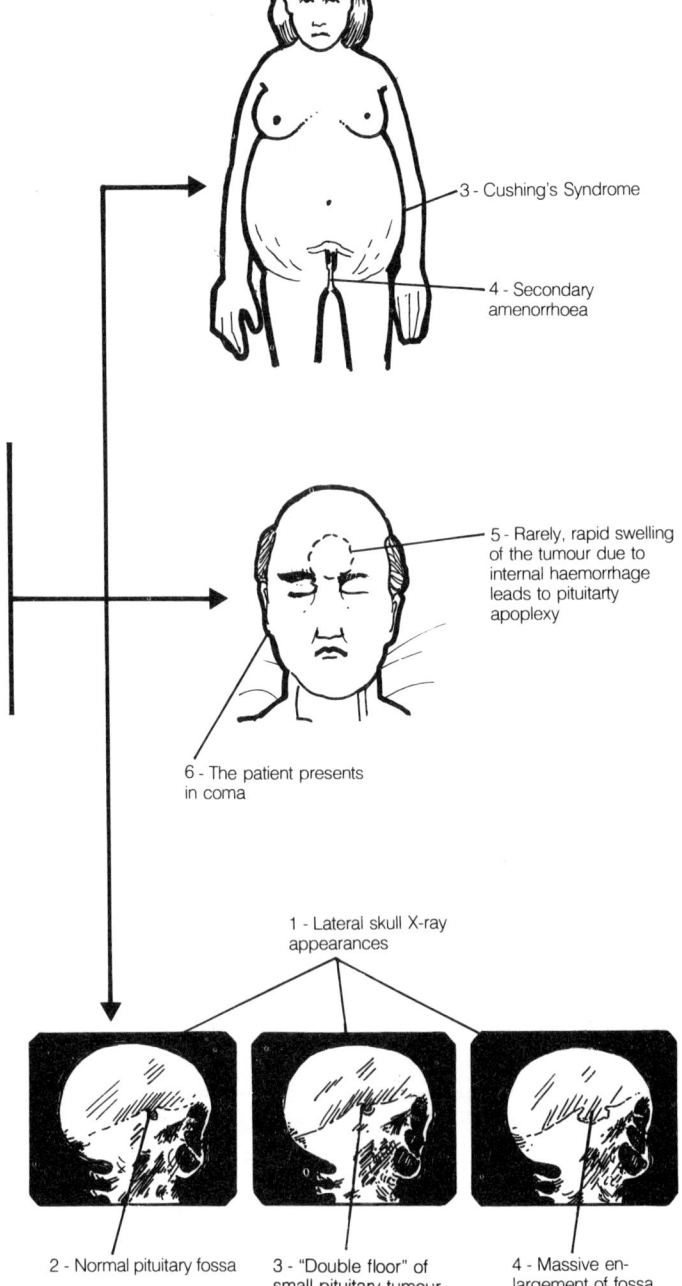

pituitary tumour due to internal haemorrhage leads to presentation in coma – **pituitary apoplexy**. Diagnosis is by plain skull X-rays showing an expanded pituitary fossa, C.T. scanning showing the intrasellar tumour and hormone assays. Pituitary tumours are almost invariably adenomas (carcinomas are very rare).

3 - Cushing's Syndrome

4 - Secondary amenorrhoea

5 - Rarely, rapid swelling of the tumour due to internal haemorrhage leads to pituitarty apoplexy

6 - The patient presents in coma

1 - Lateral skull X-ray appearances

2 - Normal pituitary fossa

3 - "Double floor" of small pituitary tumour

4 - Massive enlargement of fossa

Brain Tumours

Large pituitary tumours that are compressing the optic chiasm require neurosurgical decompression followed by radiotherapy. Radiotherapy alone is sufficient for many smaller tumours, but should be performed in a modern unit. Bromocriptine (a dopamine agonist) has a role in the management of some acidophil adenomas and prolactinomas but its use should be left to experts, and the medical therapy of large tumours causing visual problems without recourse to a neurosurgical opinion is to be deplored.

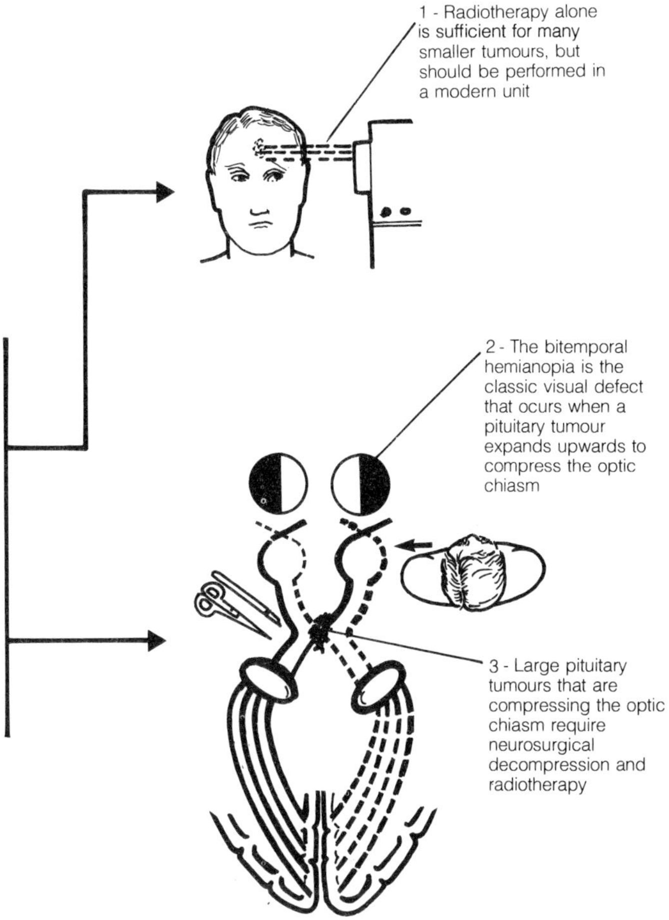

1 - Radiotherapy alone is sufficient for many smaller tumours, but should be performed in a modern unit

2 - The bitemporal hemianopia is the classic visual defect that ocurs when a pituitary tumour expands upwards to compress the optic chiasm

3 - Large pituitary tumours that are compressing the optic chiasm require neurosurgical decompression and radiotherapy

Craniopharyngiomas arise in the suprasellar region, although much of their presenting symptomatology may resemble pituitary tumours. They are often cystic and round, encapsulated masses but are difficult to resect in toto, have a propensity to recur, and radiotherapy should follow neurosurgery.

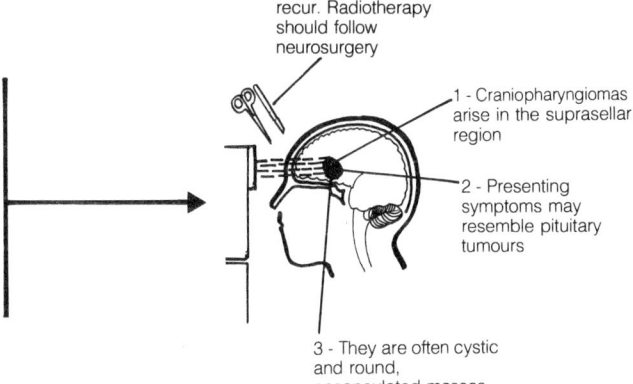

4 - They are difficult to resect in toto and may recur. Radiotherapy should follow neurosurgery

1 - Craniopharyngiomas arise in the suprasellar region

2 - Presenting symptoms may resemble pituitary tumours

3 - They are often cystic and round, encapsulated masses

Acoustic neuromas are benign schwannomas that have a peculiar tendency to form on the VIIIth nerve; they are entirely benign and neurosurgical resection is curative.

In conclusion, brain tumours are usually suspected from the history and examination, often diagnosed by the imaging tests (notably C.T. scanning) and confirmed by biopsy. Surgery and radiotherapy are the main forms of treatment.

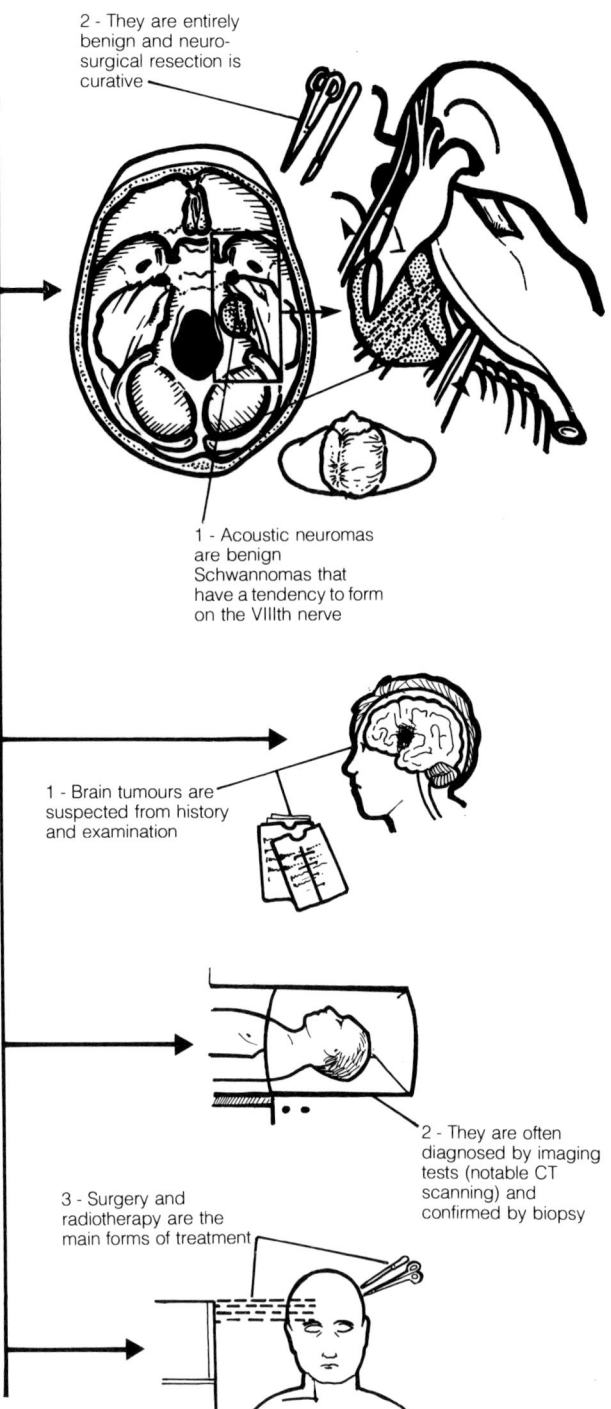

INTRACRANIAL HAEMORRHAGE

Extradural Haemorrhage – Extradural haemorrhage is caused by a head injury and the source of bleeding is most commonly the middle meningeal artery. This arterial bleeding leads to an increasing pool between the skull and dura, forming a space-occupying mass here and this compresses the brain. In the typical case, consciousness has been briefly lost following a head injury but the patient has apparently recovered; some hours may elapse,(the 'lucid interval') before there is drowsiness and then coma with constriction and later dilatation of the ipsilateral pupil and progressive contralateral hemiplegia.

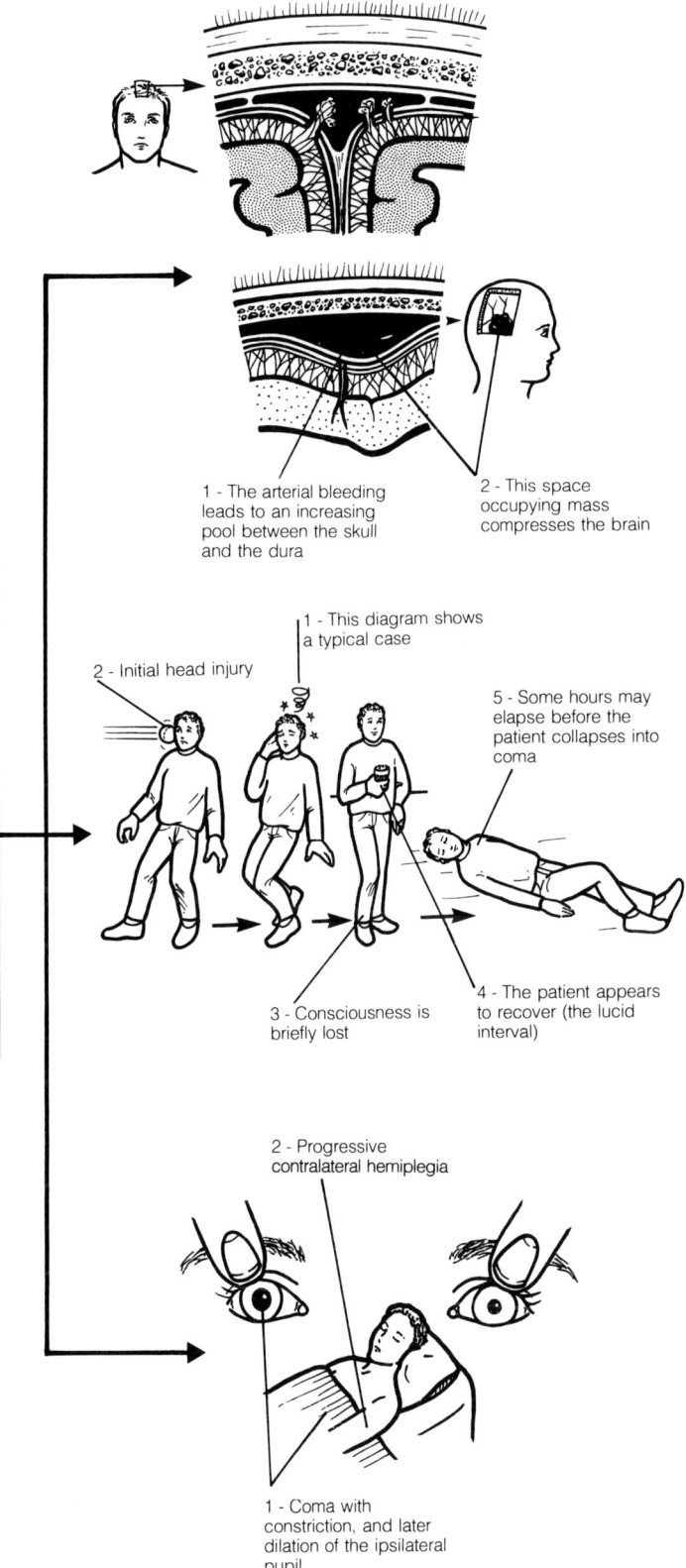

1 - The arterial bleeding leads to an increasing pool between the skull and the dura

2 - This space occupying mass compresses the brain

1 - This diagram shows a typical case

2 - Initial head injury

3 - Consciousness is briefly lost

4 - The patient appears to recover (the lucid interval)

5 - Some hours may elapse before the patient collapses into coma

2 - Progressive contralateral hemiplegia

1 - Coma with constriction, and later dilation of the ipsilateral pupil

Intracranial Haemorrhage

Patients who have sustained head injuries with loss of consciousness require careful observation with particular regard to the level of consciousness, and size, reactivity and symmetry of pupils, (see also section on Coma).

A skull X-ray series must be performed in all cases on admission and reviewed for fractures. Although an extradural haemorrhage may be well demonstrated on C.T. scan or angiography, the condition must be regarded as requiring **urgent treatment** – indeed there is not usually time for a lengthy ambulance journey to a distant neurosurgical centre and immediate surgical trephining of the skull with simple evacuation of blood clot must be within the remit of a surgeon at every hospital.

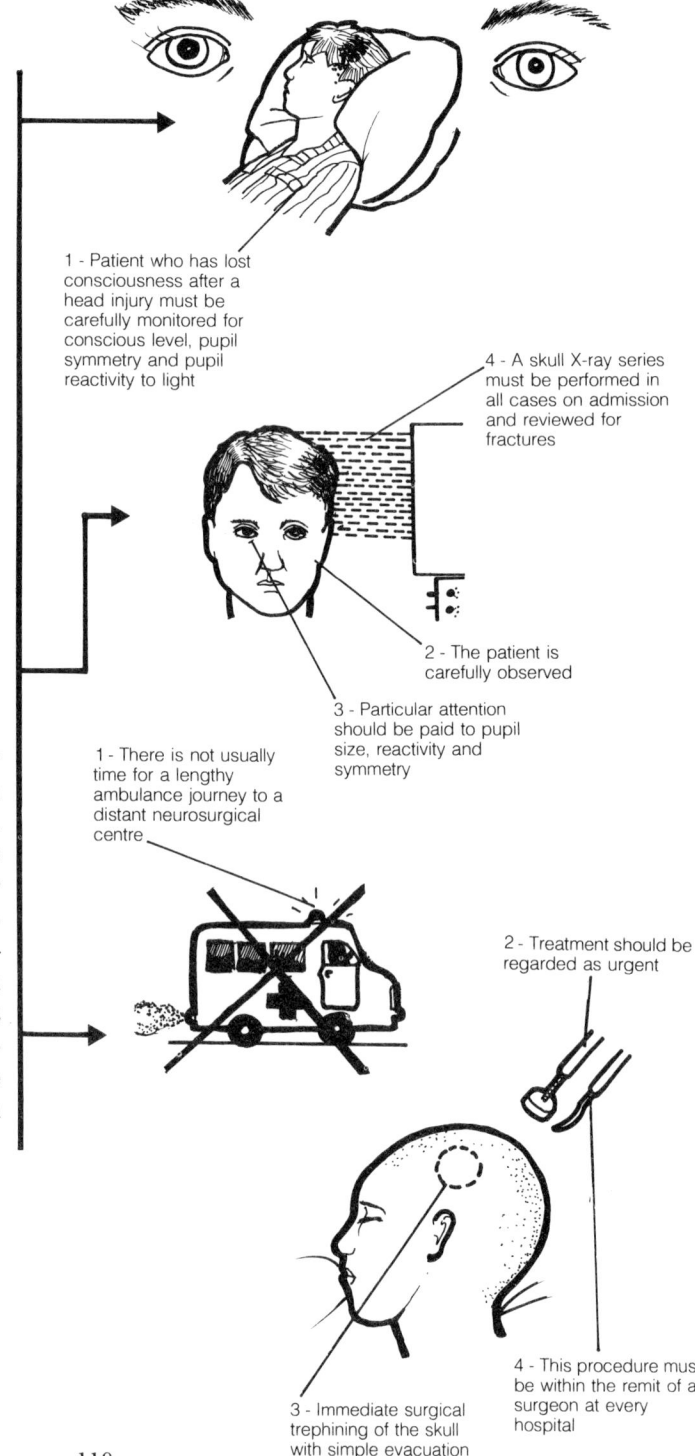

1 - Patient who has lost consciousness after a head injury must be carefully monitored for conscious level, pupil symmetry and pupil reactivity to light

4 - A skull X-ray series must be performed in all cases on admission and reviewed for fractures

2 - The patient is carefully observed

3 - Particular attention should be paid to pupil size, reactivity and symmetry

1 - There is not usually time for a lengthy ambulance journey to a distant neurosurgical centre

2 - Treatment should be regarded as urgent

3 - Immediate surgical trephining of the skull with simple evacuation of blood clot

4 - This procedure must be within the remit of a surgeon at every hospital

Subdural Haemorrhage – Subdural haematomas also follow head trauma but the bleeding usually follows more minor head trauma in the elderly, (or young children), and is from subdural veins. The oozing of venous blood leads to a much slower accumulation of the space occupying haematoma. The **symptoms** may commence some weeks after the injury with drowsiness which may fluctuate at first, personality change or psychosis and then coma with focal neurological signs (eg. hemiparesis). Papilloedema is not common. The haematoma is more diffuse than an extradural haematoma.

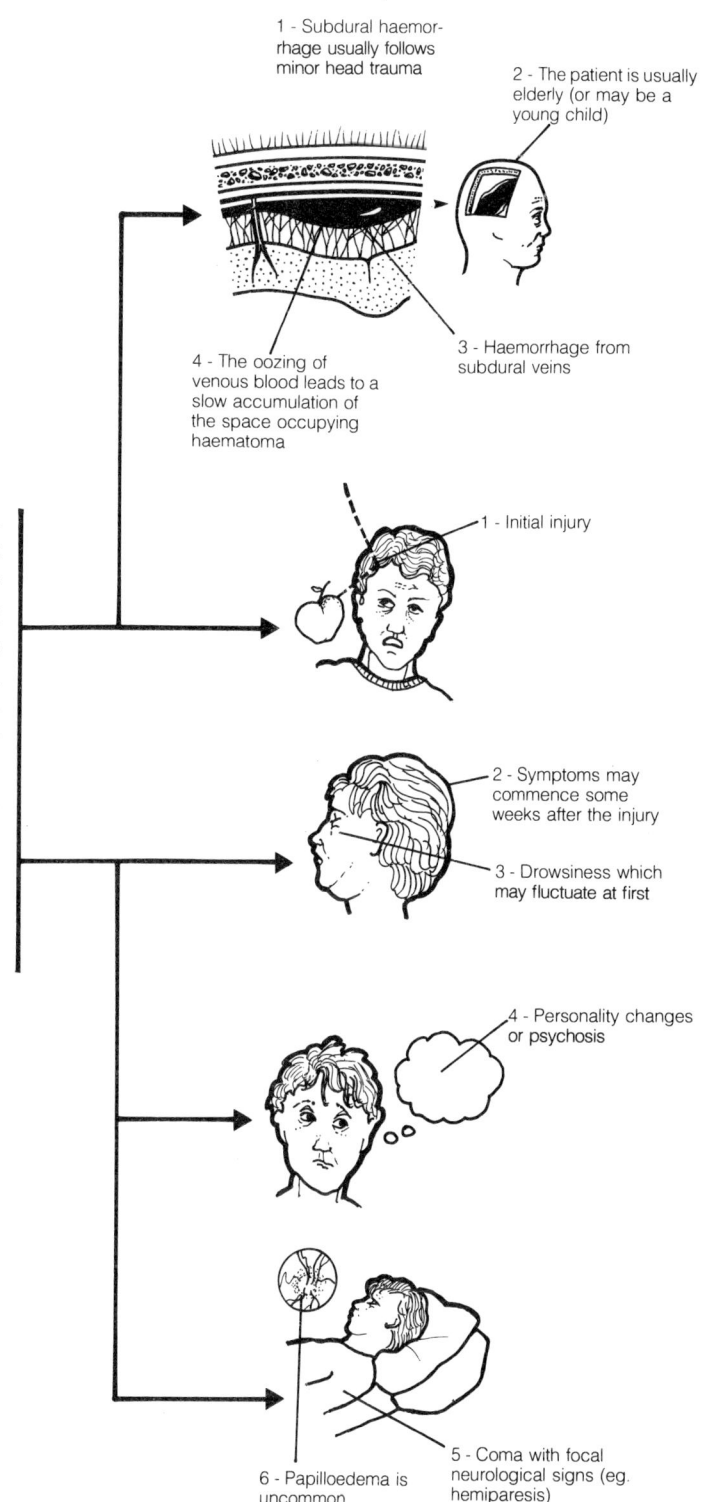

Intracranial Haemorrhage

The history of head injury in an elderly person with headache and coma, hemiparesis or brainstem signs suggest subdural haematoma. A C.T. scan or angiography are usually the most helpful diagnostic tests and all large subdural haematomas require neurosurgical evacuation.

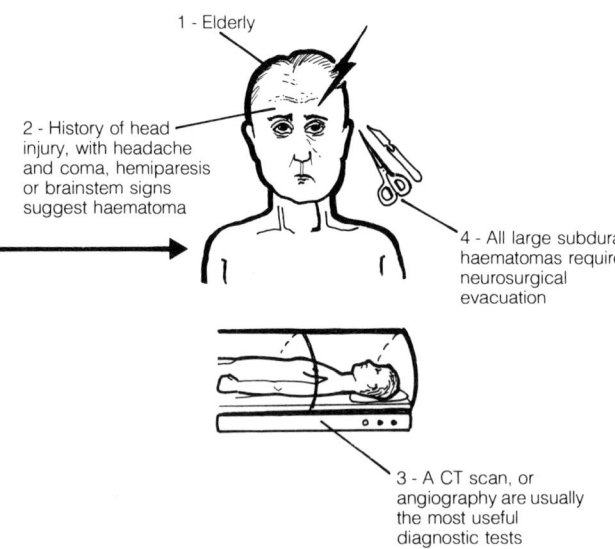

Subarachnoid Haemorrhage – In approximately 85% of cases of subarachnoid haemorrhage, the cause is a ruptured **berry aneurysm**. These aneurysms occur almost invariably at points of arterial bifurcation on the arterial circle of Willis and where, for unknown reasons, there are congenital defects in the arterial walls in these patients. In a minority

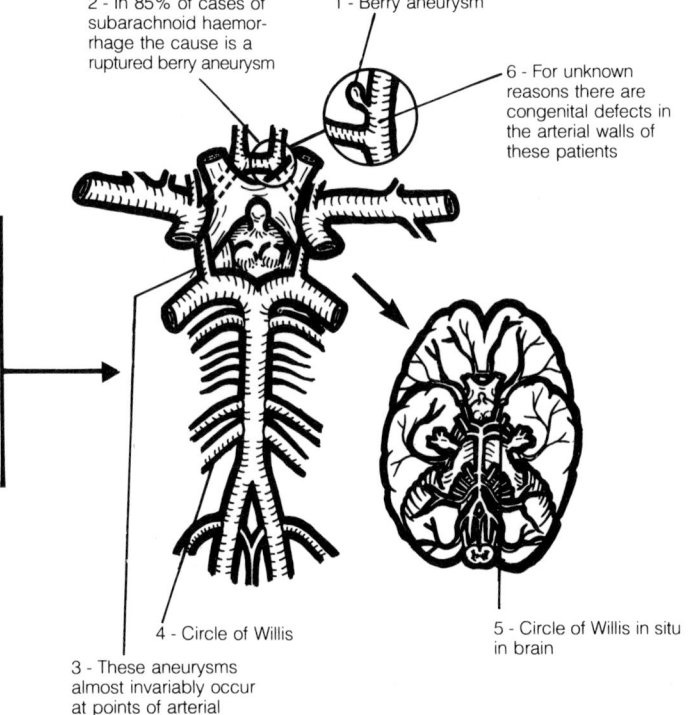

of patients, subarachnoid haemorrhage occurs from a congenital cerebral arteriovenous malformation, (angioma). In a few cases a blood dyscrasia may be the cause and in other cases no cause is found.

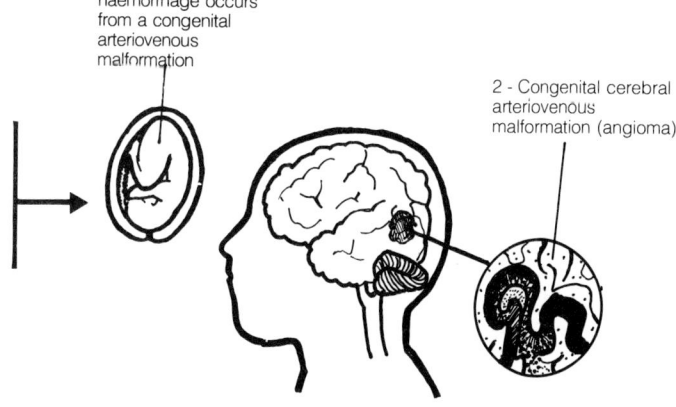

Hypertension predisposes to rupture of berry aneurysm and this is commonest in middle age. The onset is sudden with severe headache and perhaps loss of consciousness. If the patient recovers consciousness, then severe occipital headache and vomiting are common. In the physical examination there may be marked neck stiffness, (**meningism**) and subhyaloid haemorrhages seen on fundoscopy – as well as other focal neurological signs. The **diagnosis** is made by lumbar puncture:- the CSF is under increased pressure and all three serial samples are equally bloody and xanthochromic.

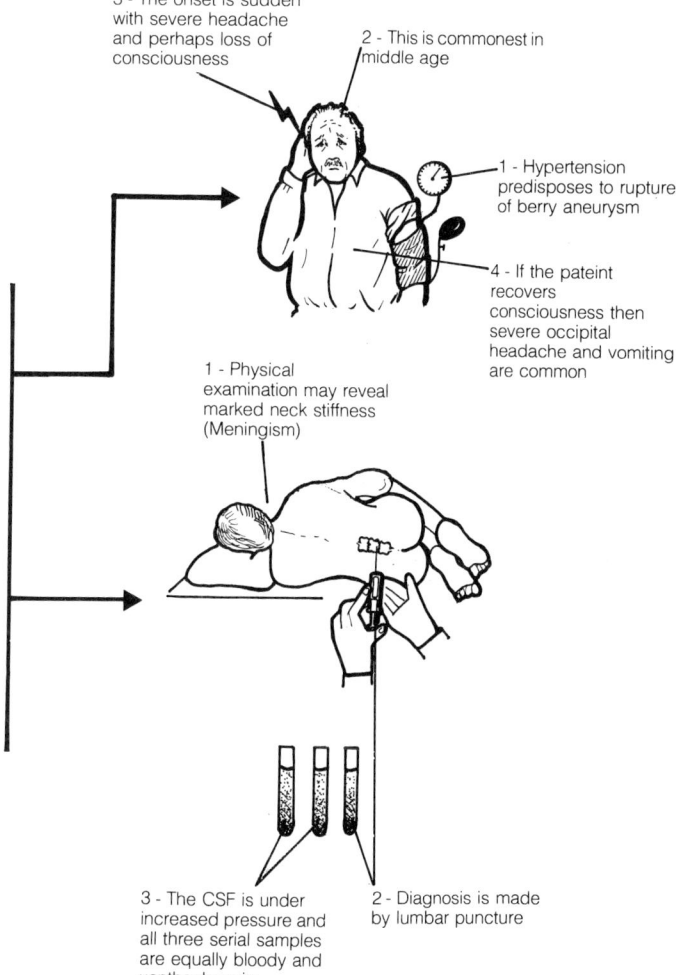

If the patient recovers sufficiently from the bleeding episode, angiography is an important investigation. If a focal bleeding source (eg. berry aneurysm) can be identified, then neurosurgery is indicated. All patients should be rested supine and hypertension treated if the blood pressure is extemely high. There is a serious risk of further and fatal bleeds in these patients and not all cases are operable.

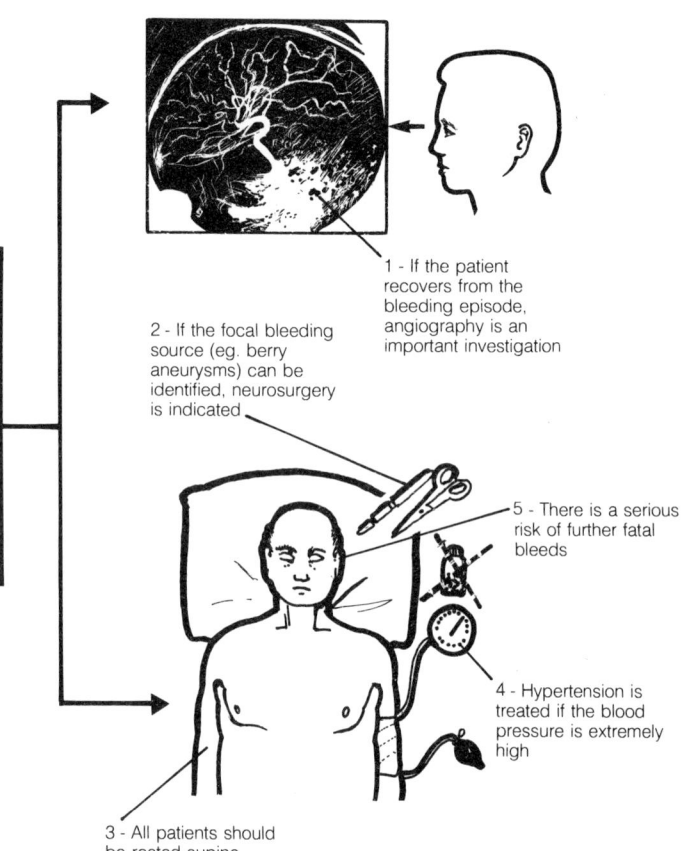

1 - If the patient recovers from the bleeding episode, angiography is an important investigation

2 - If the focal bleeding source (eg. berry aneurysms) can be identified, neurosurgery is indicated

5 - There is a serious risk of further fatal bleeds

4 - Hypertension is treated if the blood pressure is extremely high

3 - All patients should be rested supine

Intracerebral Haemorrhage – Hypertension also predisposes to intracerebral haemorrhage which most commonly afflicts the elderly and those with cerebrovascular atheroma. The most common site of haemorrhage is from branches of the middle cerebral artery in the region of the internal capsule.

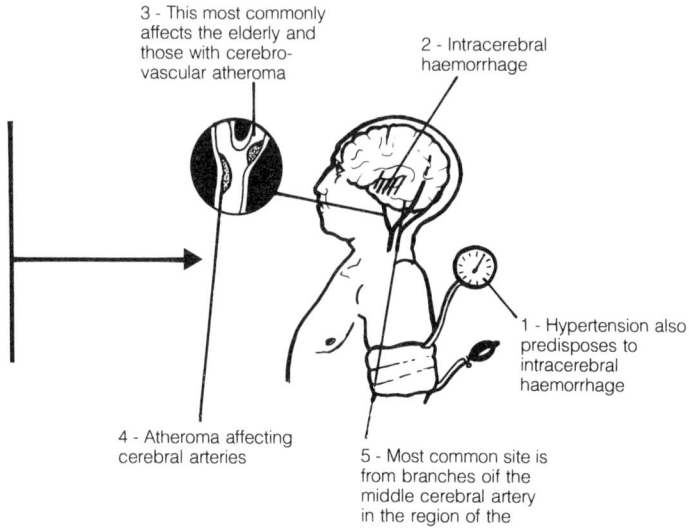

3 - This most commonly affects the elderly and those with cerebrovascular atheroma

2 - Intracerebral haemorrhage

1 - Hypertension also predisposes to intracerebral haemorrhage

4 - Atheroma affecting cerebral arteries

5 - Most common site is from branches oif the middle cerebral artery in the region of the internal capsule

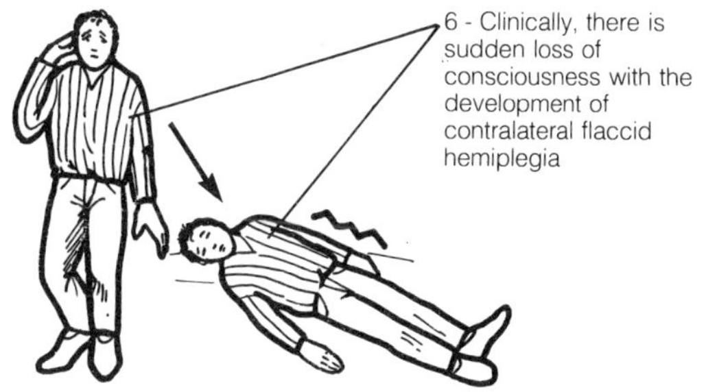

Clinically, there is a sudden loss of consciousness with the development of a contralateral flaccid hemiplegia. Immediate death is unusual.

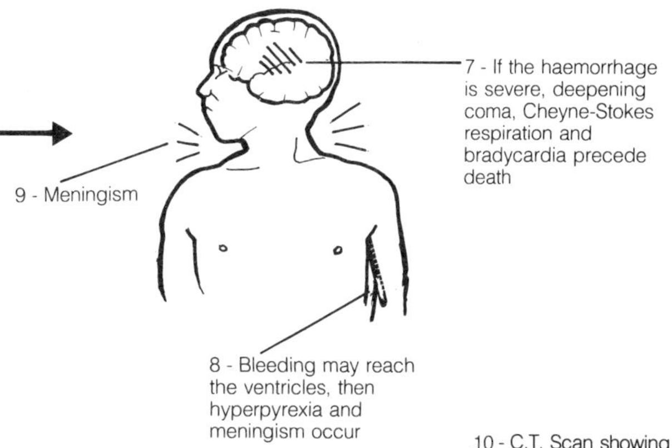

6 - Clinically, there is sudden loss of consciousness with the development of contralateral flaccid hemiplegia

If the haemorrhage is severe, deepening coma and Cheyne-Stokes respiration and bradycardia precede death. If the bleeding reaches the ventricles, then hyperpyrexia and meningism occur.

7 - If the haemorrhage is severe, deepening coma, Cheyne-Stokes respiration and bradycardia precede death

9 - Meningism

8 - Bleeding may reach the ventricles, then hyperpyrexia and meningism occur

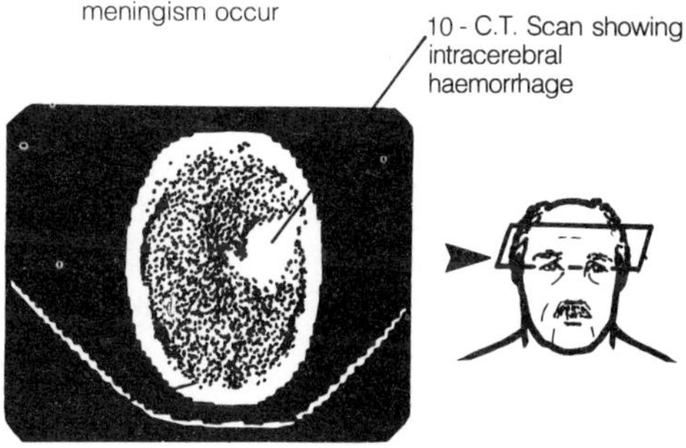

10 - C.T. Scan showing intracerebral haemorrhage

In less severe cases, consciousness will be regained and with time the hemiplegia become typically spastic (UMN). In the more extensive capsular lesions,

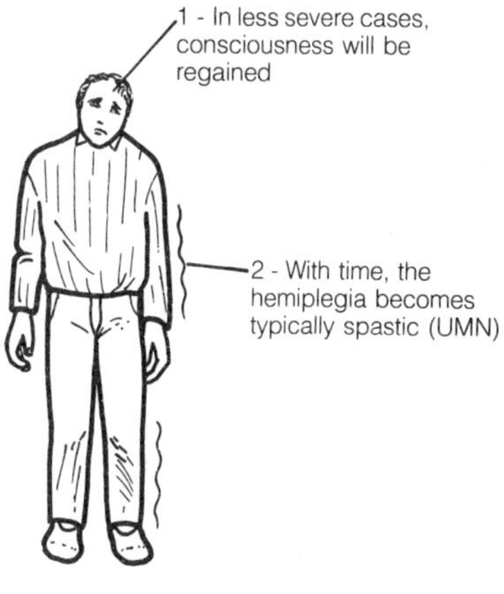

1 - In less severe cases, consciousness will be regained

2 - With time, the hemiplegia becomes typically spastic (UMN)

Intracranial Haemorrhage

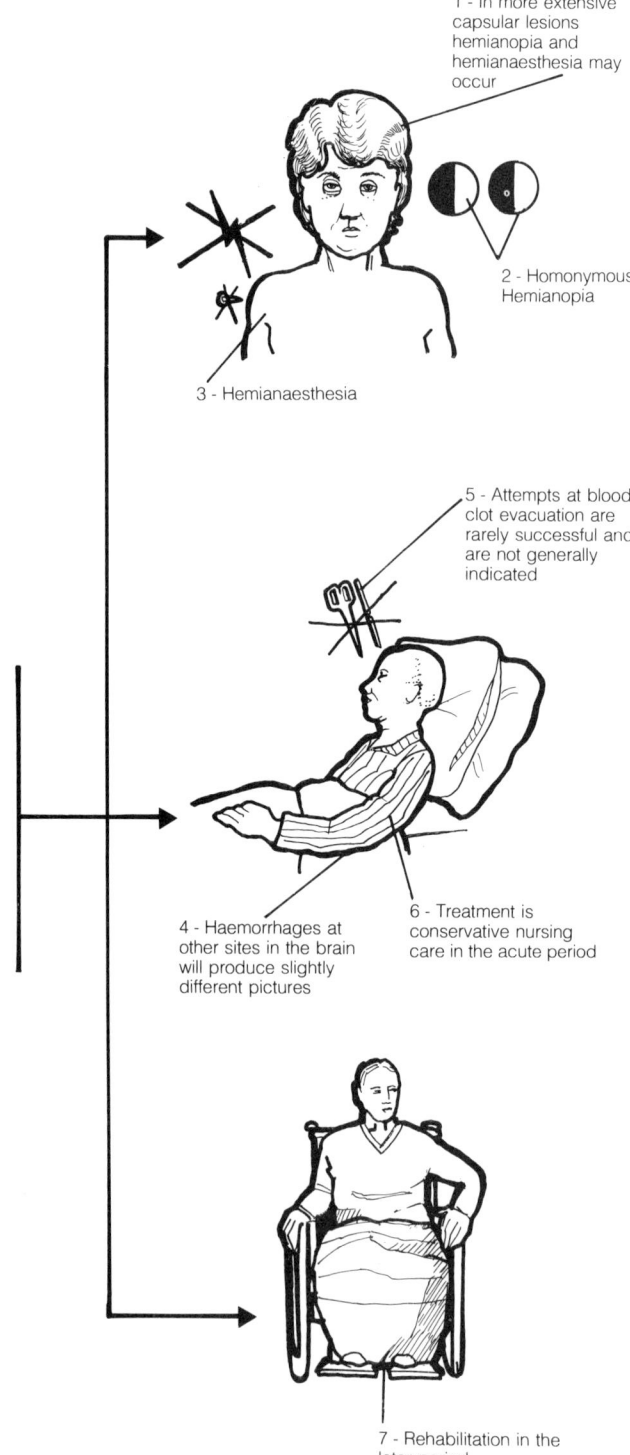

1 - In more extensive capsular lesions hemianopia and hemianaesthesia may occur

2 - Homonymous Hemianopia

3 - Hemianaesthesia

4 - Haemorrhages at other sites in the brain will produce slightly different pictures

5 - Attempts at blood clot evacuation are rarely successful and are not generally indicated

6 - Treatment is conservative nursing care in the acute period

7 - Rehabilitation in the later period

hemianopia and hemianaesthesia may occur. Cerebral haemorrhages at other sites or brain stem bleeds will produce slightly different pictures, but it is generally true that neurosurgical attempts at blood clot evacuation are rarely successful and not generally indicated. Treatment is thus conservative nursing care in the acute period and rehabilitation in the later period.

Occlusive Cerebrovascular Disease

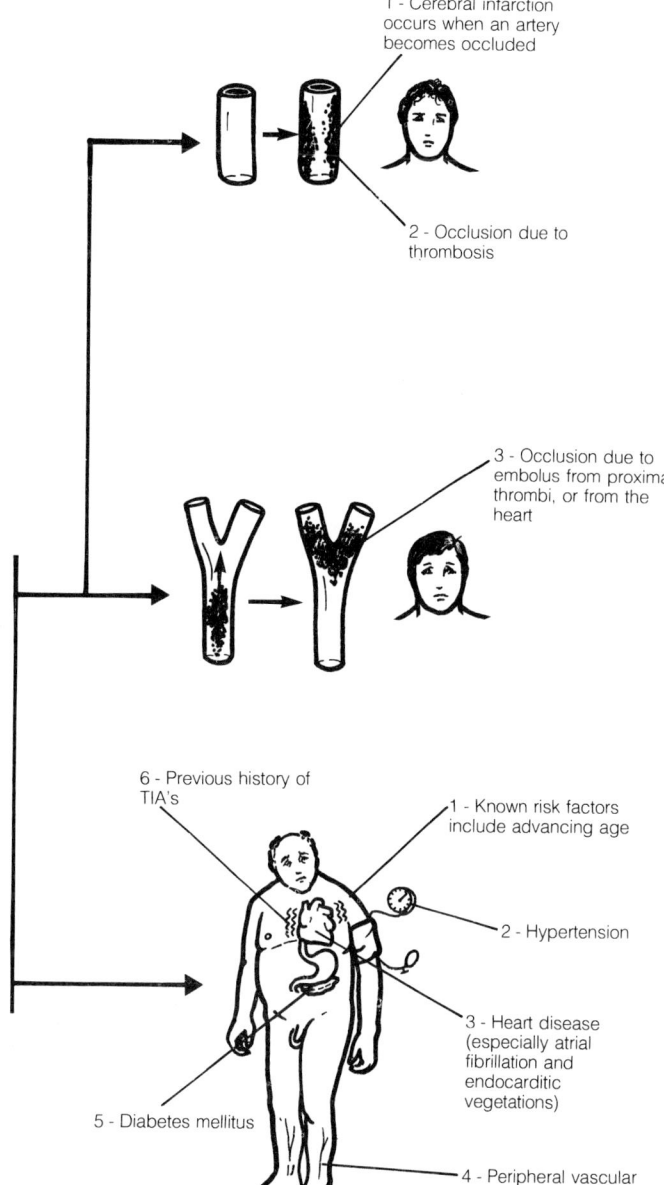

OCCLUSIVE CEREBROVASCULAR DISEASE

Cerebral infarction occurs when a cerebral artery becomes occluded in the absence of an adequate collateral circulation. Occlusion is due to thrombosis or embolism from proximal thrombi or from the heart. Known risk factors include advancing age, hypertension, heart disease (especially atrial fibrillation and endocarditic vegetations), a previous of history of **transient ischaemic attacks (TIA's)** or carotid bruit (both indicating carotid atheroma), peripheral vascular disease, diabetes mellitus, polycythaemia and hyperviscosity.

Occlusive Cerebrovascular Disease

Hyperlipidaemia and some forms of contraceptive pill may predispose. A "stroke" is an event of neurological dysfunction due to vascular disease, whose clincial symptoms last for more than 24 hours. A TIA is defined similarly but the features resolve within 24 hours and usually much more rapidly, (within a few minutes).

The syndrome of internal carotid artery occlusion includes ipsilateral blindness and contralateral hemiplegia (stroke). More recently, it has been recognised that TIA's due to temporary internal carotid

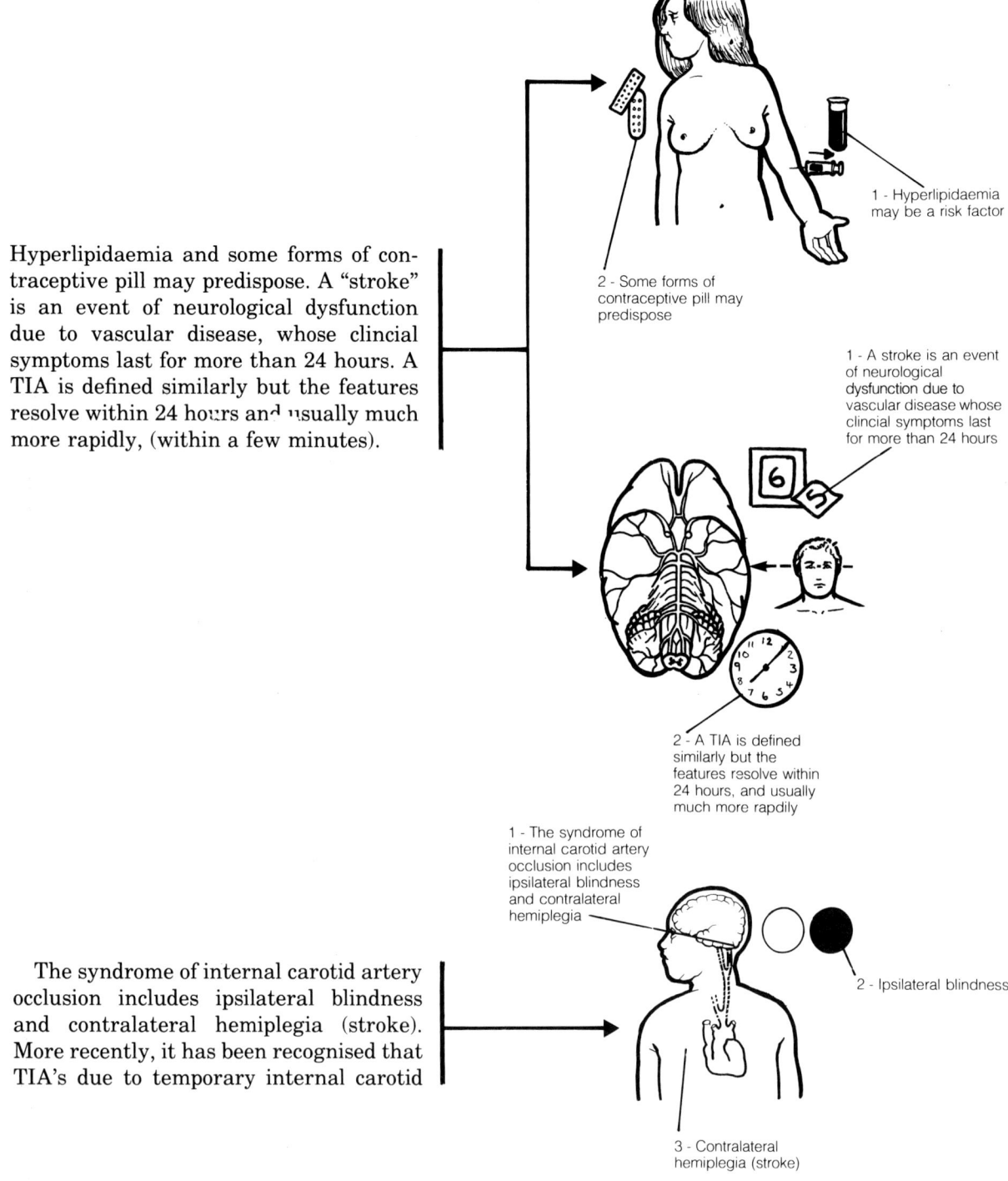

1 - Hyperlipidaemia may be a risk factor

2 - Some forms of contraceptive pill may predispose

1 - A stroke is an event of neurological dysfunction due to vascular disease whose clincial symptoms last for more than 24 hours

2 - A TIA is defined similarly but the features resolve within 24 hours, and usually much more rapdily

1 - The syndrome of internal carotid artery occlusion includes ipsilateral blindness and contralateral hemiplegia

2 - Ipsilateral blindness

3 - Contralateral hemiplegia (stroke)

Occlusive Cerebrovascular Disease

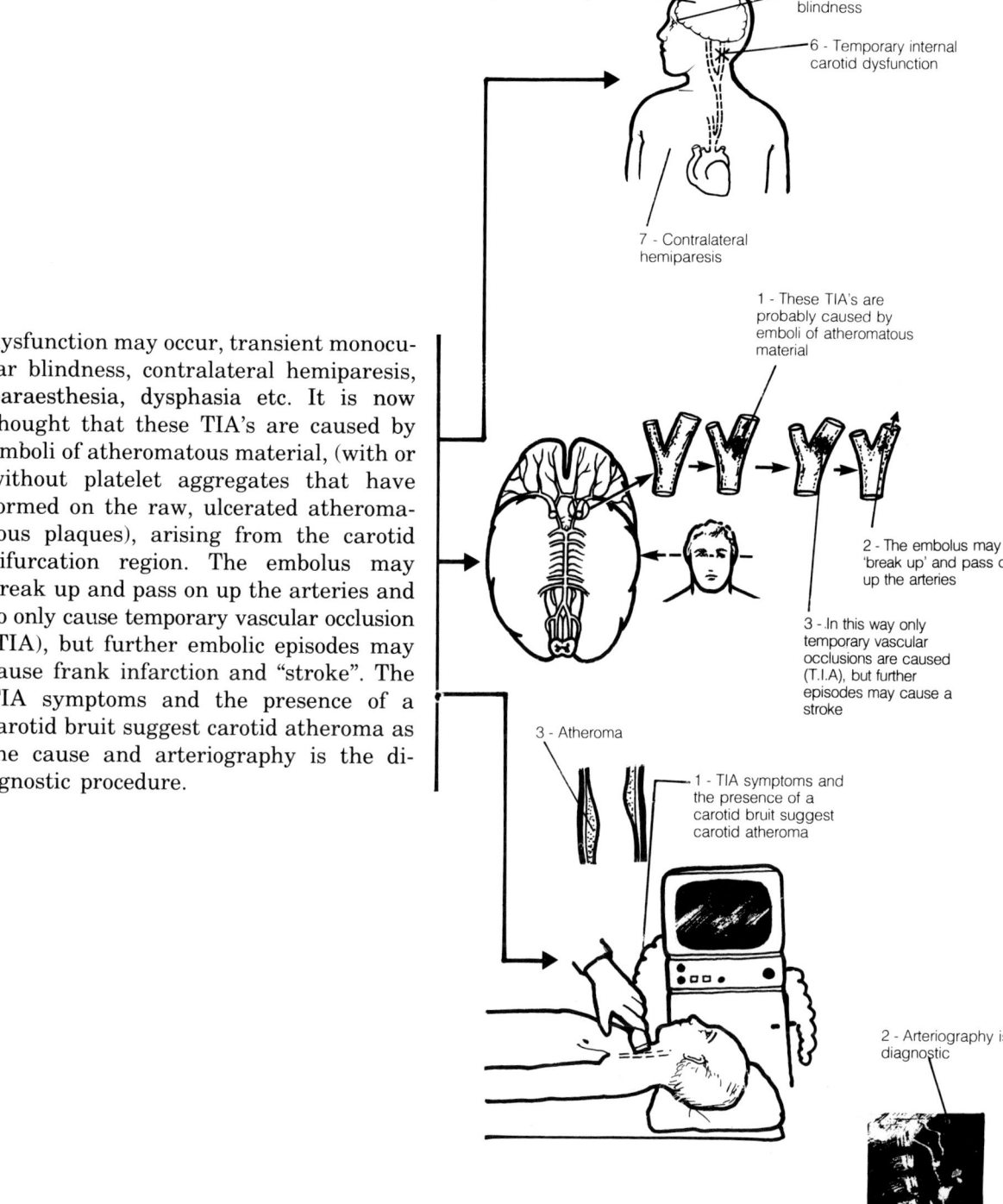

dysfunction may occur, transient monocular blindness, contralateral hemiparesis, paraesthesia, dysphasia etc. It is now thought that these TIA's are caused by emboli of atheromatous material, (with or without platelet aggregates that have formed on the raw, ulcerated atheromatous plaques), arising from the carotid bifurcation region. The embolus may break up and pass on up the arteries and so only cause temporary vascular occlusion (TIA), but further embolic episodes may cause frank infarction and "stroke". The TIA symptoms and the presence of a carotid bruit suggest carotid atheroma as the cause and arteriography is the diagnostic procedure.

Occlusive Cerebrovascular Disease

Conservative management includes antiplatelet drugs (eg. aspirin 600 mg bd) and perhaps anticoagulation (controversial), and cautious antihypertensive therapy if appropriate. Carotid endarterectomy may be indicated for localised stenotic lesions at the bifurcation of the common carotid artery. TIA's may also occur in the vertebrobasilar region and similar brief episodes eg. diplopia, vertigo, dysarthria, hemiparesis tingling sensations etc may occur. The vertebrobasilar system is less amenable to surgery, and therapy is usually conservative. Stroke may be caused by cerebral

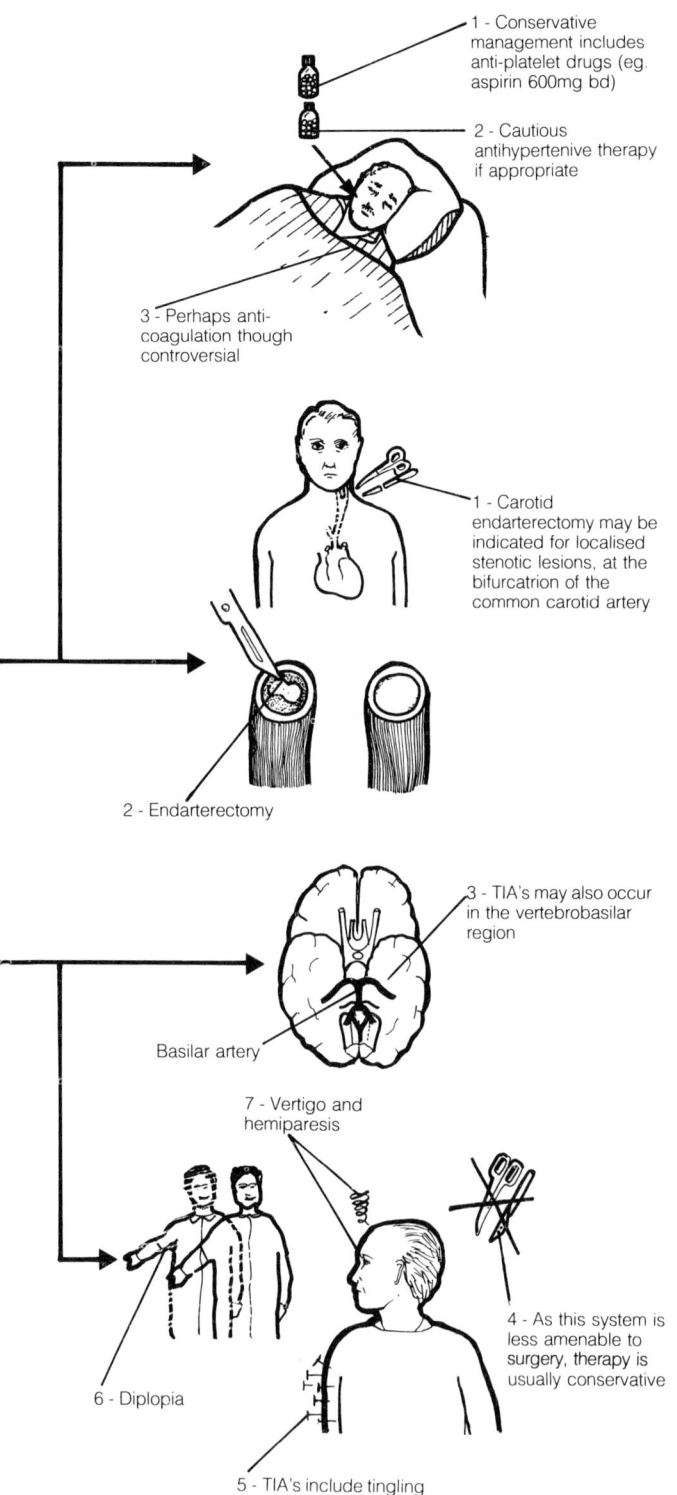

artery thrombosis, embolism or haemorrhage, the last of these three having already been discussed. There is some value in distinguishing thrombosis from embolism particularly if anticoagulation is contemplated.

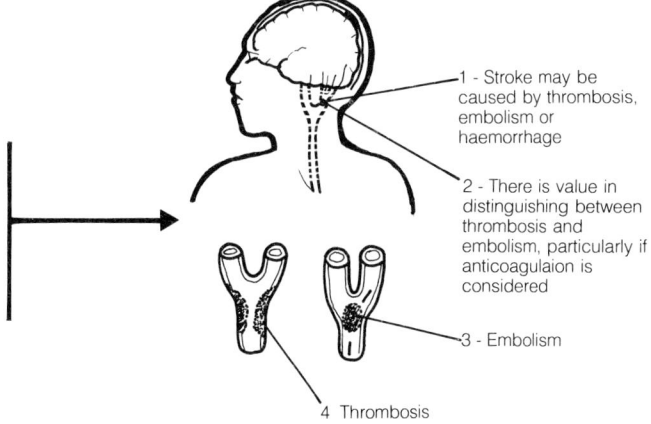

1 - Stroke may be caused by thrombosis, embolism or haemorrhage

2 - There is value in distinguishing between thrombosis and embolism, particularly if anticoagulaion is considered

3 - Embolism

4 Thrombosis

The stroke that occurs due to cerebral thrombosis develops more gradually than the clinical features of other cerebrovascular catastrophes. In children the thrombosis may occur with febrile illness and dehydration, in old people atheroma predisposes. Meningovascular neurosyphilis

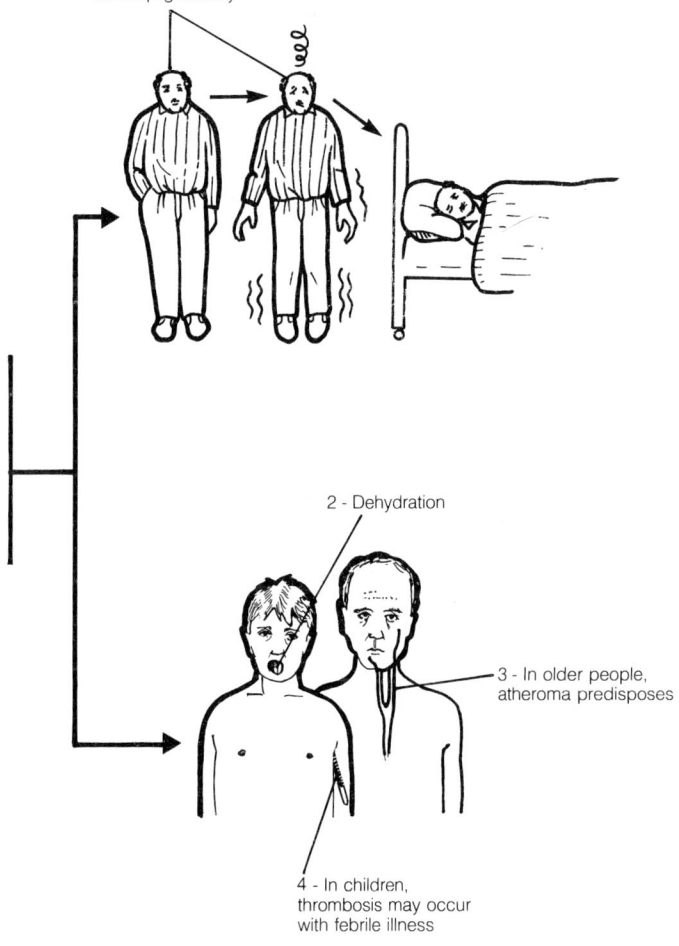

1 - Strokes due to cerebral thrombosis develop gradually

2 - Dehydration

3 - In older people, atheroma predisposes

4 - In children, thrombosis may occur with febrile illness

Occlusive Cerebrovascular Disease

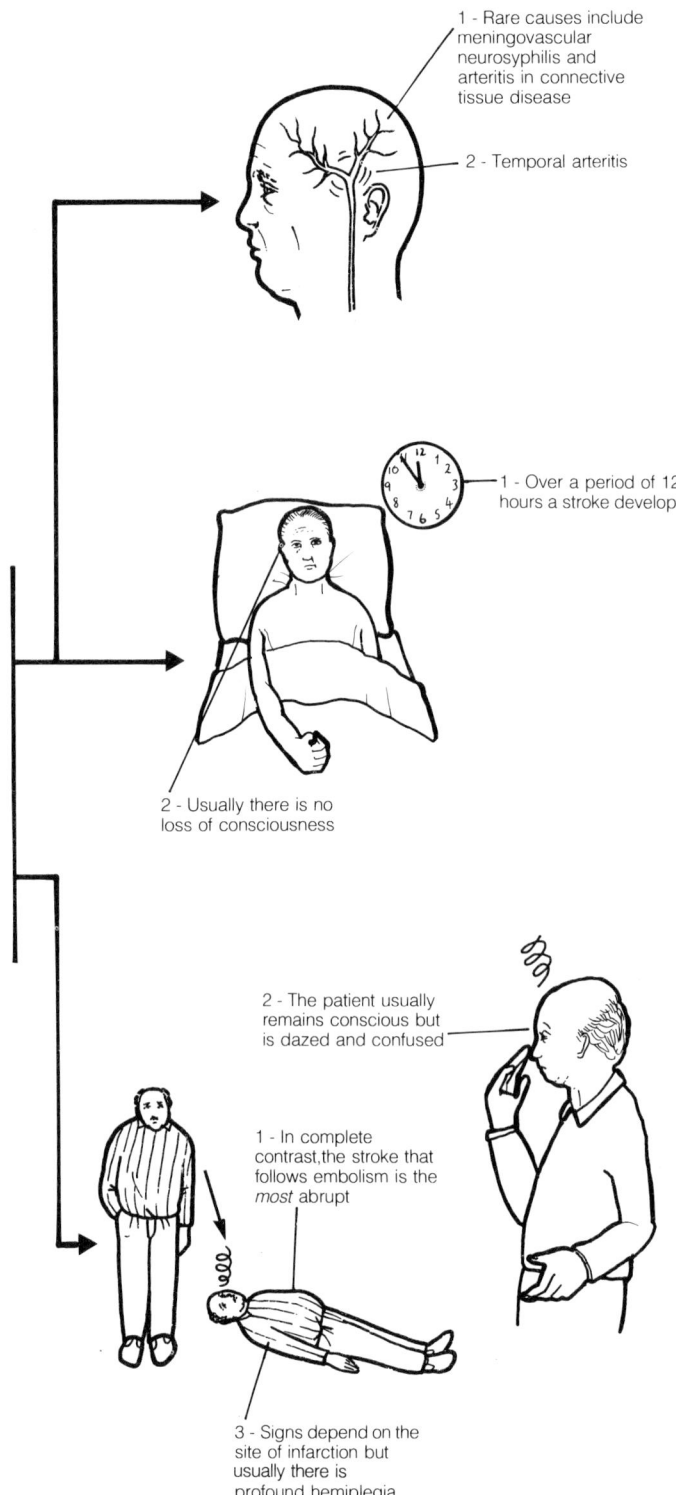

and arteritis in connective tissue disease, (temporal arteritis, PAN, SLE) are rare causes. Over a period of hours (perhaps 12 hours) a stroke develops, usually without loss of consciousness. In complete contrast, the stroke that follows embolism has the most abrupt onset of all cerebrovascular lesions. The patient usually remains conscious but is dazed and confused and (although the signs depend on the site of infarction) he usually has the most profound motor deficit (hemiplegia) from this time.

The source of the embolus, (eg. fibrillating heart, atheromatous carotid, septic source etc) may be obvious. Approximately half these stroke patients will make a reasonable recovery with good nursing care in the acute period and good rehabilitation in the longer term. Specific therapy, (eg. antiplatelet drugs, anticoagulants) are probably not indicated for the stroke *per se*. The blood pressure is often high at the time of the acute stroke and may settle spontaneously with time.

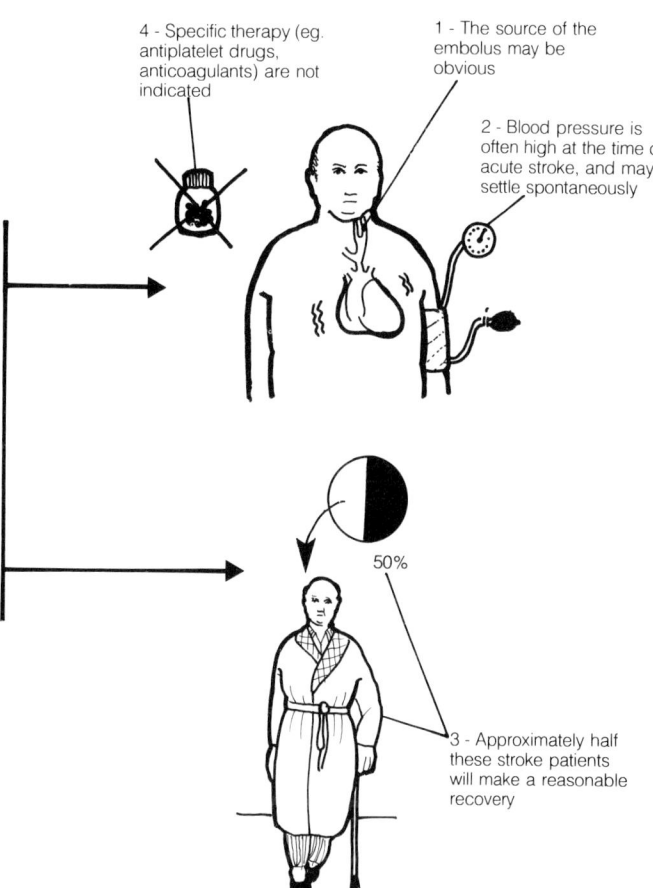

VENOUS SINUS THROMBOSIS

This may occur adjacent to a cerebral abscess or skull fracture or over a suppurative mastoiditis extensively involving the temporal bone. There is a slightly

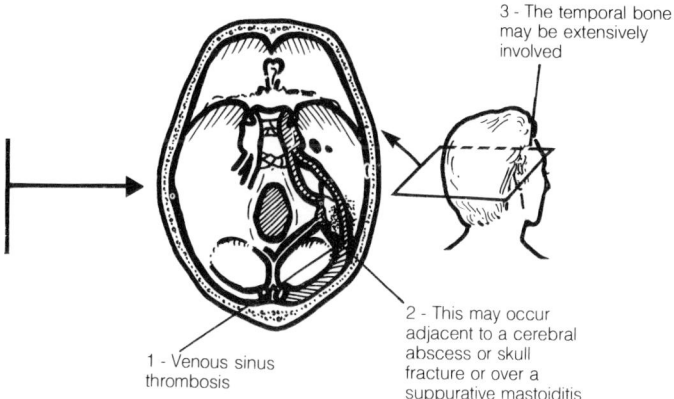

higher risk of venous sinus thrombosis during pregnancy and with the old, high oestrogen pill. Venous cerebral infarction, (perhaps with haemorrhage), may occur and anticoagulation is then frankly dangerous. Treatment is thus conservative, but dexamethasone may reduce cerebral oedema.

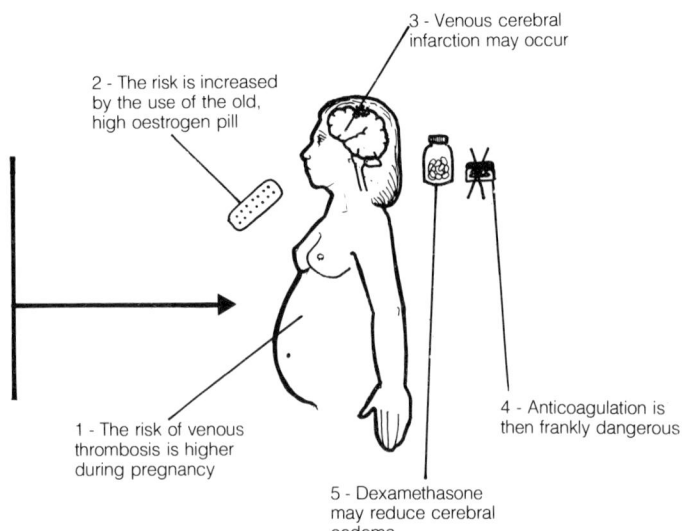

EPILEPSY

An epileptic fit is a transitory disturbance of brain function due to an abnormal discharge of neurones, occurring usually for no apparent reason. The fit usually is of sudden onset, of brief duration and ceasing spontaneously, although with a tendency to recur. A patient who has one, single fit does not warrant the diagnostic label 'epileptic', but the clinician's suspicions are aroused and investigations performed. Careful history taking will usually distinguish a fit from a syncopal attack (eg. vaso-vagal faint, cardiac dysrhythmia, vertebro-basilar insufficiency etc).

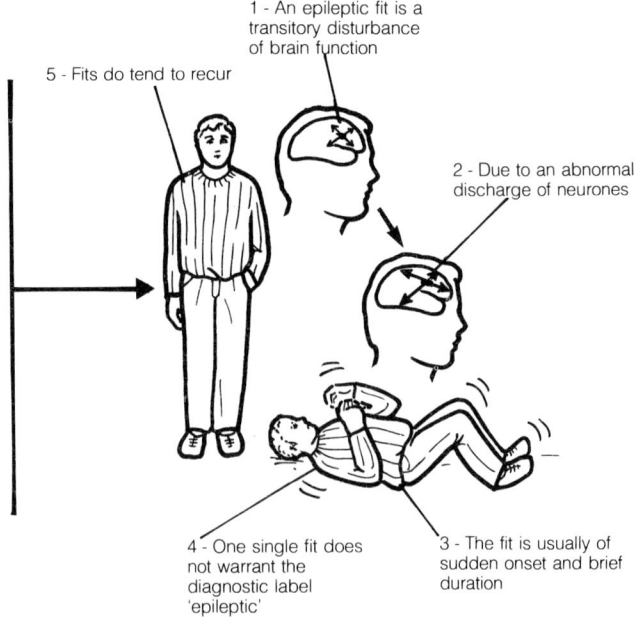

Epilepsy

Syncopal attacks usually give more warning of the attack and, (unless a fit follows the faint), there are usually no motor manifestations (tongue biting, tonic/clonic convulsions) during a syncopal episode.

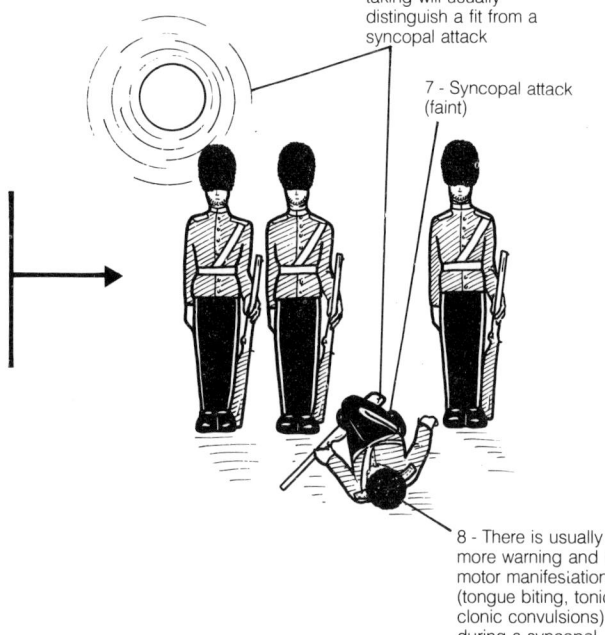

6 - Careful history taking will usually distinguish a fit from a syncopal attack

7 - Syncopal attack (faint)

8 - There is usually more warning and no motor manifestations (tongue biting, tonic/clonic convulsions) during a syncopal episode

Particularly in young people, there is often no discoverable cause for the fit and recurrent seizures in these patients lead to a diagnosis of idiopathic epilepsy; a positive family history may be obtained in up to one-third of these patients. Local brain lesions predispose to epileptic attacks (eg. brain trauma, brain tumours – primary or secondary, cerebrovascular disease, infections, brain abscess, tuberculoma, cystercercosis, encephalitis or even late meningitis, or degenerative brain conditions such as presenile dementia). The

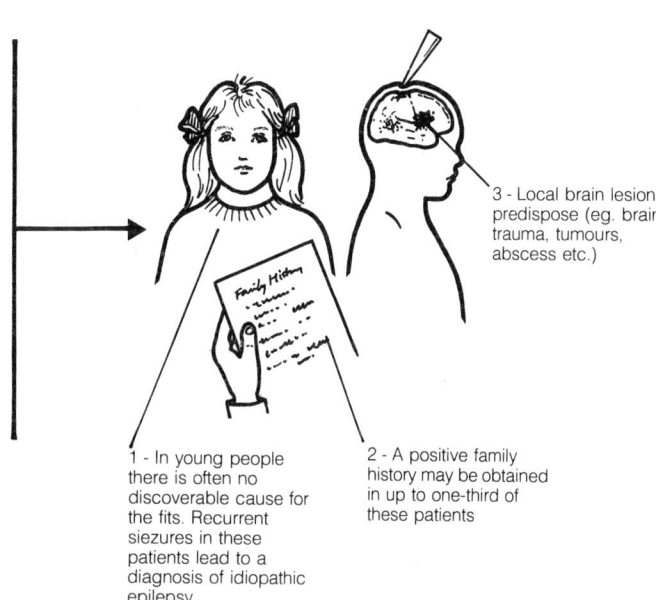

1 - In young people there is often no discoverable cause for the fits. Recurrent siezures in these patients lead to a diagnosis of idiopathic epilepsy

2 - A positive family history may be obtained in up to one-third of these patients

3 - Local brain lesions predispose (eg. brain trauma, tumours, abscess etc.)

Epilepsy

onset of fits in a previously fit middle-aged or elderly person makes one particularly suspicious of local brain pathology and brain tumours and cerebrovascular diseases are the commonest causes of 'symptomatic epilepsy' in this age group. An epilepsy which changes its clinical pattern (eg. successive fits becoming more severe) is very suggestive of an underlying local brain lesion. Focal epilepsies always suggest a local lesion.

1 - Onset of fits in a previously healthy middle aged person

2 - This should alert the clinician to search for local brain pathology

3 - Brain tumours and cerebrovascular disease are the commonest causes of 'symptomatic epilepsy' at this age

4 - Changes in the clinical pattern of fits is very suggestive of an underlying brain lesion

5 - Focal epilepsies always suggest a local lesion

There are systemic upsets which predispose to and, indeed, may present with fitting. These include: hypoglycaemia, hypocalcaemia, hypo- or hypertension, anoxia, liver or renal failure, alcohol intoxication or withdrawal states (drugs), and febrile convulsions are well recognised in young children. Systemic causes for fitting should be ruled out in the new epileptic.

1 - Certain systemic upsets predispose to, and may present with fitting

2 - Hypo or hypertension

3 - Alcohol intoxication or withdrawal

4 - Liver or renal failure

5 - Hypocalcaemia and anoxia

6 - In a new epileptic, systemic causes should be ruled out

Epilepsy

The **investigations** that are performed in the patient with fits include a skull X-ray series and an electroencephalogram (E.E.G.). However, it should be noted that both these tests may be normal in epileptic patients and only an EEG during an attack may be diagnostic. In adults in whom a local brain lesion is likely, a C.T. brain scan is also necessary.

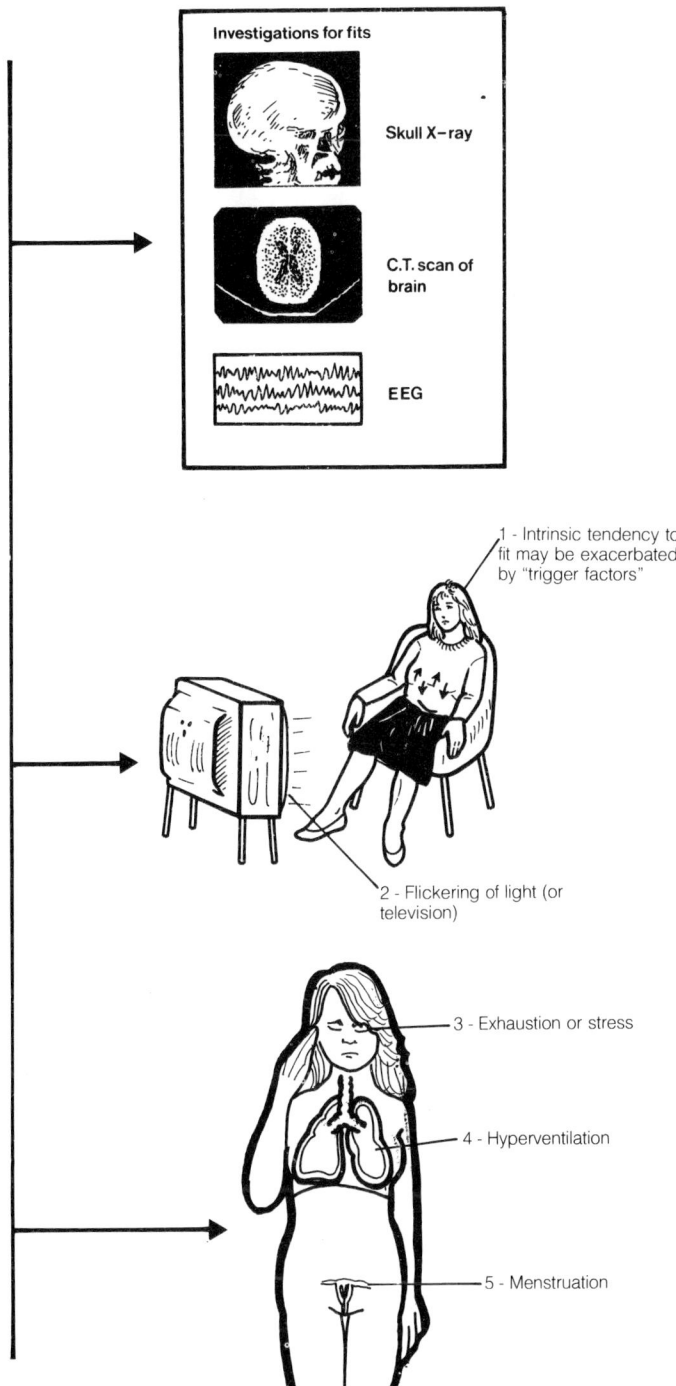

Just prior to describing the various types of epilepsy, it should be emphasied that an intrinsic tendency to fits may be exacerbated by many factors which include stress or exhaustion, menstruation, hyperventilation, alkalosis, watching a flickering light (or television) – all these may promote the occurrence of a fit in a patient with an innate tendency to fit; although not epileptogenic *per se* – they are known as "trigger factors".

The simple distinction into generalised or focal (partial) epileptic fits is still most useful:

GENERALISED EPILEPSY

In these patients there is loss of consciousness during an attack and there are symmetrical and synchronous EEG abnormalities. The discharges originate from deep, mid-line structures.

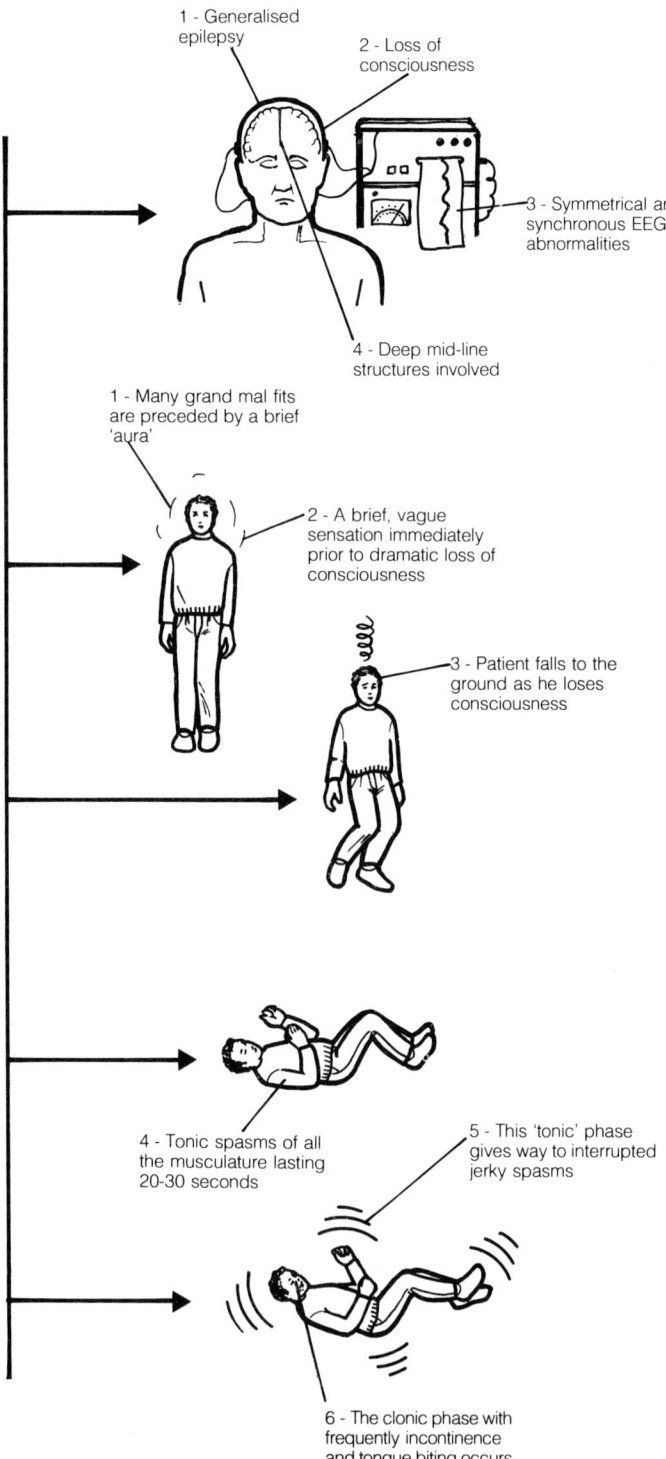

GRAND MAL

Many grand mal fits are preceded by a brief 'aura' which is usually a brief and vague, peculiar sensation immediately prior to the dramatic and sudden loss of consciousness with tonic spasms of all the musculature. The patient falls to the ground, gripped in spasm and becoming cyanosed; this tonic phase lasts perhaps 20-30 seconds. Following this, the sustained tonic contraction gives way to interrupted jerky spasms (clonic phase).

In this phase, the patient is frequently incontinent, and biting the tongue and foaming at the mouth is common. Slowly, the clonic spasms die down and a phase of relaxation occurs, usually with a period of post-ictal sleep. After regaining consciousness, the patient is commonly confused and headache is common. Rarely, there is the phenomenon of post-epileptic automatism in which the patient commits anti-social acts.

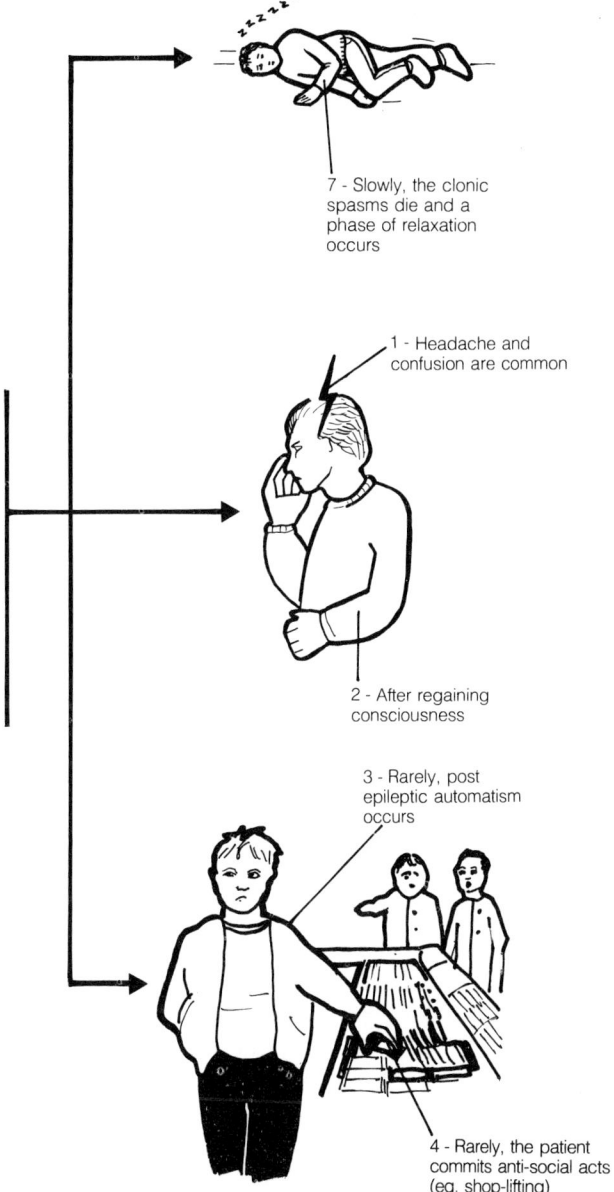

7 - Slowly, the clonic spasms die and a phase of relaxation occurs

1 - Headache and confusion are common

2 - After regaining consciousness

3 - Rarely, post epileptic automatism occurs

4 - Rarely, the patient commits anti-social acts (eg. shop-lifting)

PETIT MAL

Petit mal commences in infancy or childhood and the attacks tend to cease or be replaced by grand mal seizures in adolescence. In a typical attack, the child suddenly appears to pause in his daily activity, remaining still and gazing in a dazed fashion. The child does not fall nor convulse. The attack usually lasts only 10-15 seconds and the child then resumes his activity again. In some children, the petit mal attacks may occur many times (perhaps one hundred or more) each day. The EEG in petit mal epilepsy is characteristic with 'spike' and 'wave' discharges at 3 per second.

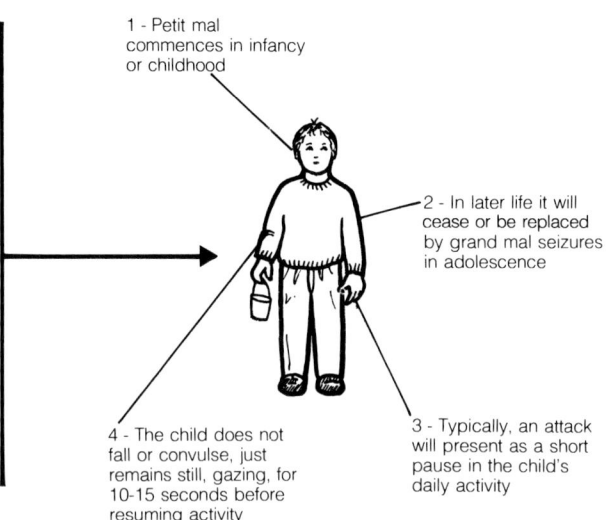

1 - Petit mal commences in infancy or childhood

2 - In later life it will cease or be replaced by grand mal seizures in adolescence

3 - Typically, an attack will present as a short pause in the child's daily activity

4 - The child does not fall or convulse, just remains still, gazing, for 10-15 seconds before resuming activity

PARTIAL EPILEPSY (FOCAL EPILEPSY)

In these fits there is one cortical focus of abnormal neuronal discharge which at first does not lead to generalised abnormal brain discharges, and therefore consciousness is commonly maintained. The exact character of the fit depends on the site of the cortical focus. This type of fit is best exemplified by a **Jacksonian fit**. In a typical case, there is a motor seizure of a limb which begins as involuntary twitching or clonic spasms in say: the fingers,

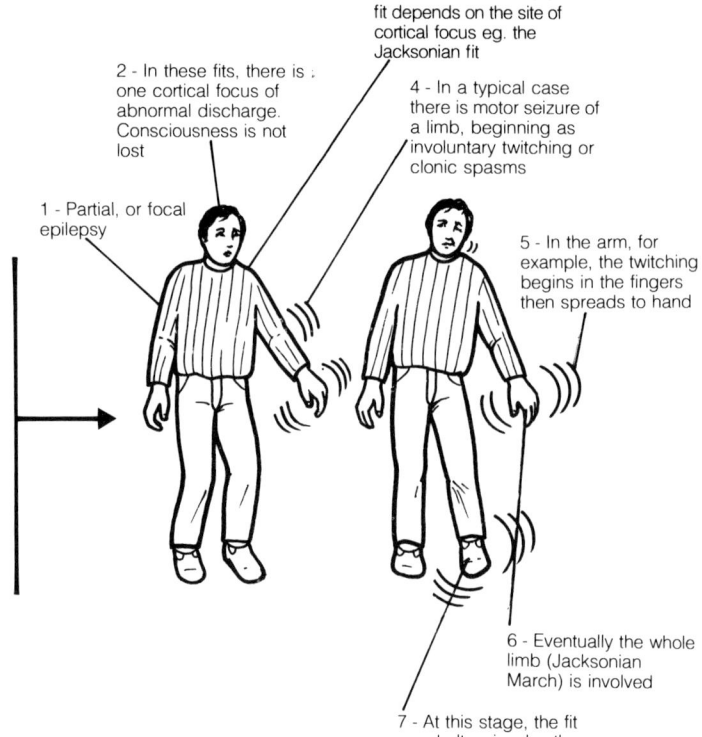

1 - Partial, or focal epilepsy

2 - In these fits, there is one cortical focus of abnormal discharge. Consciousness is not lost

3 - The character of the fit depends on the site of cortical focus eg. the Jacksonian fit

4 - In a typical case there is motor seizure of a limb, beginning as involuntary twitching or clonic spasms

5 - In the arm, for example, the twitching begins in the fingers then spreads to hand

6 - Eventually the whole limb (Jacksonian March) is involved

7 - At this stage, the fit may halt or involve the whole side of the body

which then spreads to the hand, forearm and then to involve the whole limb (Jacksonian march'). The fit may halt at this stage or progress to cause a motor seizure of the whole side of the body or spread to become a full grand mal seizure. Following recovery from a focal fit, an afflicted limb may remain temporarily paretic (**Todd's paresis**).

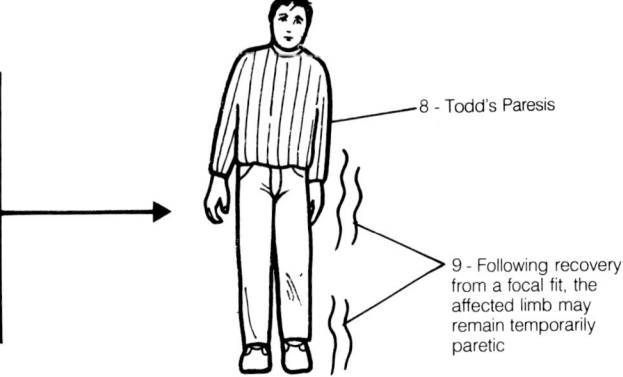

Temporal lobe epilepsy (TLE) is a distinct form of focal epilepsy. TLE may take the form of complicated auras or psychomotor attacks with illusions or hallucination, (familiarity, strangeness, micropsia, déjà-vu reminiscences) with strange emotions (eg. fears, pleasant feelings etc), with crude somatic sensations, (eg. epigastric sensation rising up to the throat, tastes or smells – often unpleasant). The patient

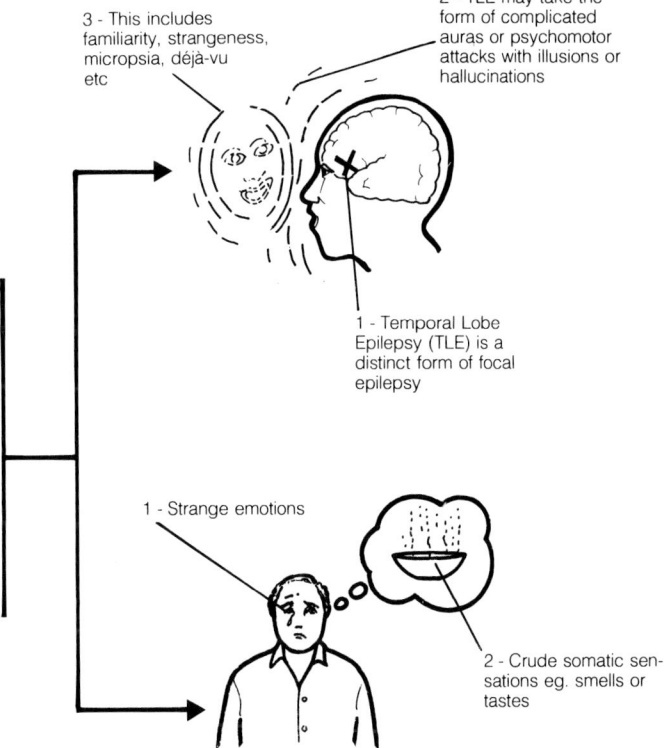

Partial Epilepsy (Focal Epilepsy)

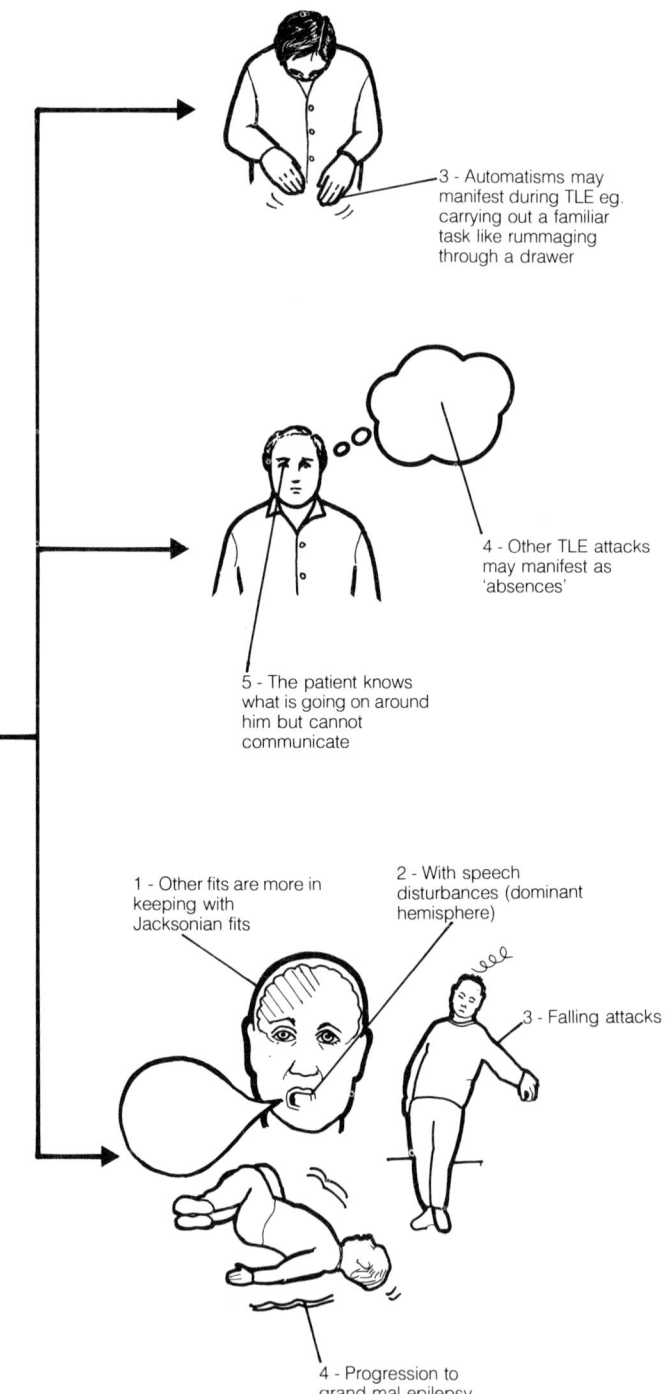

may manifest automatisms during TLE: thus he might carry out some familiar motor task (eg. dressing, rummaging through a cupboard etc). Other TLE attacks may manifest as 'absences' in which the patient knows what is going on around him in time but cannot communicate at this time. Yet other TLE attacks are more in keeping with Jacksonian fits, with speech disturbances (dominant hemisphere), falling attacks and progression to grand mal epilepsy.

TREATMENT OF EPILEPSY

If an underlying cause of epilepsy is found, it should be treated in its own right, but in the majority of cases anticonvulsant drugs will be needed. In general, idiopathic epilepsy is more easily controlled than symptomatic epilepsy (i.e. epilepsy secondary to brain disease).

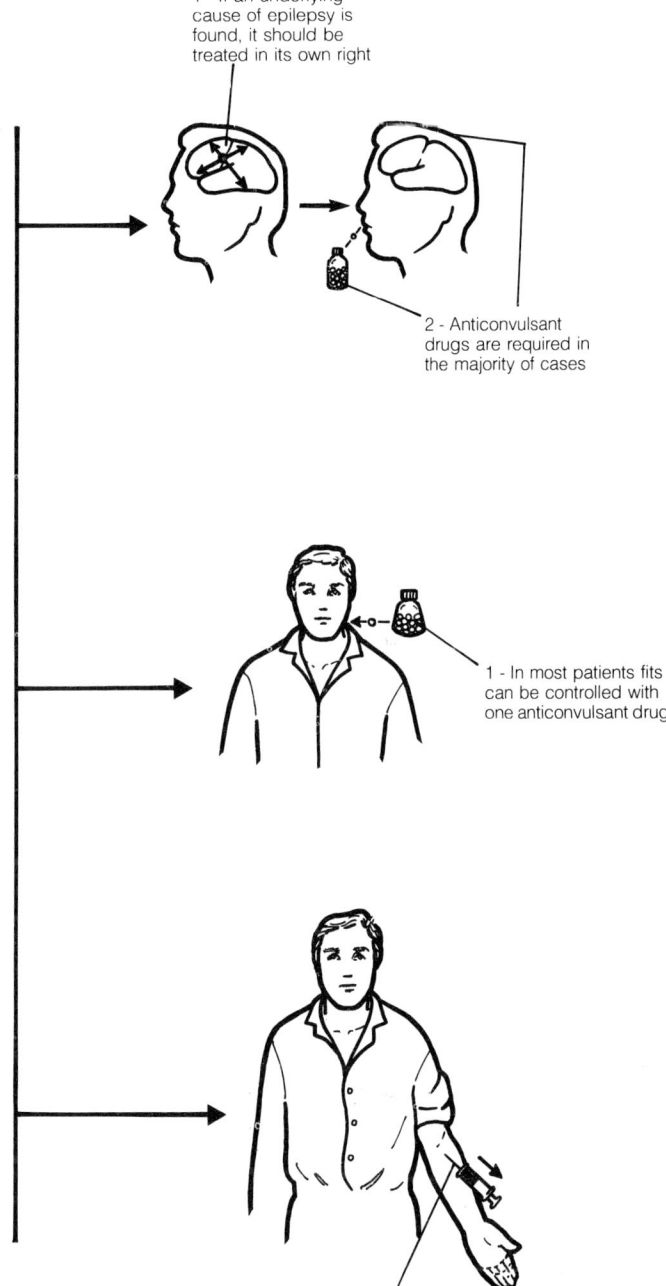

1 - If an underlying cause of epilepsy is found, it should be treated in its own right

2 - Anticonvulsant drugs are required in the majority of cases

1 - In most patients fits can be controlled with one anticonvulsant drug

In most patients, fit control can be achieved with one anticonvulsant drug, with dose adjustments such that blood levels are in the therapeutic range – and this needs to be checked a few weeks after initial stabilisation as all these drugs are hepatic enzyme inducers. The drug of first choice for grand mal attacks is phenytoin (See table). Toxic side effects of phenytoin

2 - Dose is adjusted so that blood levels are in the therapeutic range

Treatment of Epilepsy

include cerebellar ataxia, nystagmus, gum hypertrophy, megaloblastic anaemia (with low red cell folate), morbilliform rash, lymphadenopathy, lupus-like syndrome, osteomalacia and blood dyscrasia. Despite this long list of adverse effects, phenytoin is well tolerated by the majority of patients and is a powerful anticonvulsant.

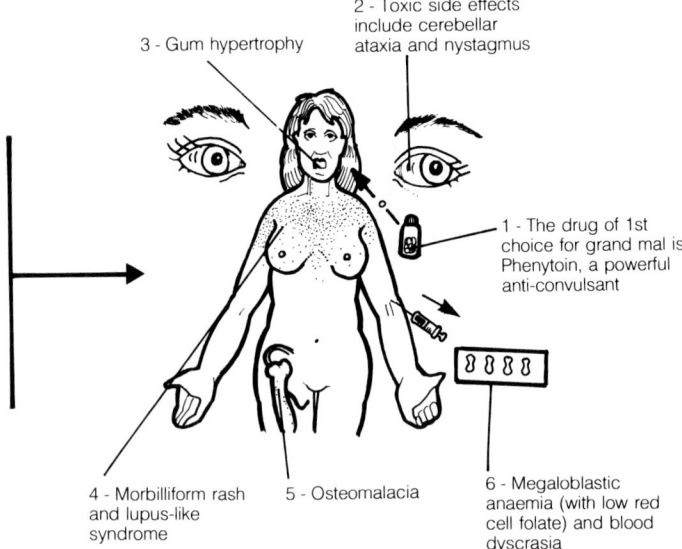

1 - The drug of 1st choice for grand mal is Phenytoin, a powerful anti-convulsant
2 - Toxic side effects include cerebellar ataxia and nystagmus
3 - Gum hypertrophy
4 - Morbilliform rash and lupus-like syndrome
5 - Osteomalacia
6 - Megaloblastic anaemia (with low red cell folate) and blood dyscrasia

Primidone, (which is partially metabolised to phenobarbitone), and phenobarbitone itself may need to be added if phenytoin, in full dosage for that individual, is not controlling the seizures. Both may cause clinically important sedation despite a night time, once per 24 hour prescription, and phenobarbitone may cause more behavioural disorders in children and the elderly. Besides these side effects, skin rashes (even Stevens-Johnson syndrome) may occur.

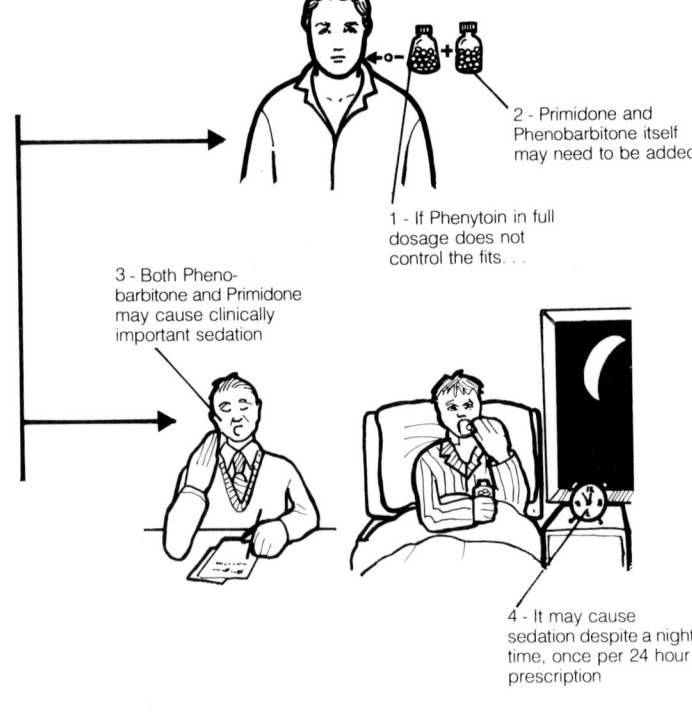

1 - If Phenytoin in full dosage does not control the fits...
2 - Primidone and Phenobarbitone itself may need to be added
3 - Both Phenobarbitone and Primidone may cause clinically important sedation
4 - It may cause sedation despite a night time, once per 24 hour prescription

Treatment of Epilepsy

All these drugs may be given once or twice daily as their half-life in plasma is long. Anti-convulsants should never be stopped abruptly.

Other useful anti-convulsants include carbamazepine and sodium valproate. Both these drugs are usually well-tolerated with few side effects but both have a short plasma half-life and require tds-qds administration. Carbamazepine

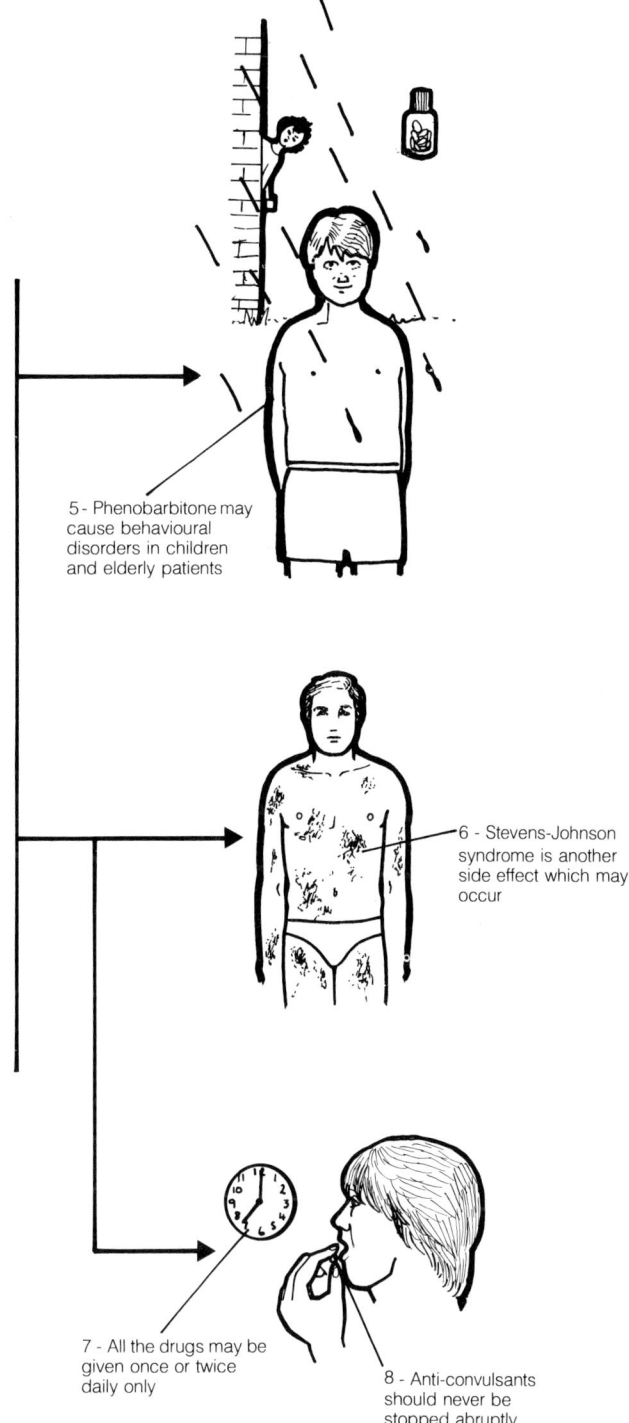

5 - Phenobarbitone may cause behavioural disorders in children and elderly patients

6 - Stevens-Johnson syndrome is another side effect which may occur

7 - All the drugs may be given once or twice daily only

8 - Anti-convulsants should never be stopped abruptly

may be particularly useful in TLE – psychomotor attacks and valproate valuable in petit mal; ethosuximide is the other first line drug for petit mal. In epilepsy with a largely myoclonic component, valproate and clonazepam are most useful

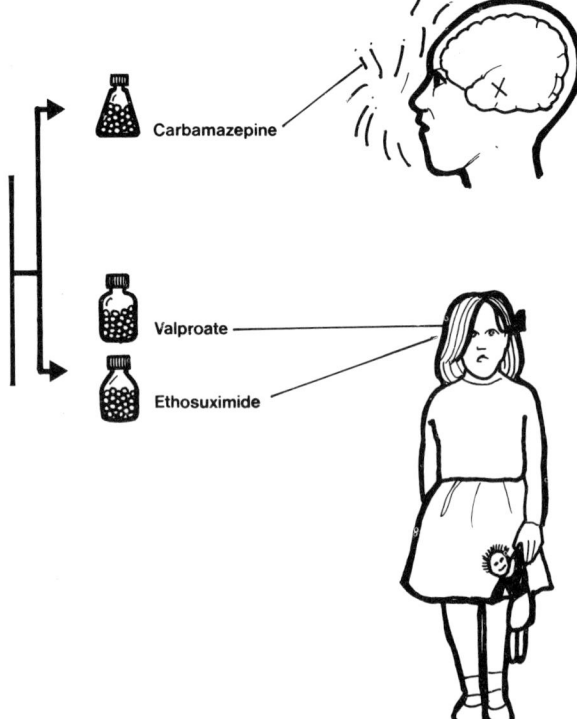

Anticonvulsant	Average adult daily dose (MG)	Therapeutic plasma range (μ mol-l)	Approx plasma T½ (Hr)	Frequency of dosage
Phenytoin	250-400	40-90	20	o.d. – b.d.
Primidone	1000	–	–	o.d. – b.d.
Phenobarbitone	90-120	60-150	80	nocte
Carbamazepine	600	17-42	12	t.d.s.
Valproate	1500	350-700	8	b.d. – tds

The addition of an anticonvulsant to the drugs taken by a patient already stabilised on another anticonvulsant, may interact to influence the blood levels of the first drug. Similarly, by enzyme induction, anti-convulsants may influence the metabolism of other drugs, (and vice versa):- all CNS sedatives, the pill, anticoagulants, some antibiotics (including antituberculous drugs) and some arthritis medications.

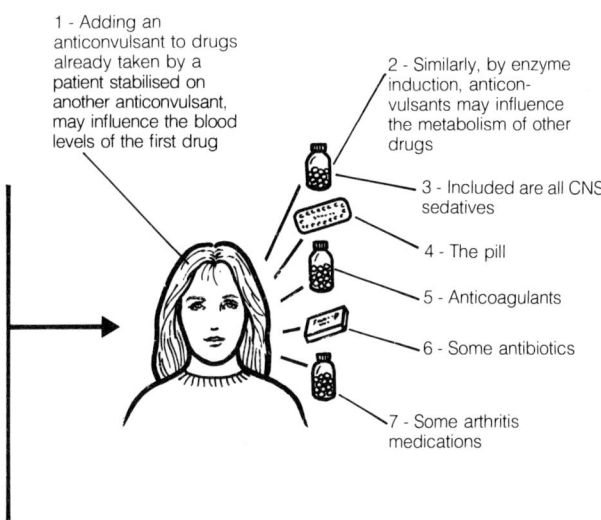

MULTIPLE SCLEROSIS (M.S., DISSEMINATED SCLEROSIS).

This disease of unknown aetiology, is characterised by the occurence of plaques or patches of demyelination of the CNS white matter. The development of these plaques, scattered at various sites and over various time periods within the CNS, gives rise to focal neurological symptoms and signs, which, (at least early in M.S.) tend to resolve as the plaques heal with only minor scarring. Whilst any site in the CNS may be affected, there is a definite predilection for: optic nerves, periventricular white matter, brain stem, cerebellum and cervical spinal cord.

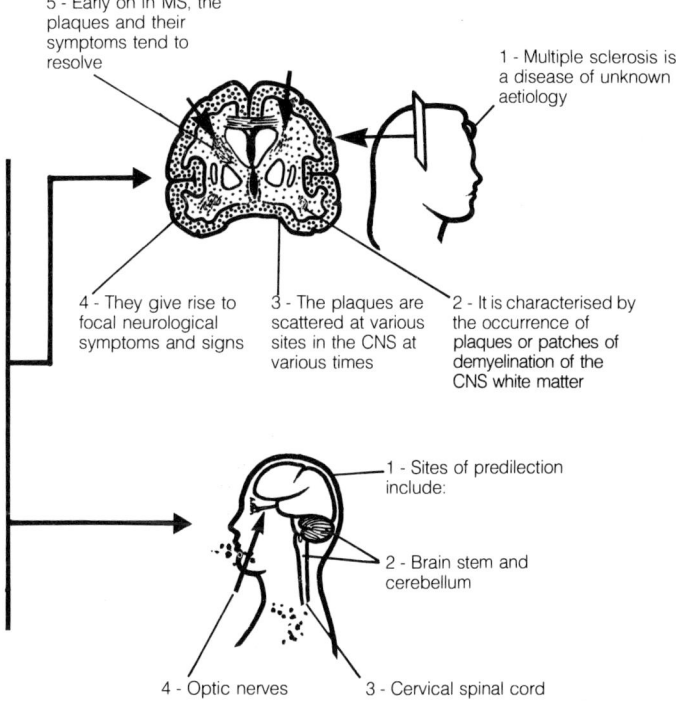

Multiple Sclerosis (M.S., Disseminated Sclerosis)

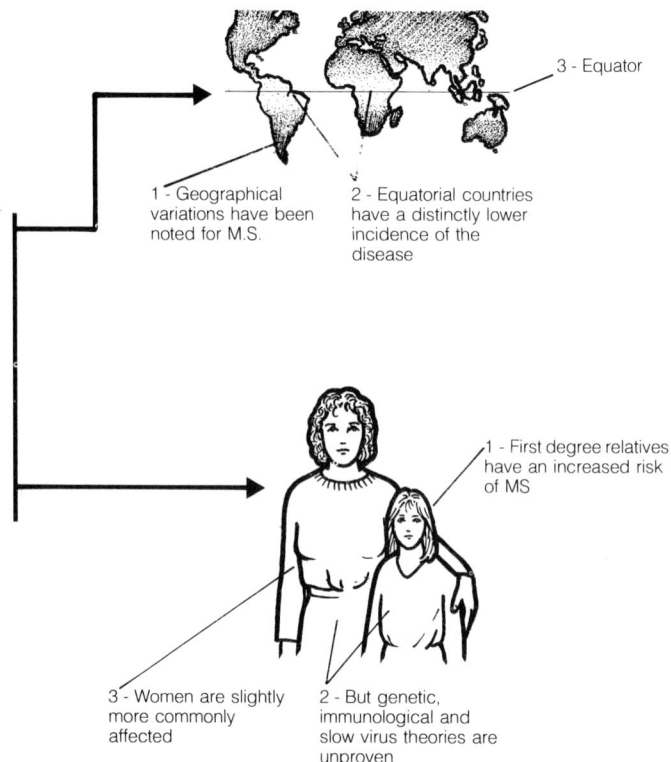

1 - Geographical variations have been noted for M.S.
2 - Equatorial countries have a distinctly lower incidence of the disease
3 - Equator

There is an interesting geographical variation in the incidence of the disease with equatorial countries having a distinctly lower incidence. There is an increased risk for first degree relatives, but no genetic basis can be elucidated and other aetiological theories, (including immunological and slow virus agents) are unproven. Women are slightly more commonly afflicted.

1 - First degree relatives have an increased risk of MS
2 - But genetic, immunological and slow virus theories are unproven
3 - Women are slightly more commonly affected

The **clinical onset** is usually between 20-40 years of age; a childhood onset is rare as is an onset at age 50 years or over. The onset may be rapid or very lengthy, in that symptoms may appear and be fully developed in hours, days or even weeks or months. The most common initial symptoms are: motor weakness in one or more limbs, retrobulbar neuritis, paraesthesiae, unsteadiness in walking, double

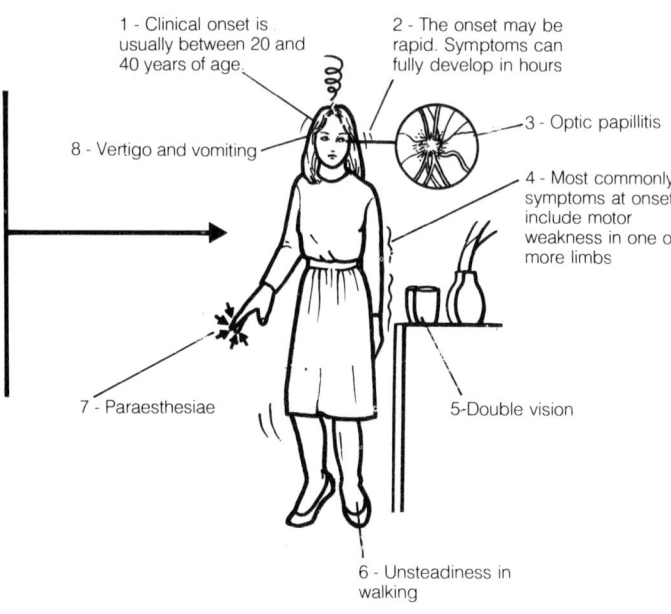

1 - Clinical onset is usually between 20 and 40 years of age
2 - The onset may be rapid. Symptoms can fully develop in hours
3 - Optic papillitis
4 - Most commonly, symptoms at onset include motor weakness in one or more limbs
5 - Double vision
6 - Unsteadiness in walking
7 - Paraesthesiae
8 - Vertigo and vomiting

Multiple Sclerosis (M.S., Disseminated Sclerosis)

vision, vertigo vomiting and micturition disturbance. It may not be possible to make the diagnosis of MS from the first attack and the diagnosis often relies on the relapsing and remitting clinical course and the development with time of evidence of multiple sites/lesions within the CNS.

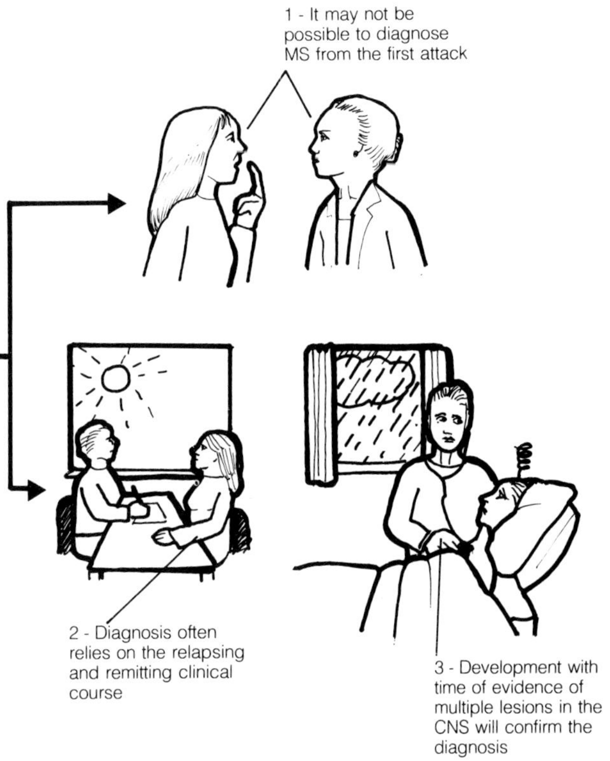

1 - It may not be possible to diagnose MS from the first attack

2 - Diagnosis often relies on the relapsing and remitting clinical course

3 - Development with time of evidence of multiple lesions in the CNS will confirm the diagnosis

Retrobulbar neuritis is the commonest presenting complaint in young adults and may be acute in onset, usually over a few days. There is blurring or loss of vision in one eye with pain on movement of the eye. The fundus is normal at this stage, (unless the plaque lies at the nerve head when "optic papillitis" appears as papilloedema in that eye).

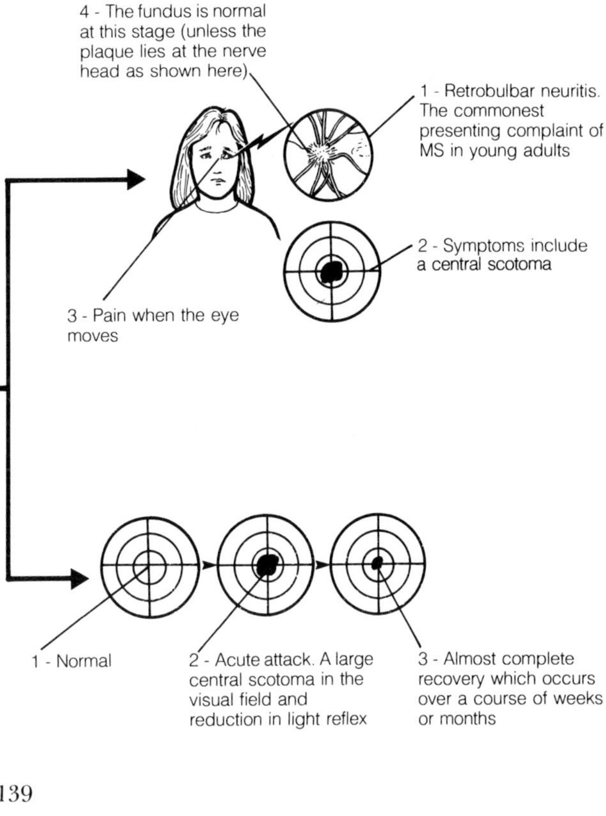

4 - The fundus is normal at this stage (unless the plaque lies at the nerve head as shown here)

1 - Retrobulbar neuritis. The commonest presenting complaint of MS in young adults

2 - Symptoms include a central scotoma

3 - Pain when the eye moves

1 - Normal

2 - Acute attack. A large central scotoma in the visual field and reduction in light reflex

3 - Almost complete recovery which occurs over a course of weeks or months

Multiple Sclerosis (M.S., Disseminated Sclerosis)

However, there is a large central scotoma in the visual field and reduction in the light reflex. Over the course of weeks or months, the clinical features partially or completely resolve. It is with the onset of the next clinical symptoms that the diagnosis of M.S. is established more firmly. In young adolescents, a rapid onset bilateral retrobulbar neuritis preceding a severe spinal cord lesion, often transverse myelitis, is recognised as a variant syndrome of M.S. (**Devic's disease**, neuromyelitis optica).

Motor weaknesses are more commonly seen in older patients and may be symmetrical. However, there may well be a differential diagnosis, and myelography, (to exclude spinal cord compression) or other tests may be indicated. Thus M.S. should be diagnosed only by exclusion at the time of the first symptoms.

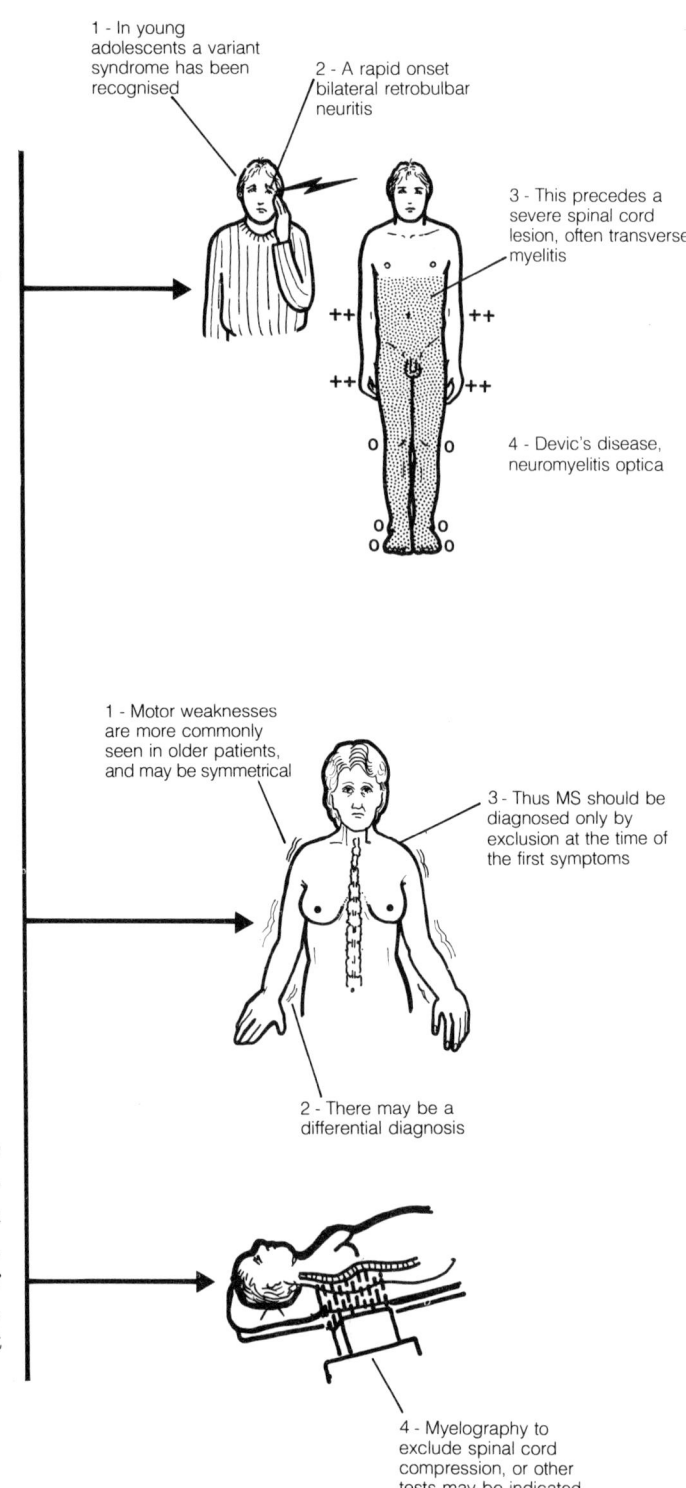

In patients with advanced M.S., the following clinical signs are frequently present: Nystagmus, other cerebellar signs (notably ataxia), pallor of the optic discs and U.M.N. limb signs; (LMN signs are rare in MS).

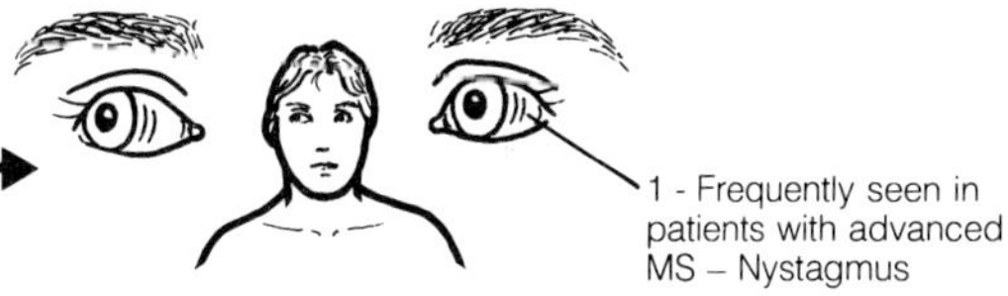

1 - Frequently seen in patients with advanced MS – Nystagmus

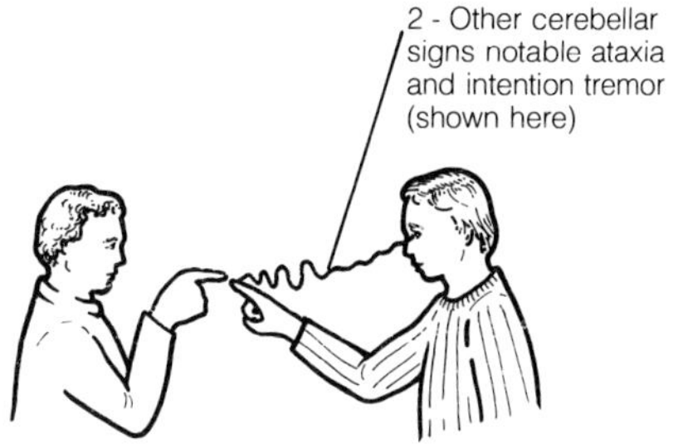

2 - Other cerebellar signs notable ataxia and intention tremor (shown here)

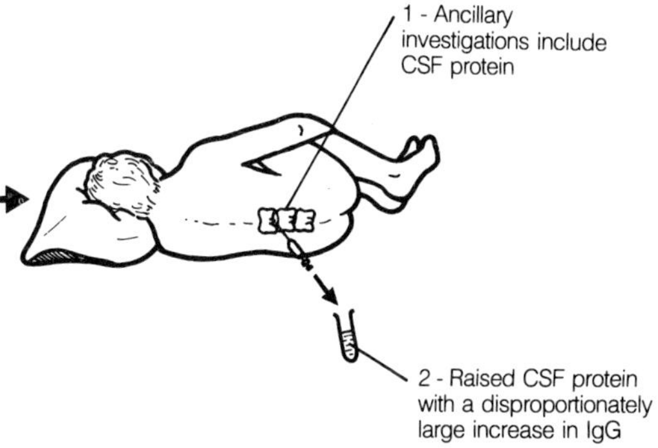

1 - Ancillary investigations include CSF protein

2 - Raised CSF protein with a disproportionately large increase in IgG

Ancillary investigations may assist in diagnosis. The C.S.F. protein may be raised with a disproportionately large increase in IgG; a mild to moderate lymphocytosis is common. The visual evoked response (V.E.R) is a valuable test in which the retina is stimulated by a flashing chequer board pattern, watched by the patient and the latency to visual cortex response measured by occipital electrodes. The V.E.R. may be delayed or distorted by subclinical M.S. plaques and, in a patient with an

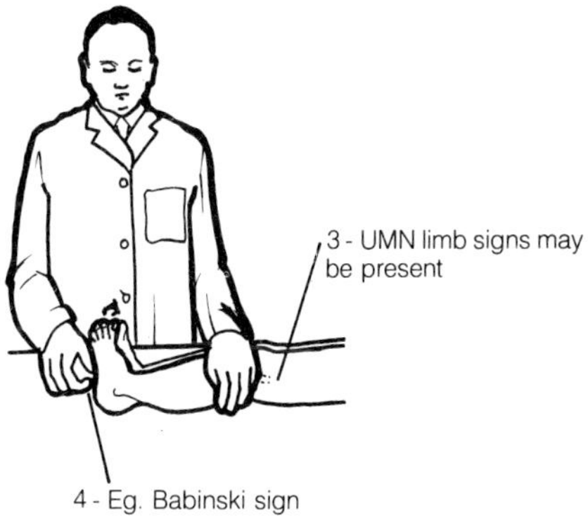

3 - UMN limb signs may be present

4 - Eg. Babinski sign

Multiple Sclerosis (M.S., Disseminated Sclerosis)

'apparently' isolated cord or brainstem clinical lesion, such an abnormal V.E.R adds credence to the diagnosis of M.S.. C.T. scanning may show large plaques as low density lesions which enhance, but NMR (MRI) scanning is probably better.

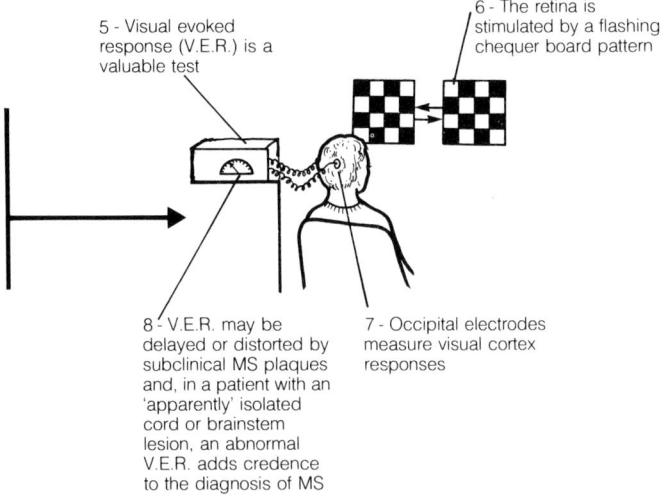

TREATMENT

A.C.T.H. gel 40 units b.d. for one week, tailing off to nothing, probably shortens the duration of the acute attack, but long courses of ACTH do not change the overall natural history of the disease and ACTH and corticosteroids are not indicated. Other forms of treatment are legion but none are of proven value; supportive measures, including physiotherapy, rehabilitation and occupational therapy are essential.

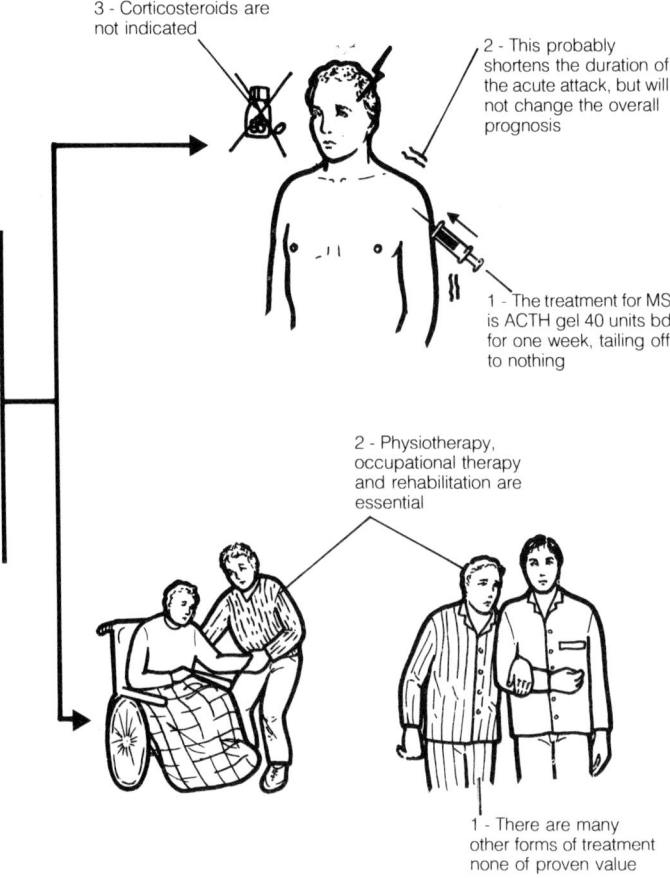

PROGNOSIS

Recovery from the initial attack may be expected, although often incomplete, but it is extremely difficult to prognosticate on the frequency and severity of future attacks/lesions. Nevertheless, long attack-free intervals are a good sign. Overall, 20-25% of patients will lead a long life with minor neurological impairment, 70% will have more severe disease not infrequently causing paralysis or other neurological features and thereby shortening life expectancy, whilst perhaps 10% will have a rapidly evolving aggressive and ultimately fatal disease.

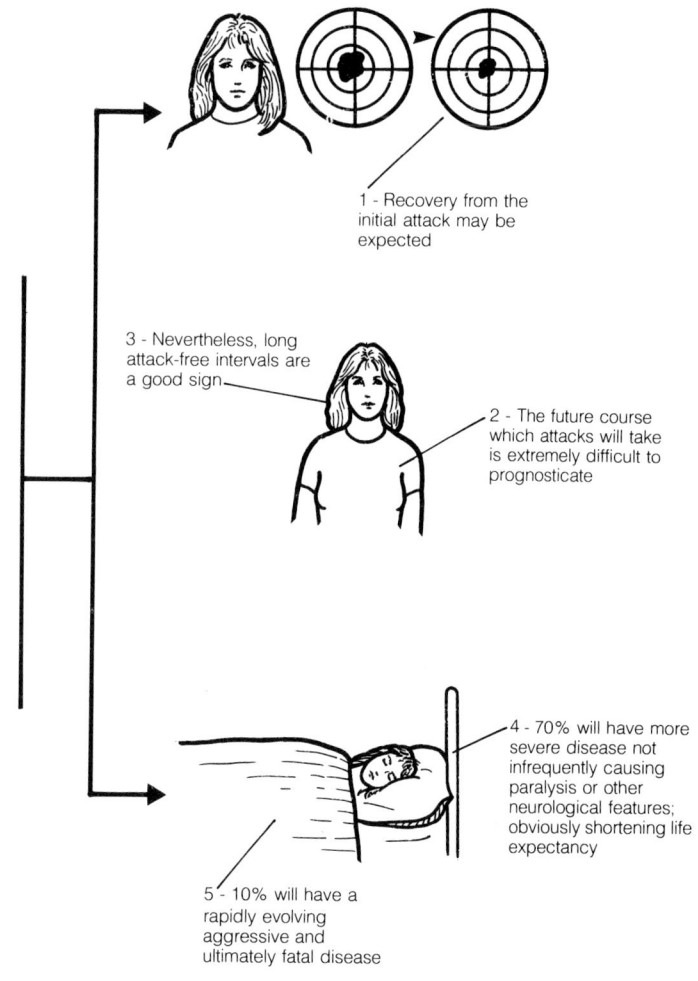

1 - Recovery from the initial attack may be expected

2 - The future course which attacks will take is extremely difficult to prognosticate

3 - Nevertheless, long attack-free intervals are a good sign

4 - 70% will have more severe disease not infrequently causing paralysis or other neurological features; obviously shortening life expectancy

5 - 10% will have a rapidly evolving aggressive and ultimately fatal disease

PARKINSONISM

Parkinsonism is a syndrome characterised by tremor, rigidity and hypokinesia, all stemming from a lesion in the basal ganglia. The commonest form of parkinsonism is the idiopathic variety (paralysis

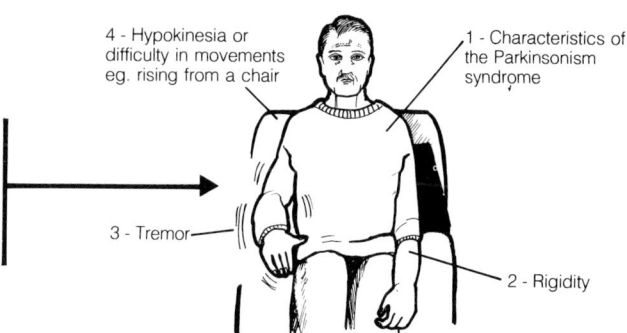

1 - Characteristics of the Parkinsonism syndrome
2 - Rigidity
3 - Tremor
4 - Hypokinesia or difficulty in movements eg. rising from a chair

agitans), where a degeneration of the basal ganglia occurs for unknown cause; this disease usually starts in middle age. Cerebrovascular disease may cause parkinsonism in the elderly as may various industrial poisons or heavy metals. Drug-induced parkinsonism (eg. as a side effect of phenothiazines) is an important iatrogenic cause in all types of parkinsonism. There is a deficiency in dopaminergic pathways in the basal ganglia. The following description is of paralysis agitans.

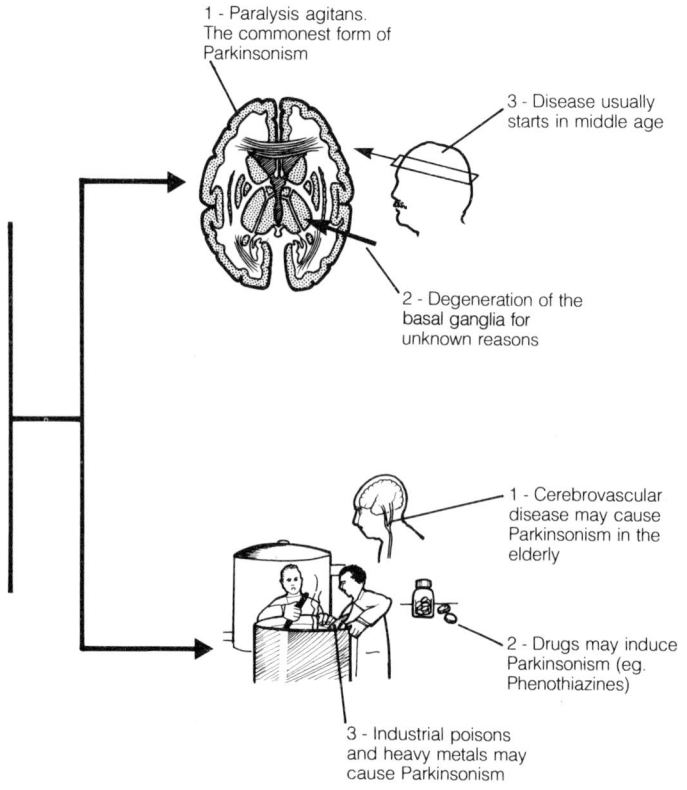

The typical parkinsonian tremor is a regular, rhythmical rest tremor at a rate of 4-8/sec, most marked in the distal muscle groups of the resting limb and exacerbated by emotion; the tremor disappears during a voluntary movement.

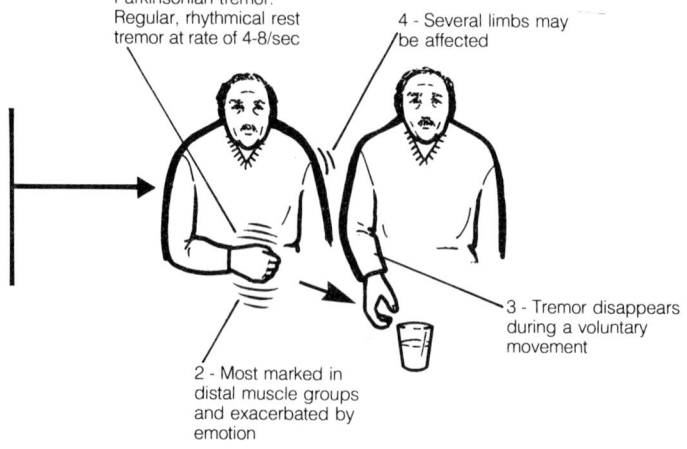

Parkinsonism

One or several limbs may be afflicted. On passive movements of the limb by the clinician, the extrapyramidal rigidity is present throughout the whole range of muscle movement, (c.f. UMN "clasp-knife" spasticity). Parkinsonian rigidity is enhanced by movement in the contralateral limb. It is the hypokinesia that is most disabling for the patient. The initiation of voluntary muscular movements is difficult and the execution of the movement is slow and laborious (eg. the cramped, little hand-writing or micrographia, and the monotonous and expressionless speech). There is a distinct poverty of automatic movements, (typical examples being the infrequency of blinking, the expressionless "mask-like" face and the absence of swinging of the arms when walking). A shuffling gait where the small footsteps and the "hurrying" to keep up with the body is called the 'festinant gait' of parkinsonism.

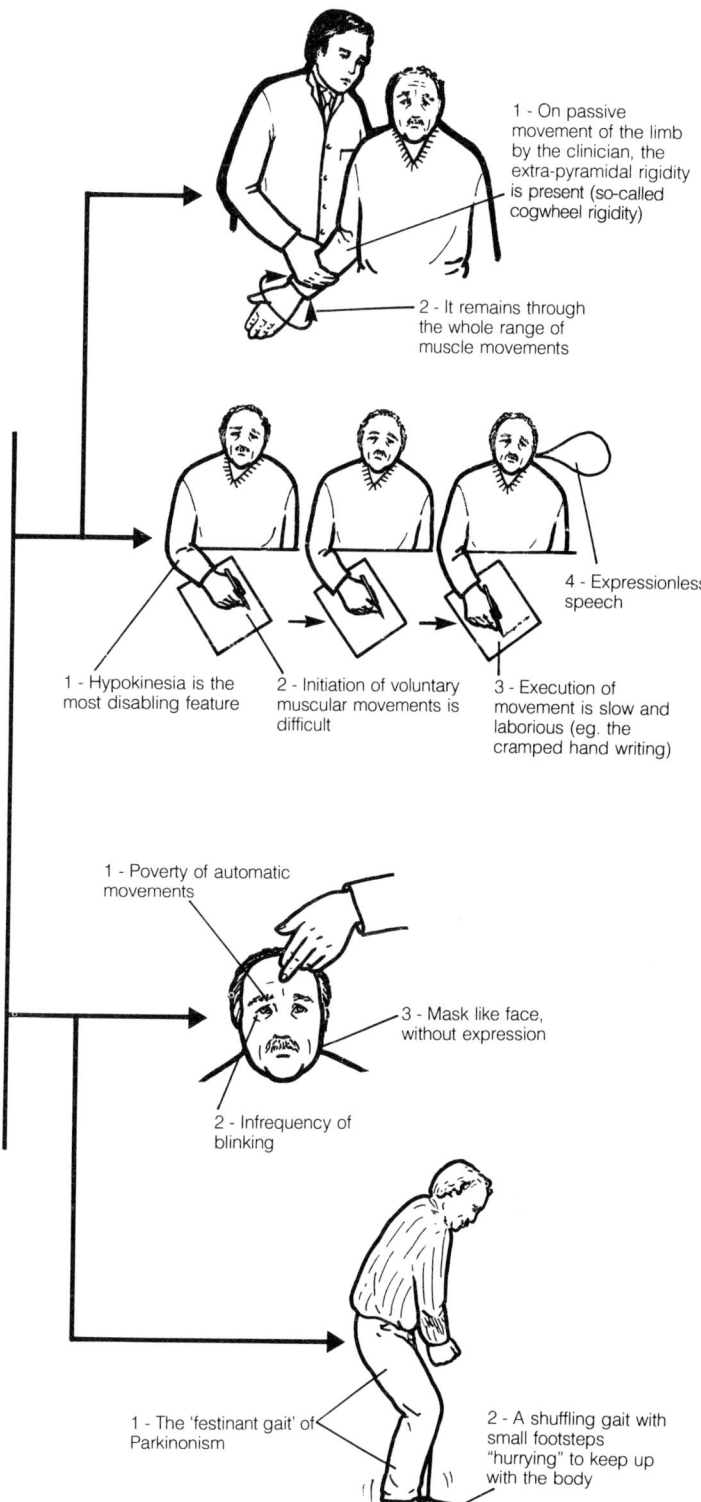

TREATMENT

Dopaminergic neuronal deficiency in the basal ganglia may be overcome by the oral administration of the dopamine precursor L-dopa. L-dopa gains access to the brain and raises dopamine levels. However, L-dopa is largely destroyed before it reaches the brain by the enzyme dopa decarboxylase, thus it is usual to prescribe L-dopa together with a decarboxylase inhibitor (eg. L-dopa 50-250mg with carbidopa 5-25mg taken tds and building up slowly from the lower dosages). The initial response to L-dopa preparations may be dramatic, in particular L-dopa reduces hypokinesia. However, in the long term, resistance to L-dopa may occur and increasing the dose may produce unwanted side effects such as involuntary movements. Indeed, L-dopa has many side effects, (particularly nausea, hypotension, palpitations, change in psyche, enhanced libido), but by starting in low dosage, most patients tolerate the drug well.

Researchers are now experimenting with the transplantation of cells from the adrenal gland into the area of the damaged basal ganglia. If this procedure produces enough dopamine, then the prognosis of Parkinsonism could be favourably changed.

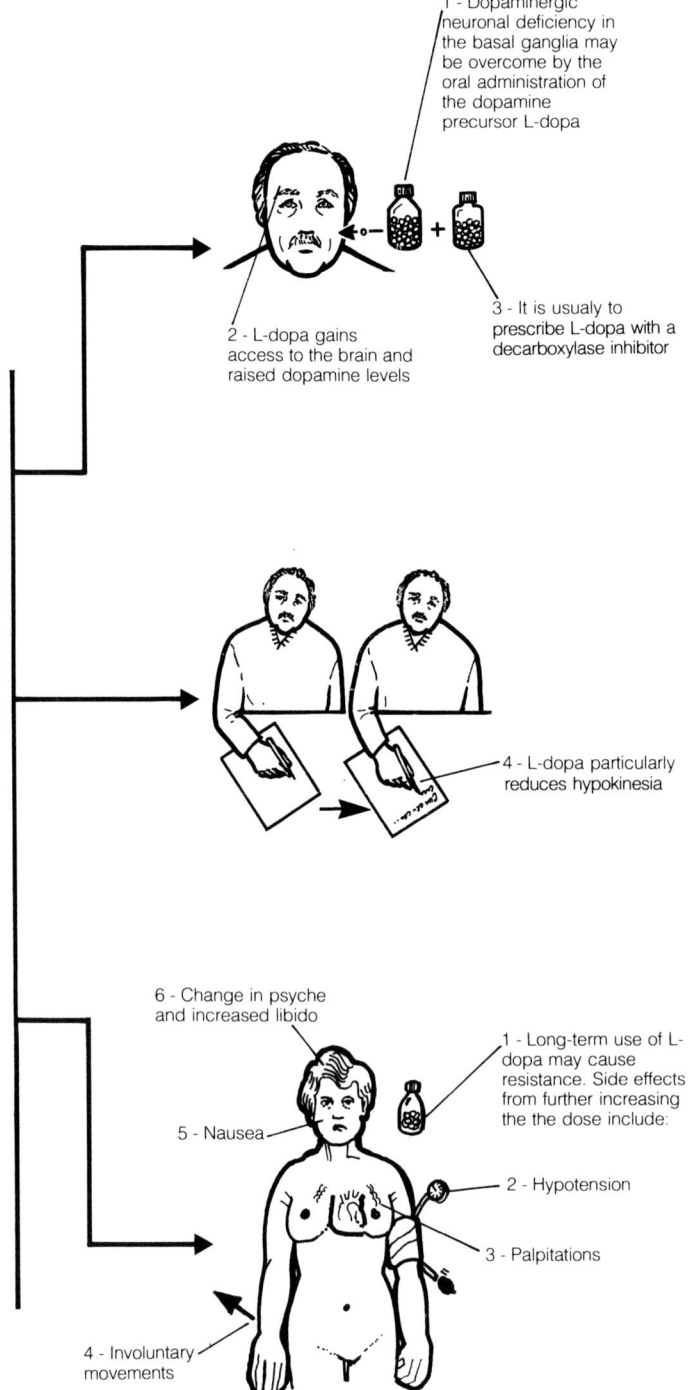

Anticholinergic drugs (eg. benzhexol 2mg tds-5mg tds) are useful either alone (particularly for rigidity and tremor) or they may be added to L-dopa preparations. Adverse effects may include confusion and hallucinations when the drugs are used in high doses, and all anticholinergics are contraindicated in glaucoma and prostatism. (L-dopa may also exacerbate glaucoma).

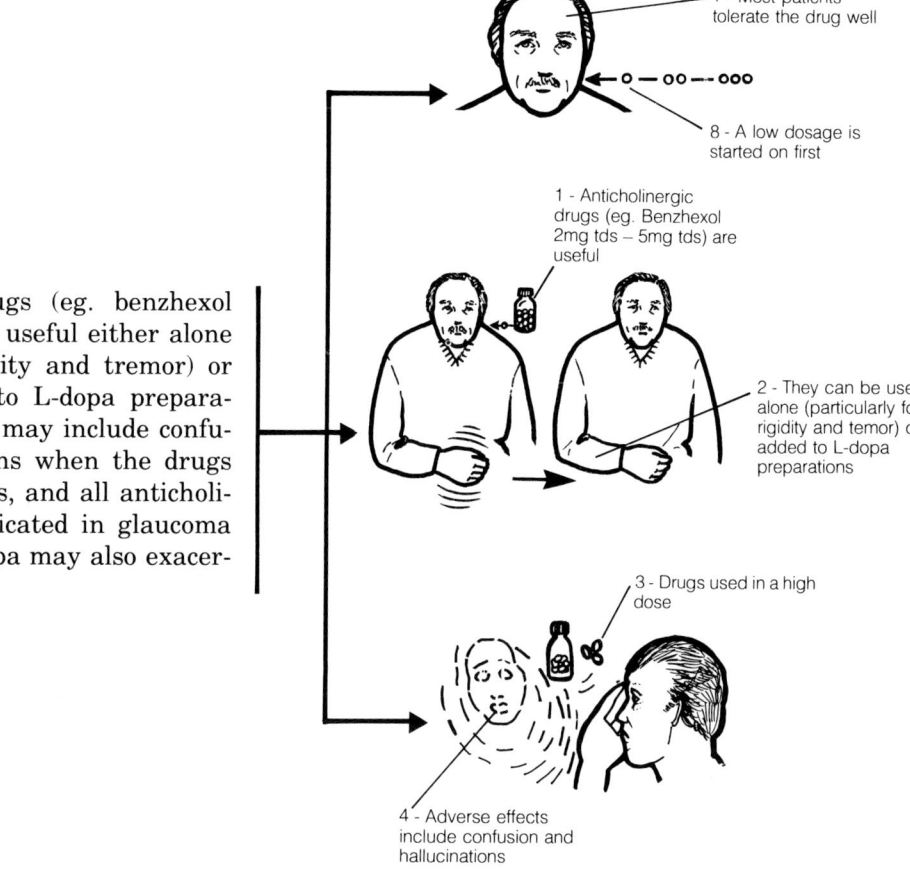

ABNORMAL MOVEMENT DISORDERS

A tremor is a rhythmical, sinusoidal movement, whereas chorea comprises a continuous flow of irregular and jerky movements that flit from one area of the body to another randomly.

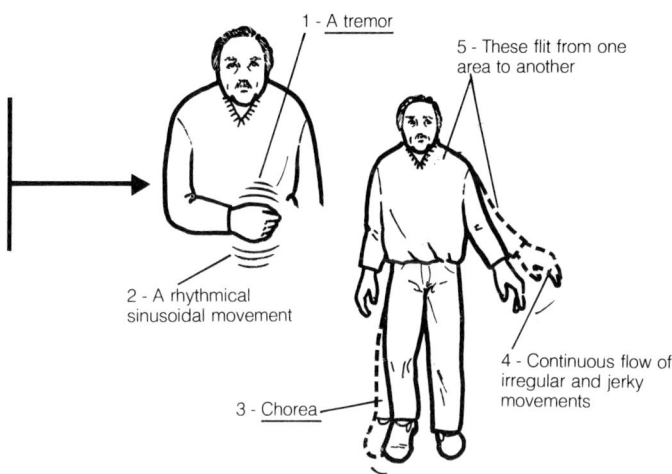

Abnormal Movement Disorders

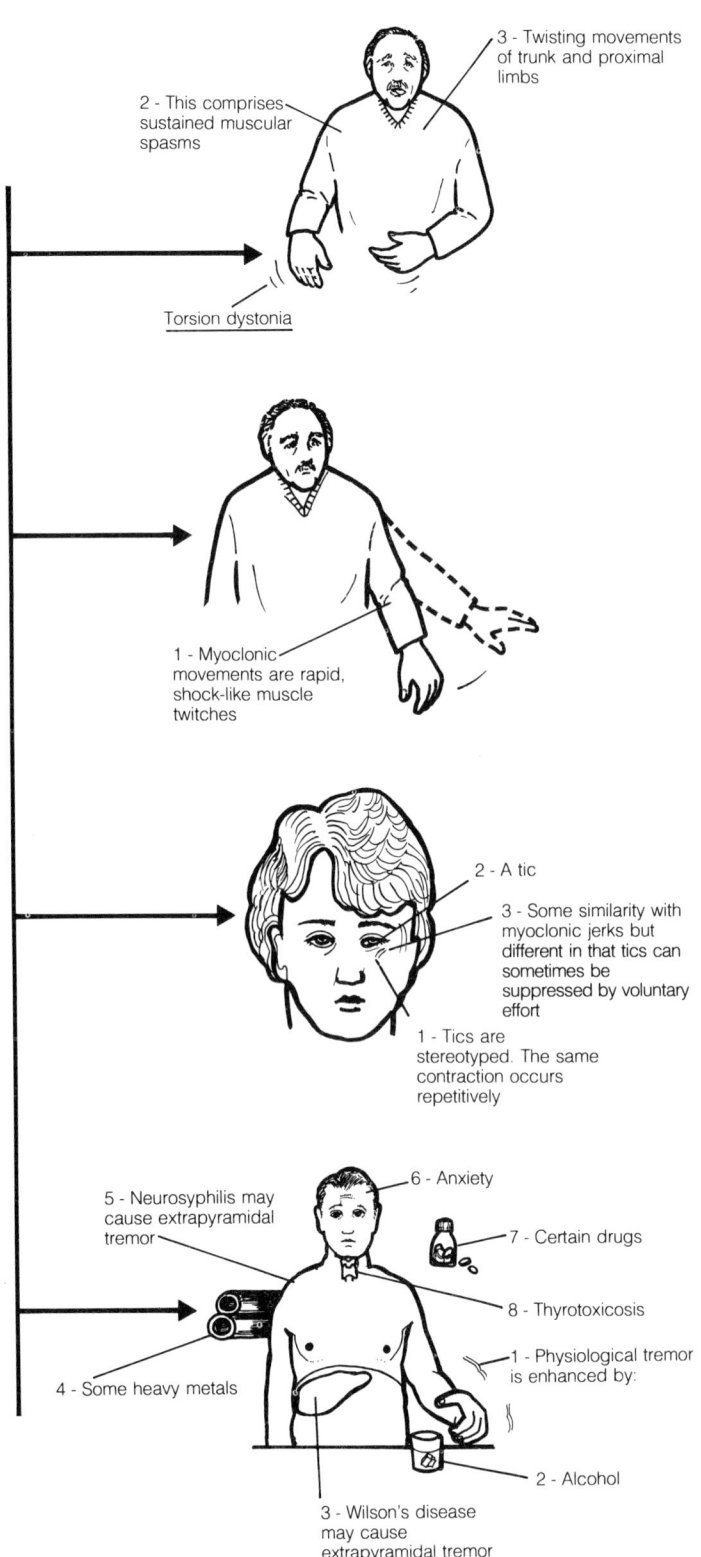

Torsion dystonia, (which includes athetosis), comprises sustained muscular spasms (eg. sustained twisting movements of the trunk or proximal limbs or the typical athetoid wavering contractions of the fingers or toes).

Myoclonic movements are rapid, shock-like muscle twitches. Tics have some similarities with myoclonic jerks but differ in that tics are sometimes suppressable by voluntary effort and are stereotyped, the same contraction occuring repetitively.

The rest tremor of parkinsonism and the intention tremor of cerebellar disease are well-known, as is the benign, essential familial tremor. Physiological tremor is enhanced in thyrotoxicosis and anxiety. Certain drugs, alcohol and some heavy metals may induce tremor. An extrapyramidal tremor may occur in neurosyphilis and **Wilson's disease**.

Abnormal Movement Disorders

Sydenham's chorea is now a rare disease and follows rheumatic fever in childhood. **Huntington's chorea** is a rare, autosomal dominant condition with the adult onset of chorea, progressive dementia and downhill clinical course progressing to death. C.T. scan shows caudate nuclear atrophy. Chorea may also occur following stroke, tumour, rarely during pregnancy or more commonly due to drugs (eg. phenothiazines). When a stroke causes chorea it is typically due to a contralateral subthalamic nuclear lesion which causes chorea (hemichorea or hemiballismus) of the contralateral side of the body. Tetrabenazine, anticholinergic drugs (eg. benztropine), diazepam, dantrolene, and other drugs may prove useful in abnormal movement disorders.

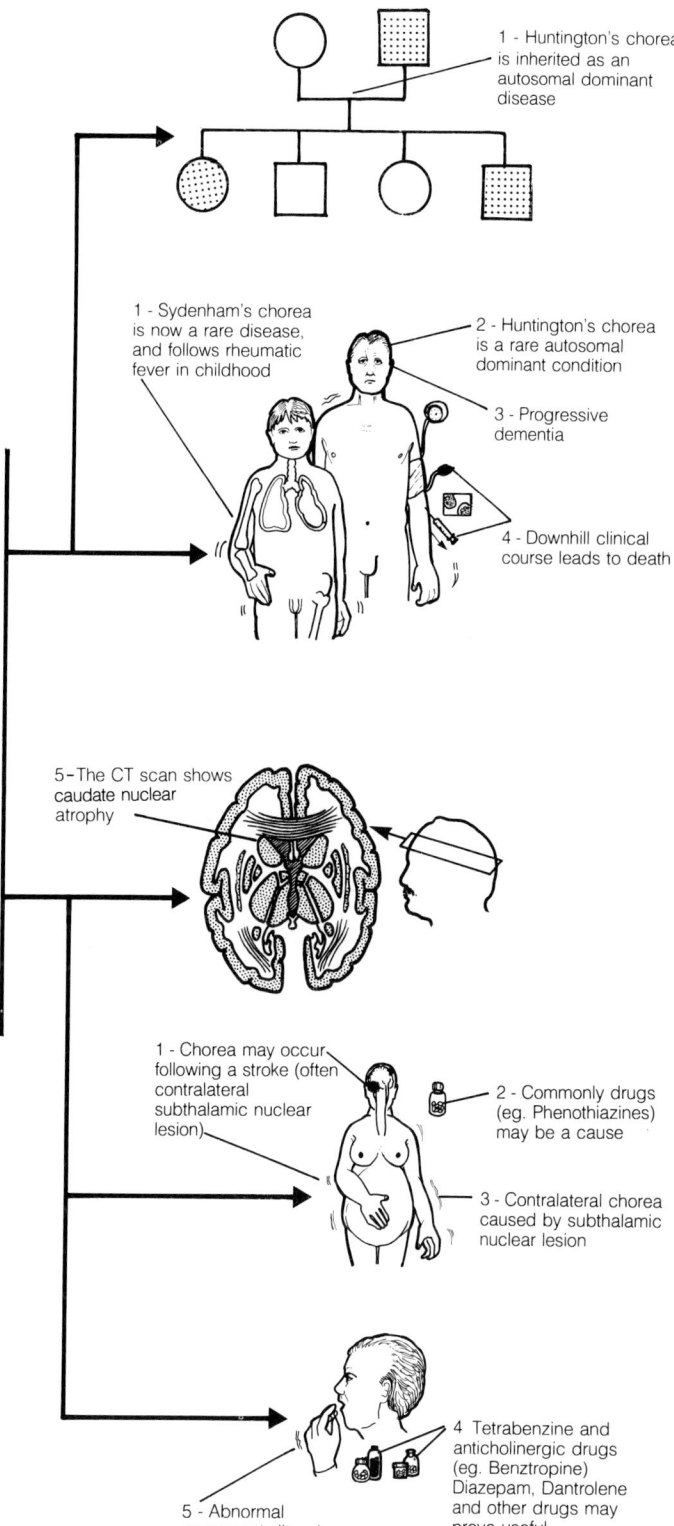

1 - Huntington's chorea is inherited as an autosomal dominant disease

1 - Sydenham's chorea is now a rare disease, and follows rheumatic fever in childhood

2 - Huntington's chorea is a rare autosomal dominant condition

3 - Progressive dementia

4 - Downhill clinical course leads to death

5 - The CT scan shows caudate nuclear atrophy

1 - Chorea may occur following a stroke (often contralateral subthalamic nuclear lesion)

2 - Commonly drugs (eg. Phenothiazines) may be a cause

3 - Contralateral chorea caused by subthalamic nuclear lesion

4 - Tetrabenzine and anticholinergic drugs (eg. Benztropine) Diazepam, Dantrolene and other drugs may prove useful

5 - Abnormal movement disorders

HEADACHE

Headache is one of the commonest symptoms bringing a patient to the doctor; more often than not there is no serious underlying cause and the headache may be no more than a pretext for reassurance. However, there are important organic causes for headaches and these must always be excluded. A careful history including psychological stresses is vital to the diagnosis and, in particular, enquiry as to when the headaches occur, where in the head, how bad they are, how long they last, any exacerbating factors and any associated features (eg. visual disturbances).

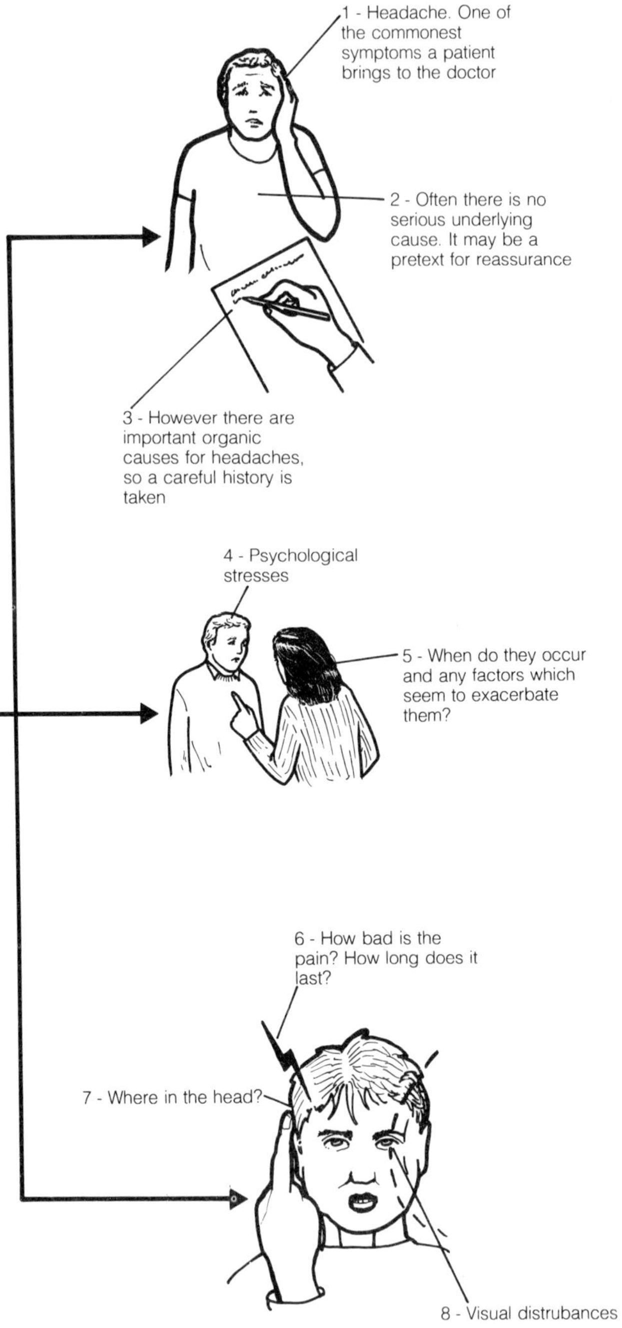

1 - Headache. One of the commonest symptoms a patient brings to the doctor

2 - Often there is no serious underlying cause. It may be a pretext for reassurance

3 - However there are important organic causes for headaches, so a careful history is taken

4 - Psychological stresses

5 - When do they occur and any factors which seem to exacerbate them?

6 - How bad is the pain? How long does it last?

7 - Where in the head?

8 - Visual distrubances

TENSION HEADACHE (PSYCHOGENIC HEADACHE)

Tension headache is very common and experienced by the majority of people at some time, especially at times of strife or severe stress. The headache is diffuse and often more like a pressure or tightness across the brow or vault. Analgesics, sedatives and tranquillisers are only of limited use. Tension headache with anxiety may be part of a mixed depressive illness and such cases are important to recognise. Enquiry should be made for the somatic accompaniments of depression – loss of appetite, weight and libido, together with disturbed sleep.

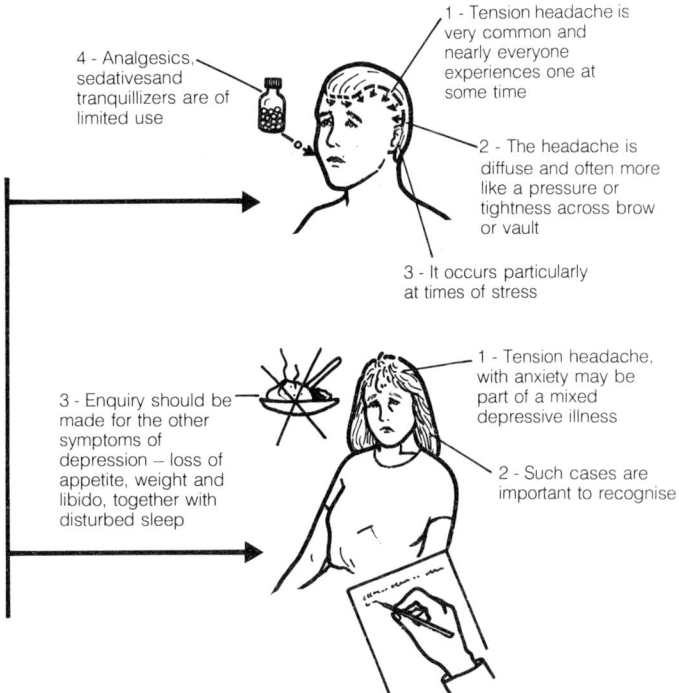

MIGRAINE

Migraine comprises recurrent paroxysmal headaches, lasting from a couple of hours to a couple of days and in the typical patient dating from an onset in adolescence. Heredity plays a role in the tendency to migraine and the condition is more common in those with obsessional personalities. The migraine attack often comes on, not during a period of concentration, but later when the patient is relaxing.

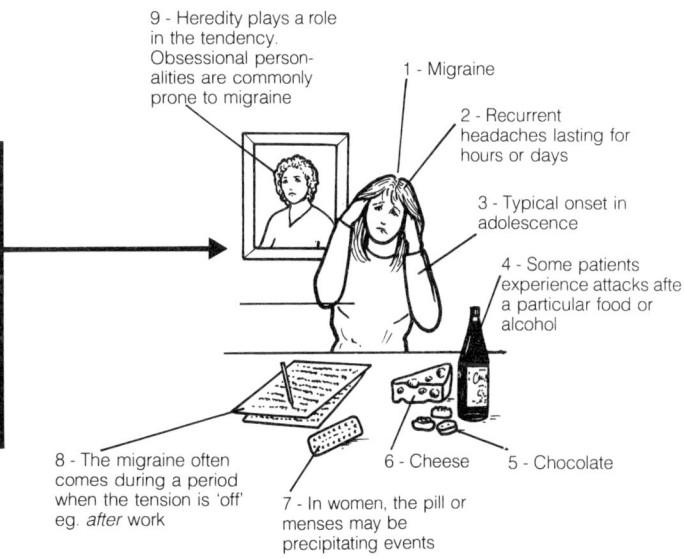

Migraine

Some patients experience attacks after a particular food (eg. chocolate, cheese, alcohol) and, in women, the attacks may be related to the menses (or the pill).

During a migraine attack, there is an initial phase of vasoconstriction causing symptoms due to local cortical or brainstem ischaemia (eg. the aura) and then there follows the period of vasodilation (of both intra- and extra-cranial arteries) with headache. An attack may commence with an aura (eg. visual aura such as flashing lights, zig-zag lines or wavy lines 'fortification phenomena', distorted images such as micropsia or macropsia or visual defects), or other focal signs (eg. peri-oral paraesthesiae, hemiparesis, dysphasia).

In the less common brainstem or basilar migraine, the initial period of vasoconstriction may be associated with diplopia, vertigo or even loss of consciousness. Fortunately, the vasoconstrictive phase is usually short (15-30 minutes) and gives way to a severe and throbbing

2 - Symptoms due to local cortical or brainstem ischaemia eg. aura

1 - The attack begins with an initial phase of vasoconstriction

3 - Then follows a period of vasodilation (both intra and extracranial arteries) with headache

1 - An attack may commence with an aura, such as flashing lights and zig zag lines

2 - Wavy lines (fortification phenomena) and distorted images

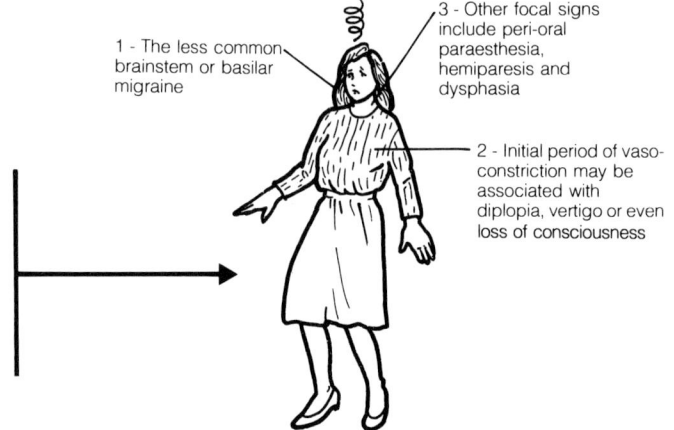

1 - The less common brainstem or basilar migraine

2 - Initial period of vasoconstriction may be associated with diplopia, vertigo or even loss of consciousness

3 - Other focal signs include peri-oral paraesthesia, hemiparesis and dysphasia

headache often unilateral fronto-temporal in site or over the whole of one side of the head (hemicrania). There may be associated vomiting, photophobia, sweating, pallor and prostration. The patient seeks a dark, quiet corner, preferably a bedroom. The headache commonly lasts 12 hours or more and leaves the patient exhausted.

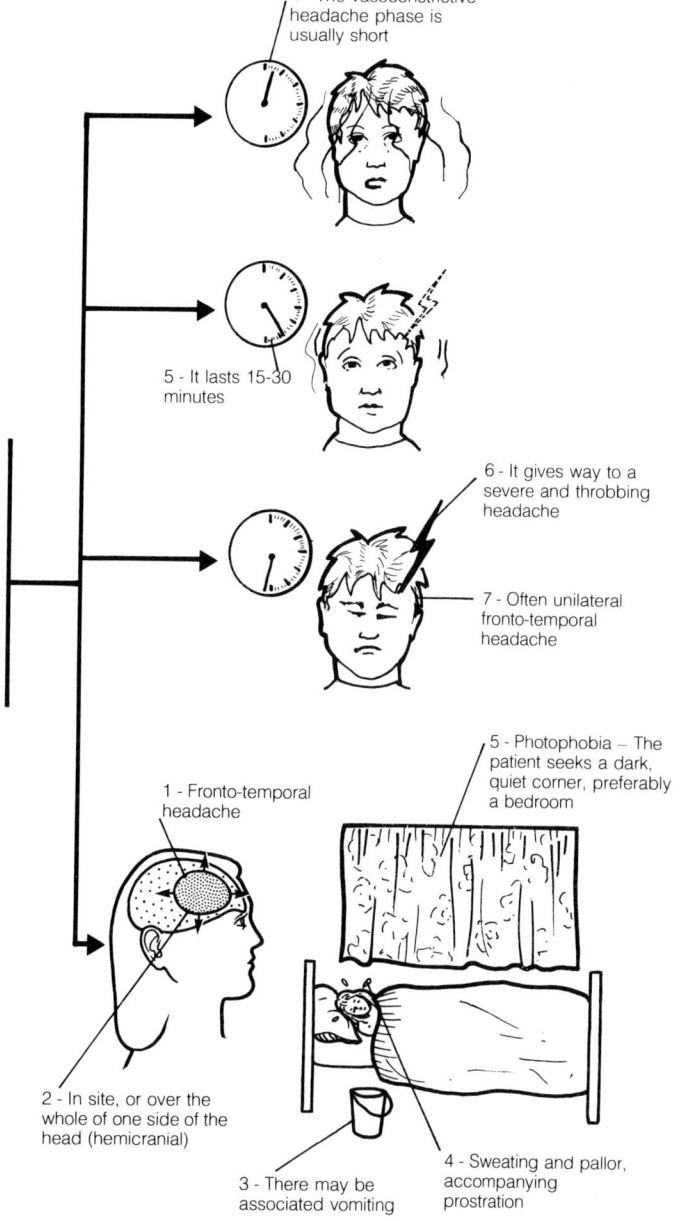

Migraine

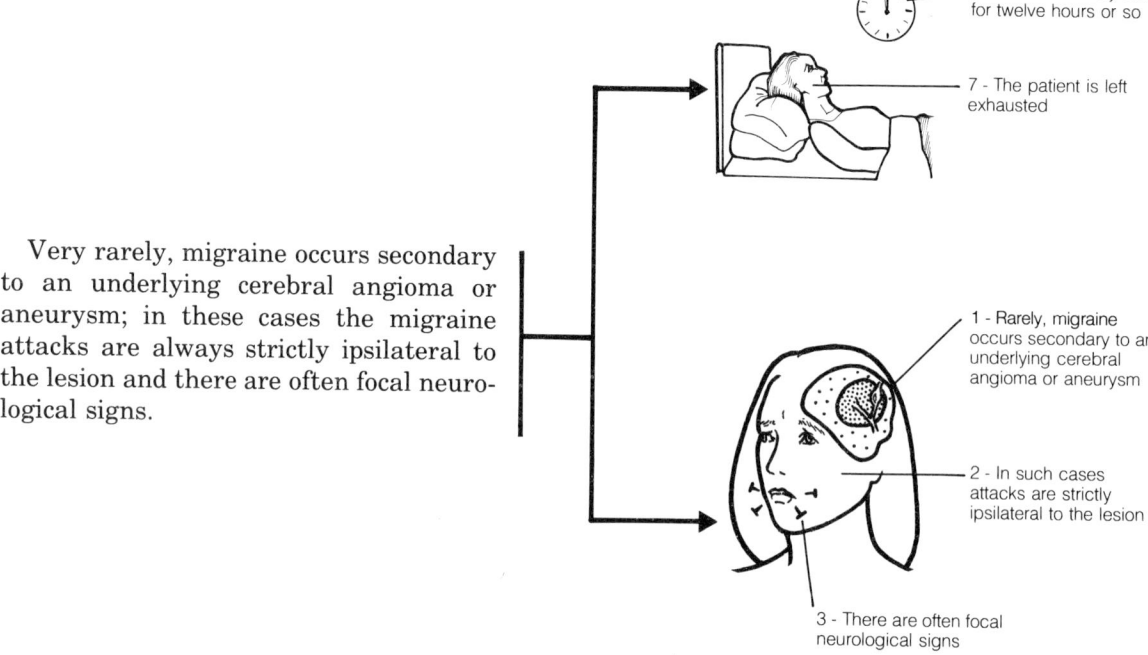

Very rarely, migraine occurs secondary to an underlying cerebral angioma or aneurysm; in these cases the migraine attacks are always strictly ipsilateral to the lesion and there are often focal neurological signs.

The secret of ameliorating an attack of migraine is early therapy with a simple analgesic such as aspirin together with a sedative anti-emetic (eg. phenergan). If the patient recognises from the prodroma that he is about to experience a severe attack, then a standard ergotamine preparation is to be recommended again, as early as possible after the onset of symptoms. Ergot derivatives have several pharmacological actions but their major role in the therapy of migraine is to cause vasoconstriction; ergotamine tartrate 0.25 - 0.50mg s.c. or i.m. is best repeated in 6 hours, (up to 1mg per 24 hours

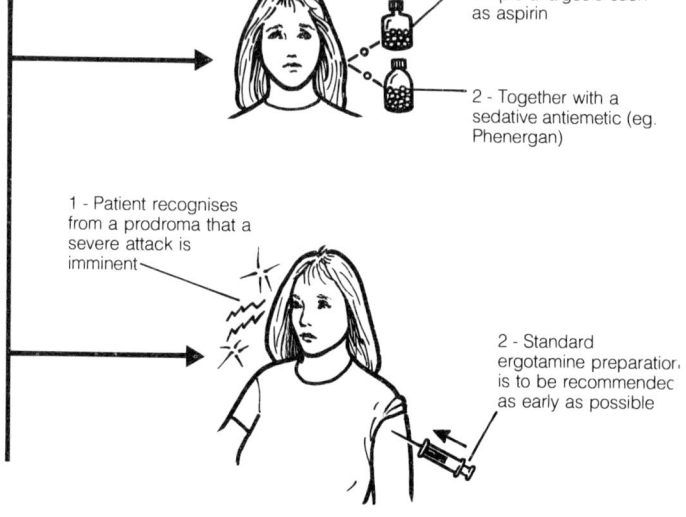

maximum). Oral preparations are useful but the absorption is more erratic, (possibly improved by the co-administration of caffeine). Ergotamine preparations are contraindicated in pregnancy, ischaemic heart disease, hypertension and peripheral vascular disease.

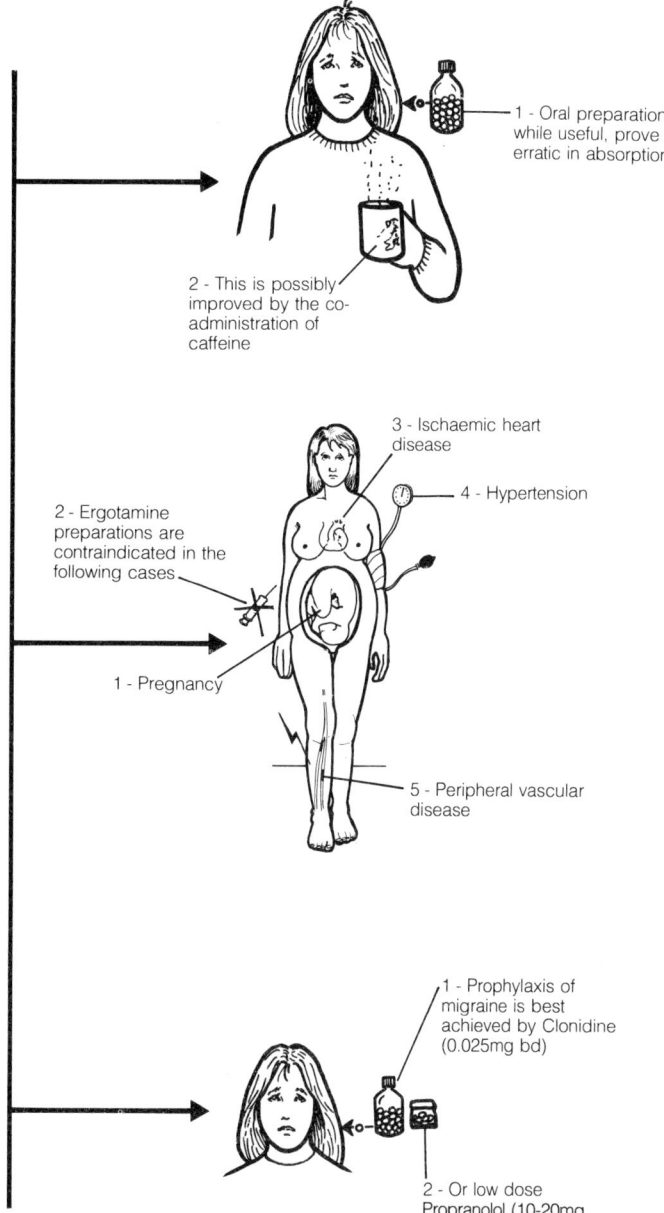

Prophylaxis of migraine is best achieved by clonidine (0.025mg b.d.) or low dose propranolol (10-20mg tds). Uncommonly low dosage methysergide is required, but this drug is known to precipitate retroperitoneal fibrosis if used in high dosage for long periods and it is not the drug of first choice. Obviously, the patient must avoid known precipitating factors.

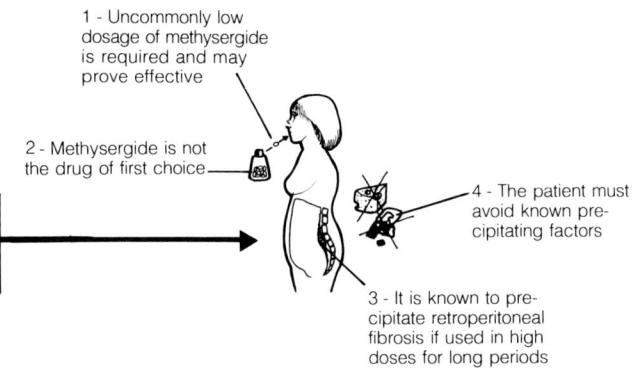

OTHER VASCULAR CAUSES OF HEADACHE

Headache is a symptom in hypertension, and in malignant hypertension the headache may be severe. In cerebrovascular disease, particularly affecting the vertebrobasilar vessels, headache may occur; cervical spondylosis often co-exists in this patient group, and this may exacerbate the headache. Arterial aneurysms are occasional causes of headache.

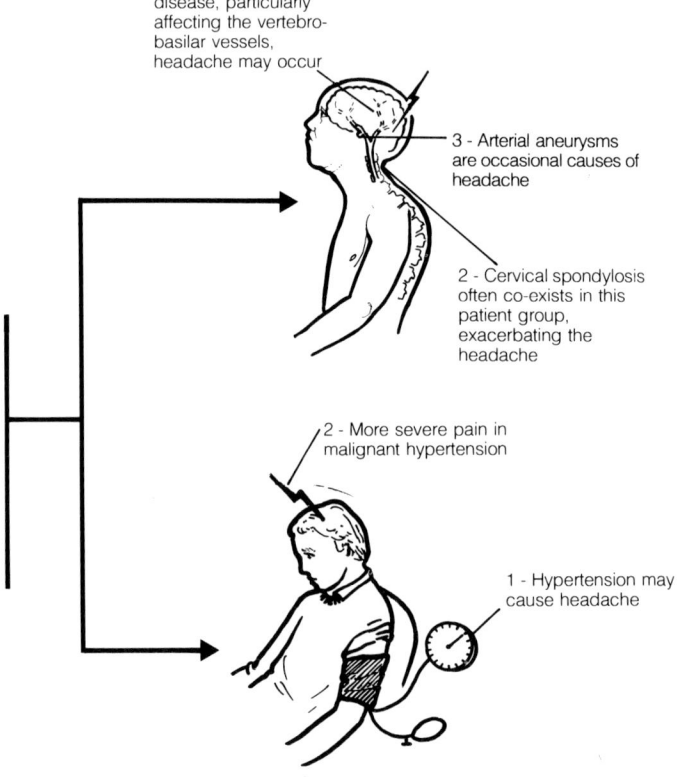

Other Vascular Causes of Headache

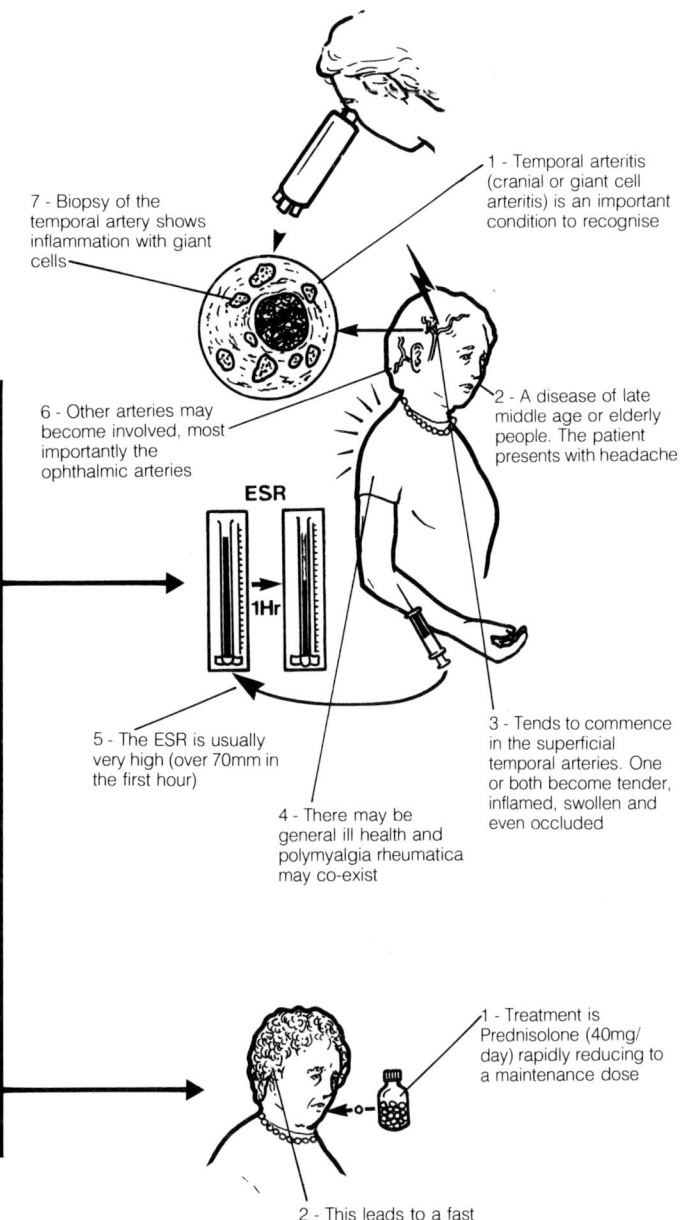

Temporal arteritis

(Cranial or giant cell arteritis), is an important condition to recognise. This is a disease of late middle age or of the elderly with a tendency to commence in the superficial temporal arteries. One or both arteries become swollen, tender, inflamed, and even occluded; the patient presents with headache often localised in that temple. There may be general ill-health and polymyalgia rheumatica may co-exist. The arteritis may spread to other arteries of which the ophthalmic arteries are often the most critical as blindness may result. The diagnosis of temporal arteritis must always be considered in an elderly patient with headache. The ESR is usually very high (over 70mm in first hour) and biopsy of the temporal artery shows inflammation with giant cells. **Treatment** with prednisolone (40mg/day) rapidly reducing to a maintenance dose leads to fast regression of symptoms and the steroids may often be stopped completely after a while, using the ESR to assess disease activity at follow-up.

HEADACHE DUE TO RAISED INTRACRANIAL PRESSURE

Headache due to raised I.C.P. is of varying severity, occurs particularly on waking in the morning, is aggravated by coughing, sneezing and straining and is often accompanied by vomiting. The physical examination will usually show papilloedema and leads to investigations as detailed under 'brain tumours'.

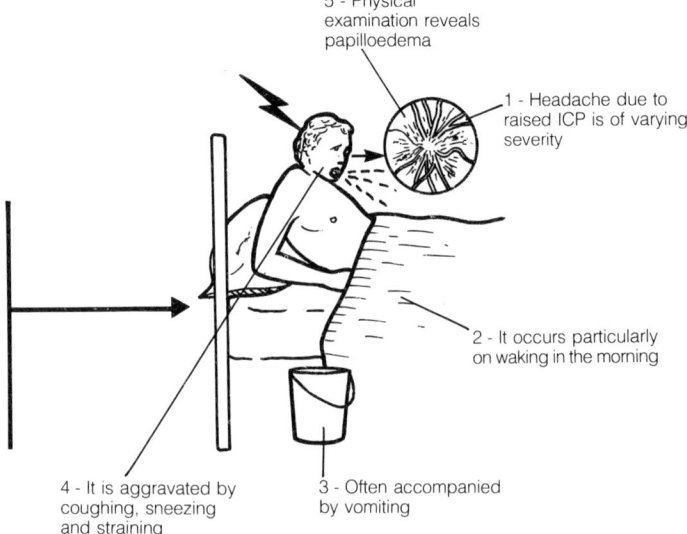

OTHER CAUSES OF HEADACHE

Trauma to the skull and referred pain from other structures in the head (eg. dental pain, sinus pain, middle ear pain, temporomandibular joint pain, ocular pain, herpetic pain particularly in the pre-eruptive phase – especially V and VII – are all cause of 'headaches'. Other occasional causes include cervical spondylosis and Paget's disease of skull with nerve entrapment. Trigeminal neuralgia ought to be easily distinguishable from 'headache'.

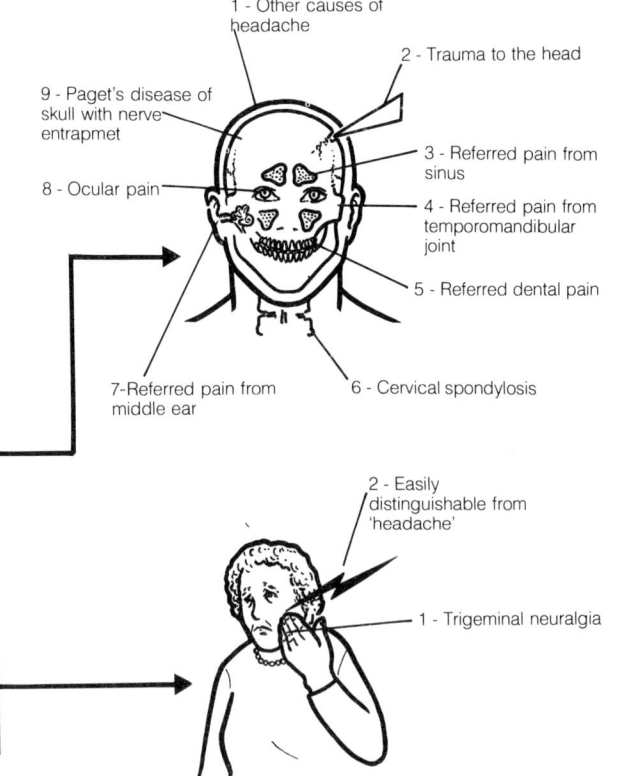

COMA

Consciousness depends upon the normal functioning of the cerebral cortex and reticular-activating formation in the brain stem. With slightly disturbed integrity of function there is obtundation in which the patient is less alert than normal, more easily distracted, unable to think rapidly, has short attention span and tends to slump into apathetic slumber. With greater degress of impairment the patient becomes progressively more difficult to arouse.

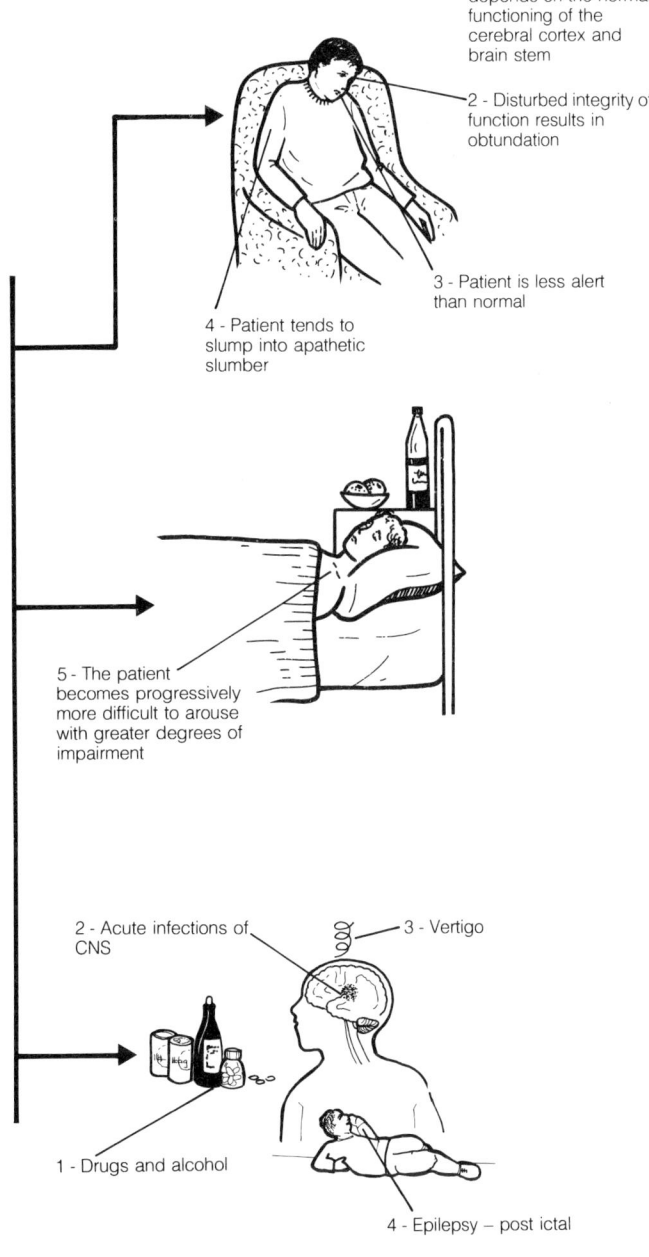

There is an important list of causes of coma which may be best remembered as DAVE PIMAH's:-

Coma

Drugs – eg. barbiturates overdose or other sedatives, alcohol, aspirin, other poisons.
Acute infections of CNS – meningitis, encephalitis, abscess.
Vascular – subarachnoid haemorrhage, 'stroke', syncope, hypertensive encephalopathy.
Epilepsy – post-ictal
Pressure – tumours, extradural and subdural haemorrhages.
Injury – depressed fracture of skull or fracture of base of skull.*
Metabolic – hyper- or hypoglycaemia, uraemia, cholaemia. Addison's disease, myxoedema, pituitary apoplexy, inappropriate ADH secretion etc.
Acute generalised infections – septicaemia, malaria.
H's – Hysteria, Hyperthermia, Hypothermia.

*All cases of head trauma with loss of consciousness merit skull X-rays and 24 hours' observation in hospital.

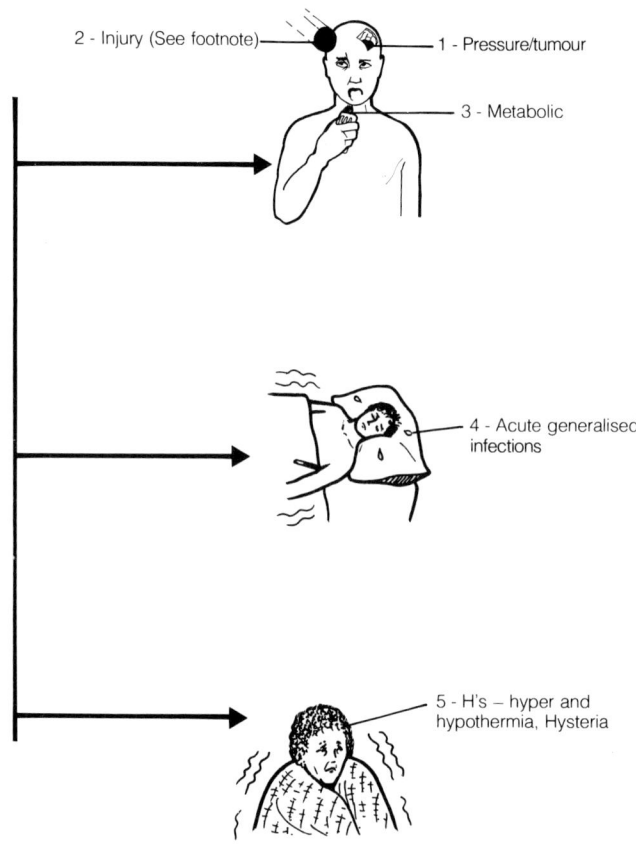

A good history from witnesses, from past medical details etc, followed by a careful examination of the patient often leads to a diagnosis, and the investigations will differ with the individual case. The

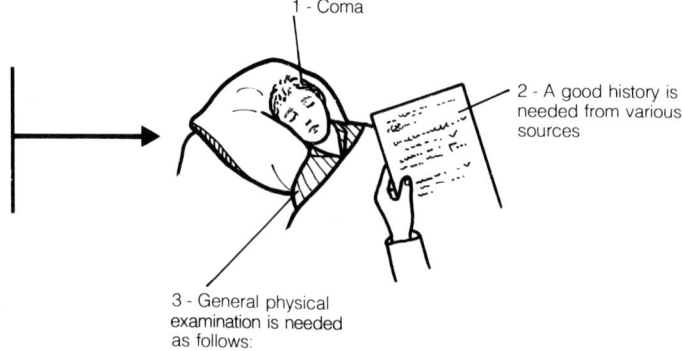

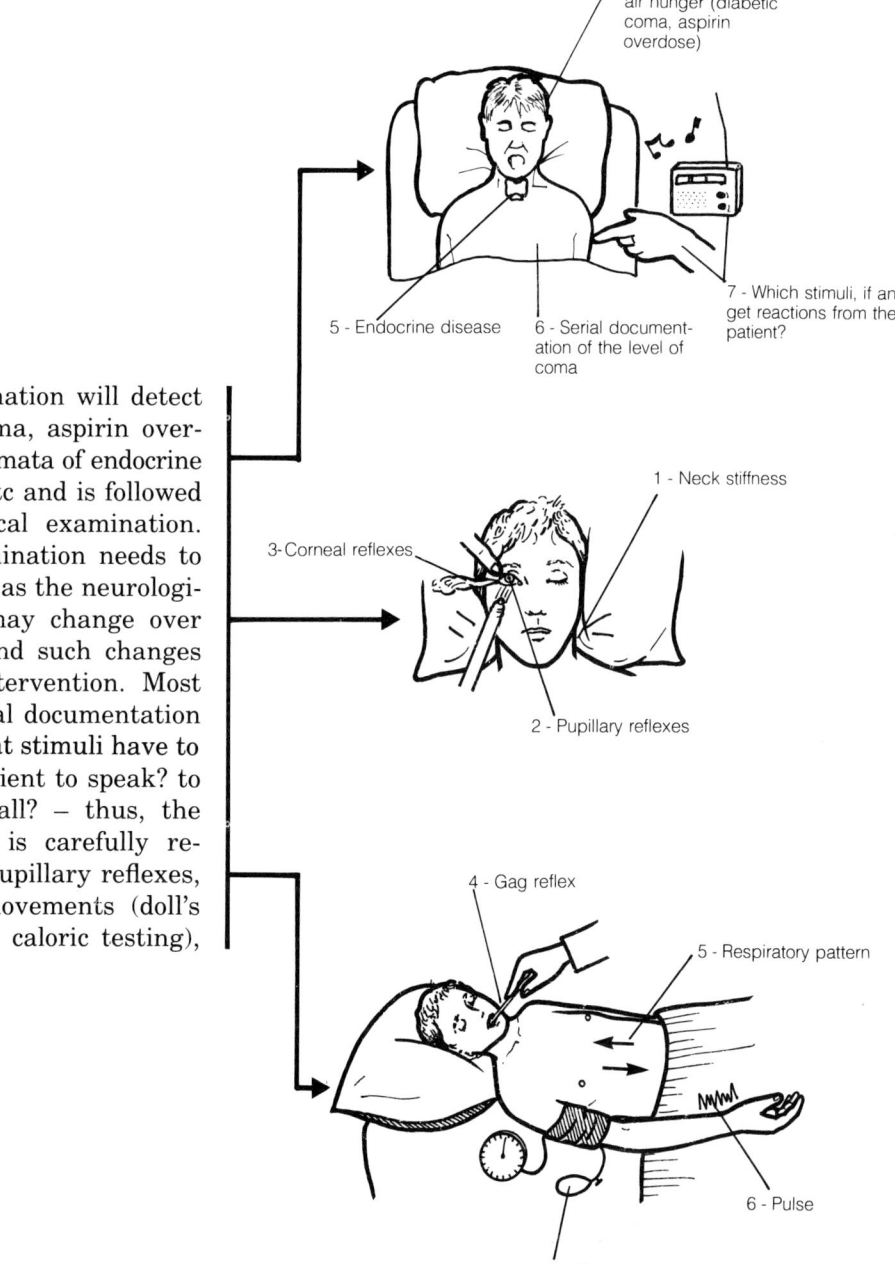

general physical examination will detect air hunger (diabetic coma, aspirin overdosage), the physical stigmata of endocrine disease, hypertension, etc and is followed by a careful neurological examination. Furthermore, this examination needs to be repeated many times as the neurological (and other signs) may change over short periods of time and such changes may demand active intervention. Most critical of all is the serial documentation of the level of coma. What stimuli have to be used to rouse the patient to speak? to flinch? or to react at all? – thus, the patient's responsivenes is carefully recorded. Neck stiffness, pupillary reflexes, corneal reflexes, eye movements (doll's head manoeuvre and to caloric testing), gag reflex, respiratory pattern, pulse and blood pressure together with limb tone and the withdrawal of each of the four limbs to noxious stimuli are serially monitored. Fundoscopy, particularly for papilloedema (but also looking for other diagnostic clues – eg. choroidal tubercles, subhyaloid haemorrhage etc) is important.

When the physical signs suggest intact brainstem pathways then diffuse brain disease or metabolic or toxic causes of coma are likely. If there is evidence of brainstem dysfunction, is this due to primary brainstem lesion (eg. infarction)?, or is it due to mechanical pressure as in a pressure cone? – (see the sections: "The Pupil" and "Extradural haemorrhage") requiring an urgent neurosurgical opinion. Again, investigations depend on the clinical situation but radiological imaging is usually appropriate and an EEG may help to establish cortical pathology.

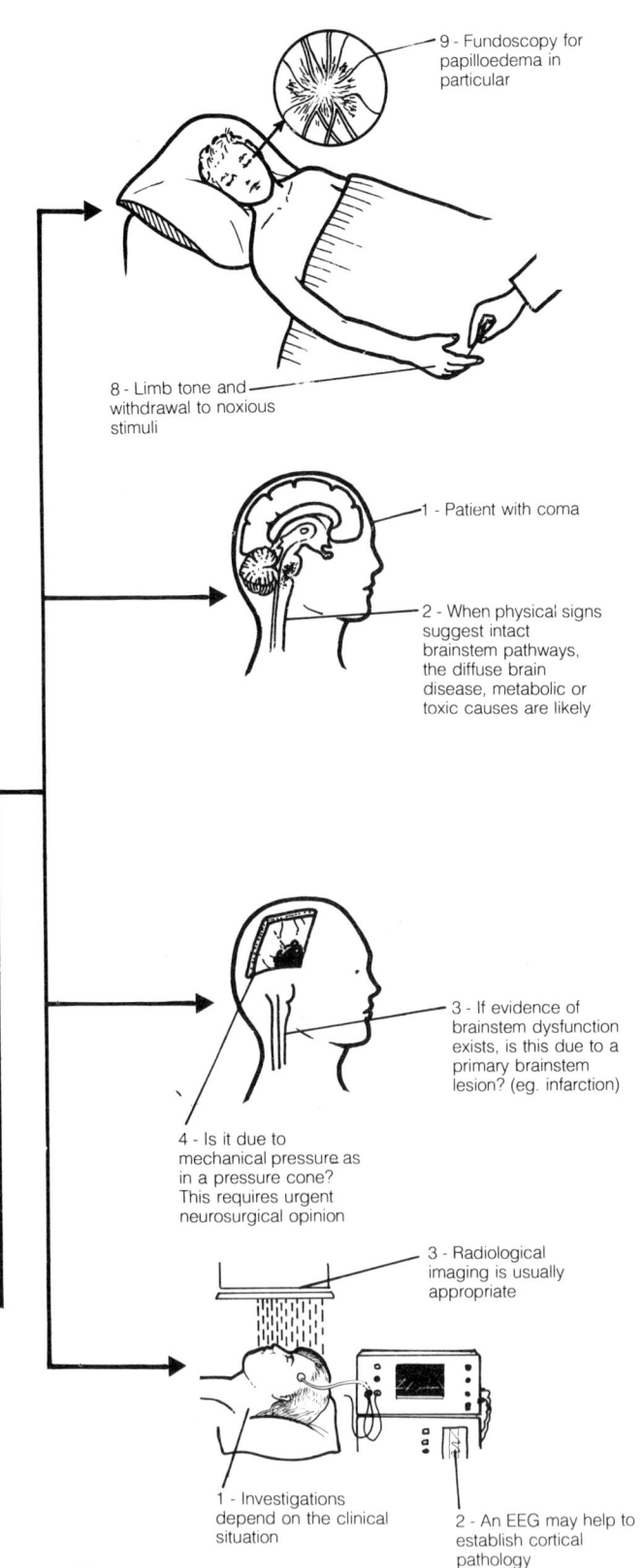

BRAIN DEATH

The United Kingdom directives on brain death (which are particularly necessary for clinicians treating comatose patients maintained by artificial ventilation), are clear, (statement by United Kingdom Medical Royal Colleges 1976): For brain death, the patient is deeply unconscious not due to metabolic or drug induced causes and there is no doubt that the patient's condition is due to irremediable structural brain damage. Spontaneous respiration is inadequate for survival and all brainstem reflexes should be absent.

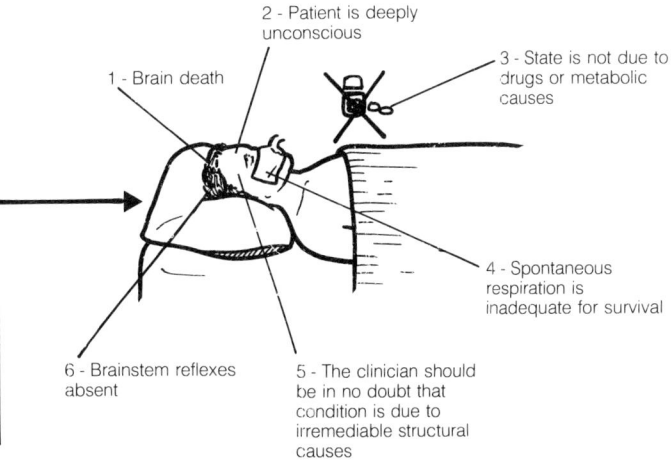

1 - Brain death
2 - Patient is deeply unconscious
3 - State is not due to drugs or metabolic causes
4 - Spontaneous respiration is inadequate for survival
5 - The clinician should be in no doubt that condition is due to irremediable structural causes
6 - Brainstem reflexes absent

SYRINGOMYELIA

Syringomyelia is characterised by dilatations or outpouchings (even rupture) of the central canal of the spinal cord, which most commonly occurs in the lower cervical region, but the dilatation may elongate and extend upwards to involve the medulla oblongata (syringobulbia). There are

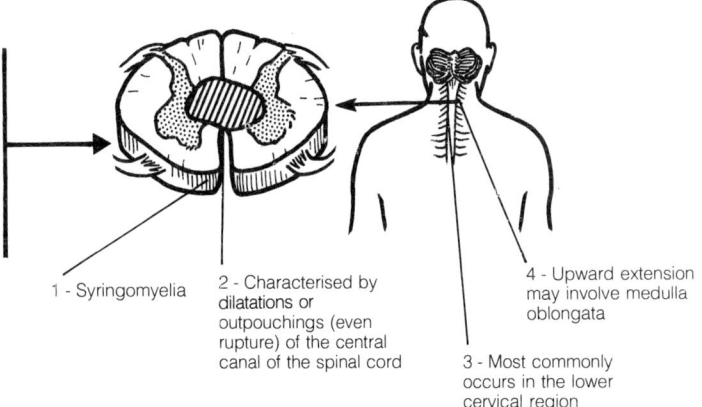

1 - Syringomyelia
2 - Characterised by dilatations or outpouchings (even rupture) of the central canal of the spinal cord
3 - Most commonly occurs in the lower cervical region
4 - Upward extension may involve medulla oblongata

Syringomyelia

many theories as the the exact mechanism that leads to the dilatation of the central canal but secondary pressure effects from an abnormal drainage of CSF from the IVth ventricle may be the underlying fault. Indeed, in many cases of syringomyelia there is a developmental abnormality in the region of the IVth ventricle (eg. the malformation of the foramina of Luschka and Magendie – the **Dandy-Walker malformation**, eg. the protrusion of the cerebellar tonsils through the foramen magnum – the **Arnold-Chiari malformation**, eg. the coexistence of cerebellar ectopia and skeletal defects such as atlanto-occipital fusion and basilar impression – **Klippel-Feil deformity**). Kyphoscoliosis is also a recognised association.

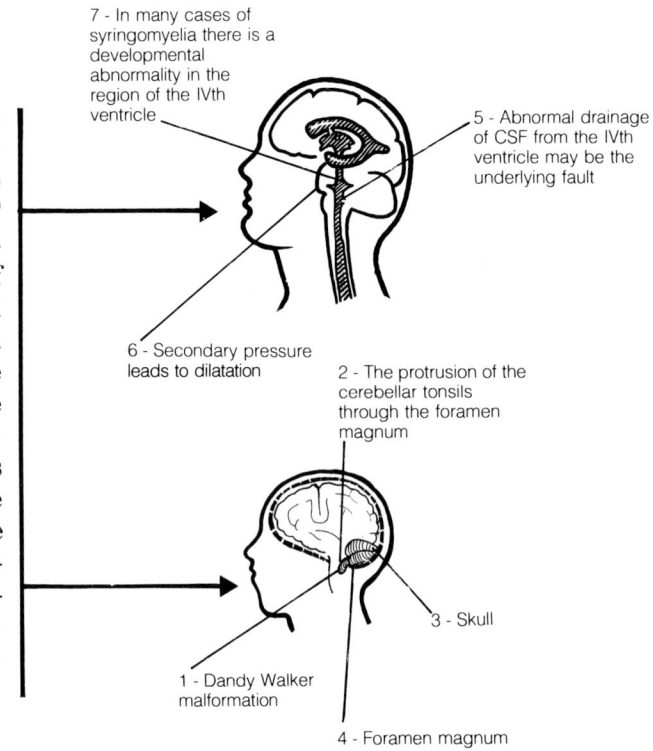

7 - In many cases of syringomyelia there is a developmental abnormality in the region of the IVth ventricle

5 - Abnormal drainage of CSF from the IVth ventricle may be the underlying fault

6 - Secondary pressure leads to dilatation

2 - The protrusion of the cerebellar tonsils through the foramen magnum

3 - Skull

1 - Dandy Walker malformation

4 - Foramen magnum

Dilatation of the spinal canal first impinges on decussating pain and temperature bearing sensory fibres that are crossing to reach the opposite lateral spinothalamic tract. As the dilatation (syrinx) most commonly occurs in the lower cervical region, this leads to absent pain and temperature sensation in the arm, hands and fingers. Next, the syrinx impinges on the anterior horn cells leading to a LMN lesion and the loss of tendon reflexes at that spinal level. The sensory modalities conveyed in the dorsal columns, (light, touch, proprioception) are preserved until late, thus clinicians refer to "dissociated sensory loss" in syringomyelia (ie. only affecting pain and temperature sense).

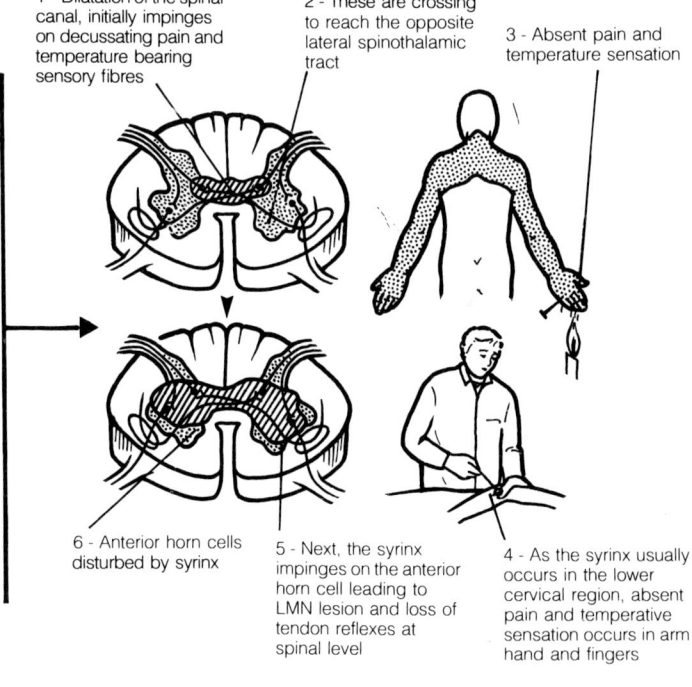

1 - Dilatation of the spinal canal, initially impinges on decussating pain and temperature bearing sensory fibres

2 - These are crossing to reach the opposite lateral spinothalamic tract

3 - Absent pain and temperature sensation

6 - Anterior horn cells disturbed by syrinx

5 - Next, the syrinx impinges on the anterior horn cell leading to LMN lesion and loss of tendon reflexes at spinal level

4 - As the syrinx usually occurs in the lower cervical region, absent pain and temperture sensation occurs in arm hand and fingers

Syringomyelia

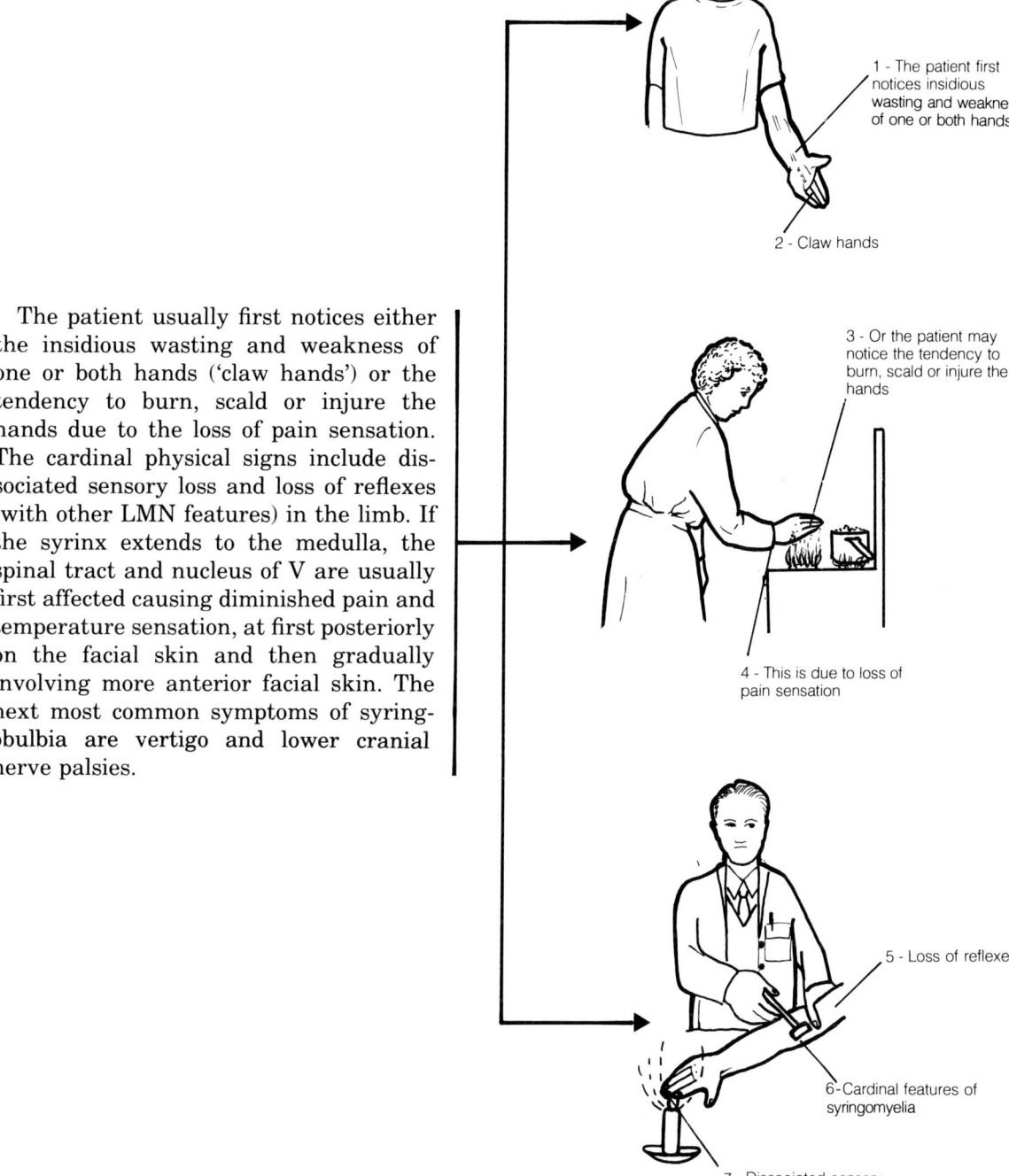

1 - The patient first notices insidious wasting and weakness of one or both hands

2 - Claw hands

3 - Or the patient may notice the tendency to burn, scald or injure the hands

4 - This is due to loss of pain sensation

5 - Loss of reflexes

6 - Cardinal features of syringomyelia

7 - Dissociated sensory loss in the limb

The patient usually first notices either the insidious wasting and weakness of one or both hands ('claw hands') or the tendency to burn, scald or injure the hands due to the loss of pain sensation. The cardinal physical signs include dissociated sensory loss and loss of reflexes (with other LMN features) in the limb. If the syrinx extends to the medulla, the spinal tract and nucleus of V are usually first affected causing diminished pain and temperature sensation, at first posteriorly on the facial skin and then gradually involving more anterior facial skin. The next most common symptoms of syringobulbia are vertigo and lower cranial nerve palsies.

Syringomyelia

Plain X-rays may diagnose skeletal abnormalities (eg. **Klippel-Feil** deformity) and myelography may be helpful. Other diagnoses include cervical rib, cervical spondylosis, peripheral neuropathy, spinal cord tumour – all of which may give rise to diagnostic confusion.

If a causative congenital lesion is discovered, surgical decompression of the IVth ventricle may be indicated.

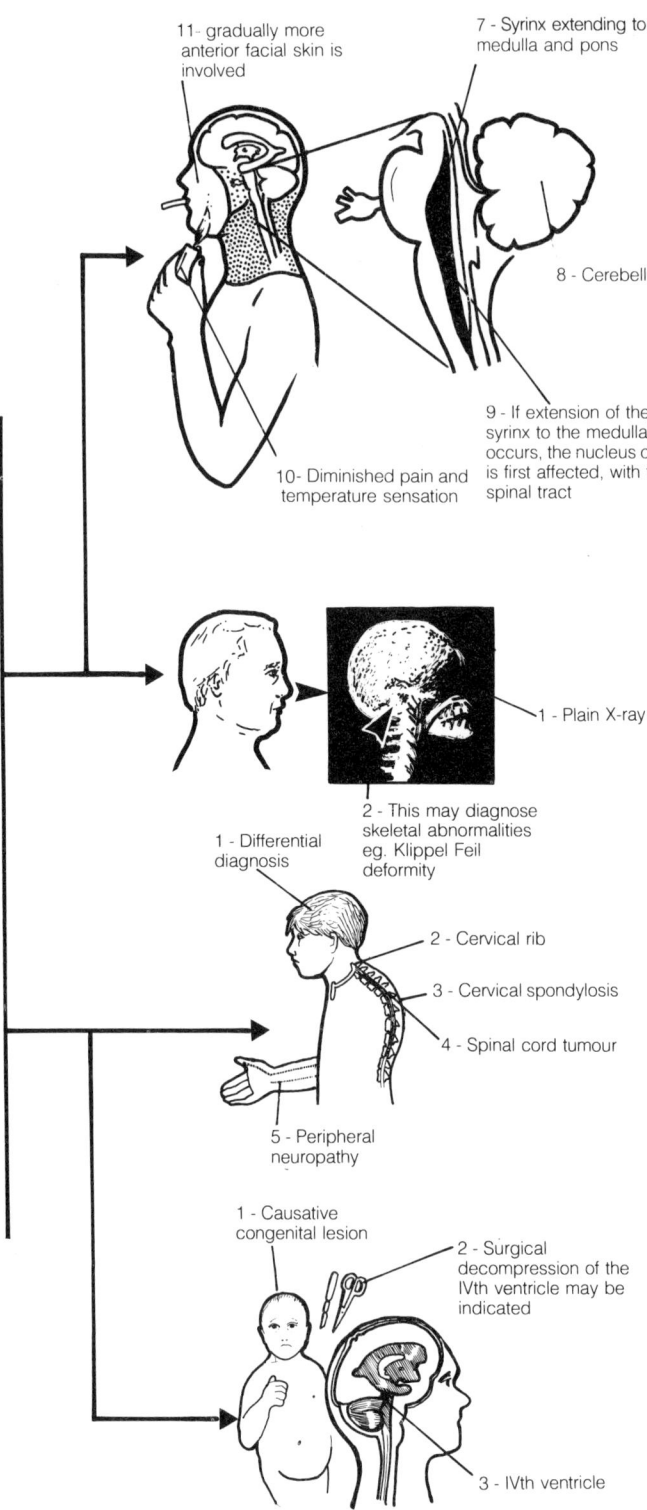

MOTOR NEURONE DISEASE

This rare disease of unknown aetiology is uncommon before middle age and most commonly presents in the fifth to sixth decade of life, being more frequent in men. There is a progressive degeneration of the anterior horn cells, the motor nuclei in the medulla and the upper motor neurones in the spinal cord and the brainstem; there are never any sensory features, (except occasional cramps in affected muscles).

In the clinical presentation termed '**progressive bulbar palsy**', there is slowly progressive wasting of the musculature of the tongue, palate and pharynx with dysphagia and slow dysarthria; the wasted, fibrillating tongue is the most noticeable clinical feature. In **Progressive muscular atrophy**, there is usually wasting, (not necessarily but frequently symmetrical, of the small hand muscles resulting in claw hand(s). The wasting spreads proximally up the arm and, following muscular exercises, (or percussion of the muscles with a tendon hammer), fasciculation of the muscles is usually demonstrable. Uncommonly, the lower limb is affected.

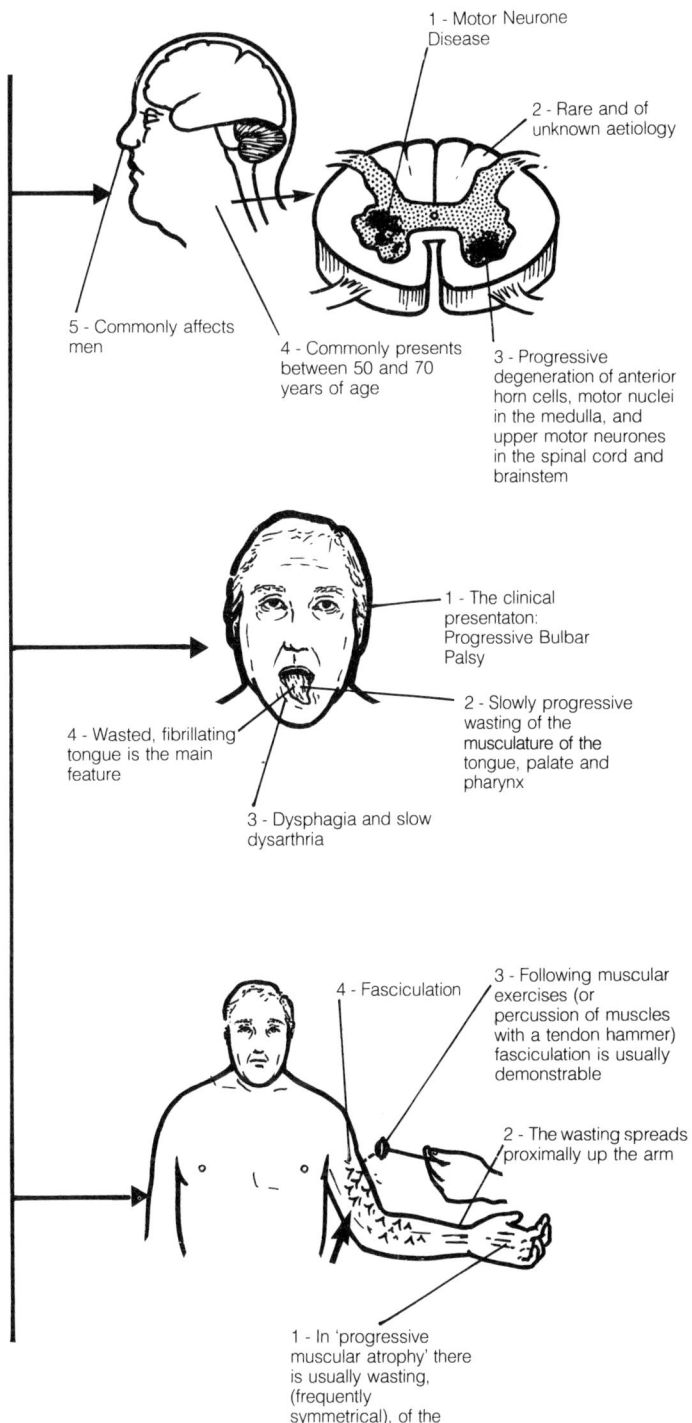

Motor Neurone Disease

In **amyotrophic lateral sclerosis**, there is degeneration of the upper motor neurone and spasticity (UMN lesion) results, perhaps in combination with LMN lesions depending on other features of motor neurone disease. However, frequently LMN arm lesions, (with most obvious wasting and weakness in the hands), is associated with UMN lesions in the legs (spastic paraparesis with upgoing plantar responses). When amyotrophic lateral sclerosis involves the medulla, bilateral pyramidal tract lesions and pseudobulbar palsy results; the jaw jerk is increased.

1 - Amyotrophic lateral sclerosis
2 - LMN lesion in arms
3 - UMN lesions in legs
4 - Spastic paraparesis with upgoing plantar responses

5 - Amyotrophic lateral sclerosis involving medulla with bilateral pyramidal tract lesions
6 - Pseudobulbar palsy results
7 - The jaw jerk is increased

In general, patients with brainstem involvement by motor neurone disease have a bad prognosis, dying within a few years. Patients with progressive muscular atrophy may survive considerably longer. There is no speciific treatment for motor neurone disease and the condition tends to be progressive.

1 - Prognosis is bad for patients with brainstem involvement in motor neurone disease
2 - There is no specific treatment and condition tends to be progressive

DISEASES OF PERIPHERAL NERVES

Various disease processes may affect peripheral nerves and indeed one method of classification of neuropathy would be by the pathological disease process, eg. where the vasculoconnective tissue or vasa nervorum were primarily diseased, or where the disease process primarily afflicted the nerve cell, axon, myelin sheath. However, the easiest classification of neuropathy is by the anatomical distribution:-

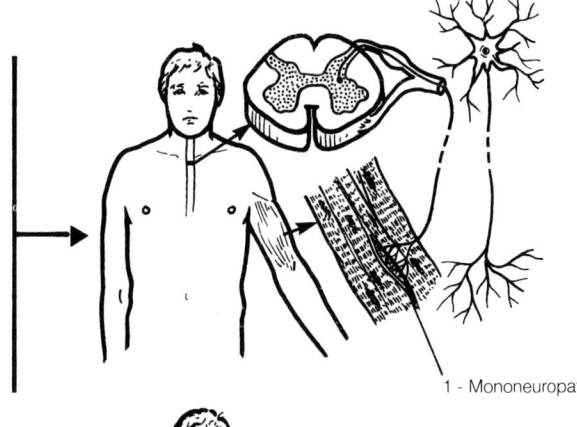

1 - Mononeuropathy

MONONEUROPATHY

A single peripheral nerve is afflicted and trauma is the commonest cause. A radial nerve palsy may result from trauma from a crutch, the ulnar nerve is vulnerable to trauma at the elbow and the common peroneal nerve on the lateral aspect of the upper fibula – traumatic lesions here produce the paralysis and anaesthesia expected from a knowledge of the anatomical supply. Nerves may be compressed as they pass through rigid and confined anatomical spaces; the commonest of these 'entrapment mononeuropathies' is the carpal tunnel syndrome.

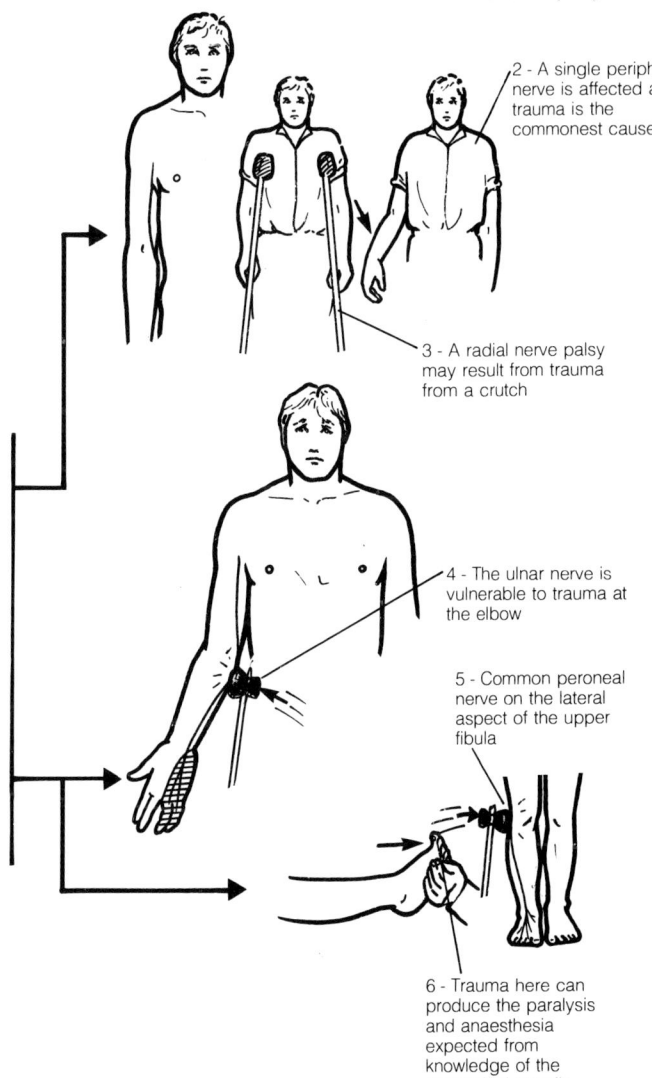

2 - A single peripheral nerve is affected and trauma is the commonest cause

3 - A radial nerve palsy may result from trauma from a crutch

4 - The ulnar nerve is vulnerable to trauma at the elbow

5 - Common peroneal nerve on the lateral aspect of the upper fibula

6 - Trauma here can produce the paralysis and anaesthesia expected from knowledge of the anatomical supplly

Mononeuropathy

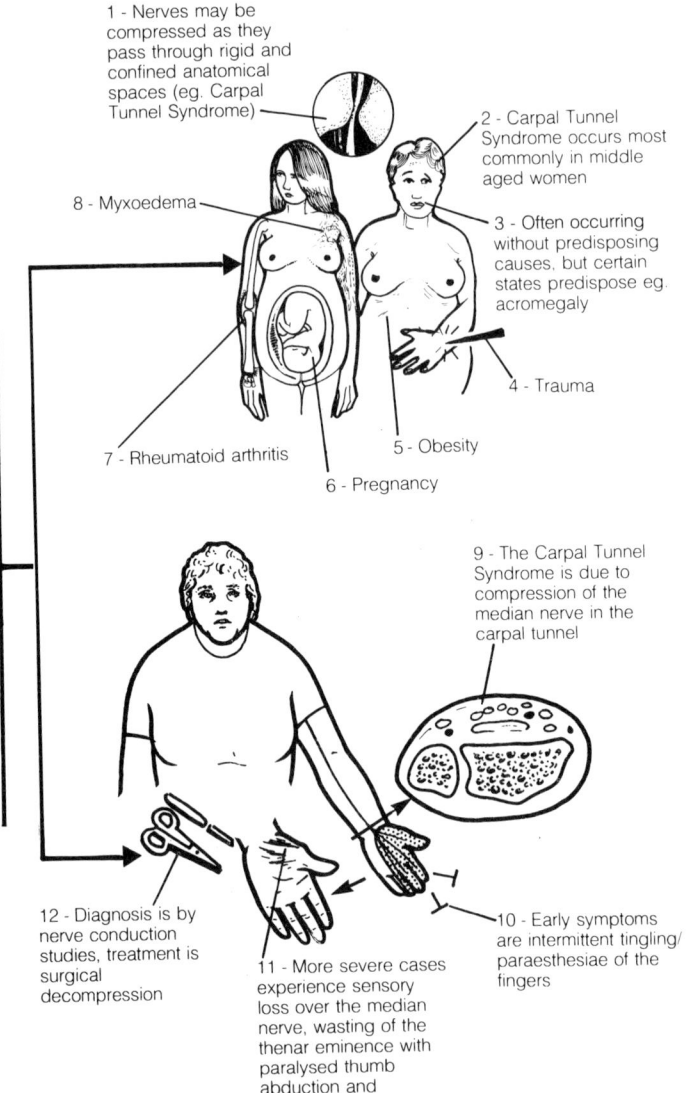

1 - Nerves may be compressed as they pass through rigid and confined anatomical spaces (eg. Carpal Tunnel Syndrome)

2 - Carpal Tunnel Syndrome occurs most commonly in middle aged women

3 - Often occurring without predisposing causes, but certain states predispose eg. acromegaly

4 - Trauma

5 - Obesity

6 - Pregnancy

7 - Rheumatoid arthritis

8 - Myxoedema

9 - The Carpal Tunnel Syndrome is due to compression of the median nerve in the carpal tunnel

10 - Early symptoms are intermittent tingling/paraesthesiae of the fingers

11 - More severe cases experience sensory loss over the median nerve, wasting of the thenar eminence with paralysed thumb abduction and opposition

12 - Diagnosis is by nerve conduction studies, treatment is surgical decompression

The **carpal tunnel syndrome** is due to compresssion of the median nerve in the carpal tunnel; it occurs most commonly in middle-aged women often without predisposing causes, although pregnancy, myxoedema, acromegaly, trauma, obesity and rheumatoid arthritis all predispose. The early symptoms are intermittent tingling/paraesthesiae of the fingers, often worse at night. In more severe cases there is sensory loss over the median nerve territory and wasting of the thenar eminence with paralysed thumb abduction and opposition. Diagnosis is by nerve conduction studies and treatment by surgical decompression.

Meralgia paraesthetica is another entrapment mononeuropathy, this time of the lateral cutaneous nerve of thigh as it passes under the inguinal ligament. The condition is commonest in the obese, and the clinical symptoms are of pain in the lateral aspect of the thigh on exercise. A **cervical rib** may cause an entrapment 'plexopathy' of the lower fibres of the brachial plexus at the thoracic inlet, causing wasting of the small muscles of the hand, (T_1 root and medial cord of plexus).

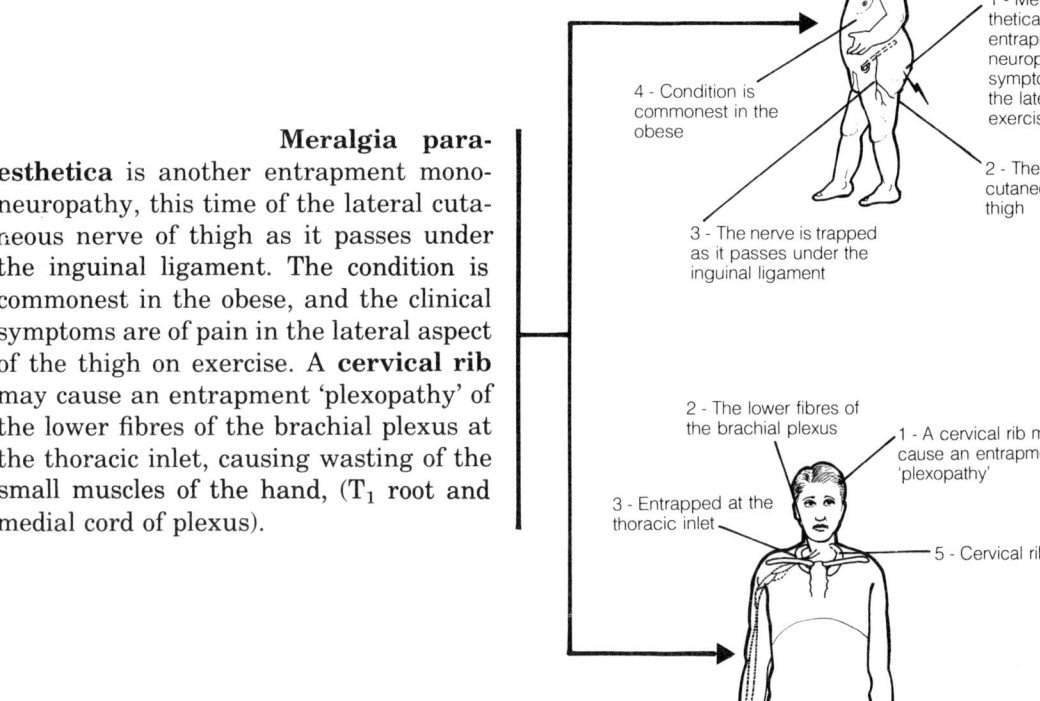

MONONEURITIS MULTIPLEX

In this condition, several unrelated peripheral nerves are diseased serially or concurrently. In diabetes mellitus and the collagenoses, (notably polyarteritis nodosa), the vasculitis affecting the vasa nervorum accounts for the haphazard affliction of various peripheral nerves. Other causes of mononeuritis multiplex include leprosy and sarcoidosis.

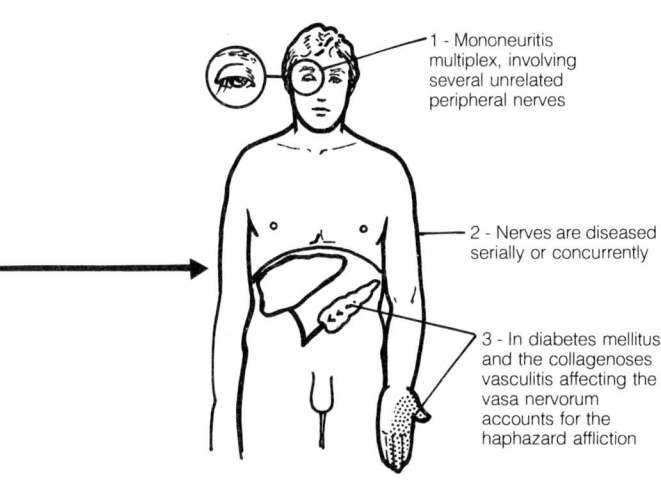

POLYNEUROPATHY

Here, there is symmetrical loss of sensation and power in the distal parts of the limbs, the legs being affected more than the arms. The distal limb anaesthesia is of "glove and stocking" distribution and includes all sensory modalities. The weakness similarly progresses proximally from the distal extremities, and muscle wasting and loss of tendon jerks are early features. However, some acute polyneuropathies may be predominantly sensory (eg. diabetes mellitus) or predominantly motor (eg. porphyria) or even commence in proximal muscles. The rate of progression of polyneuropathy is extremely variable: acute cases may develop generalised paralysis within two days whilst in chronic cases the polyneuropathy may evolve over months or longer.

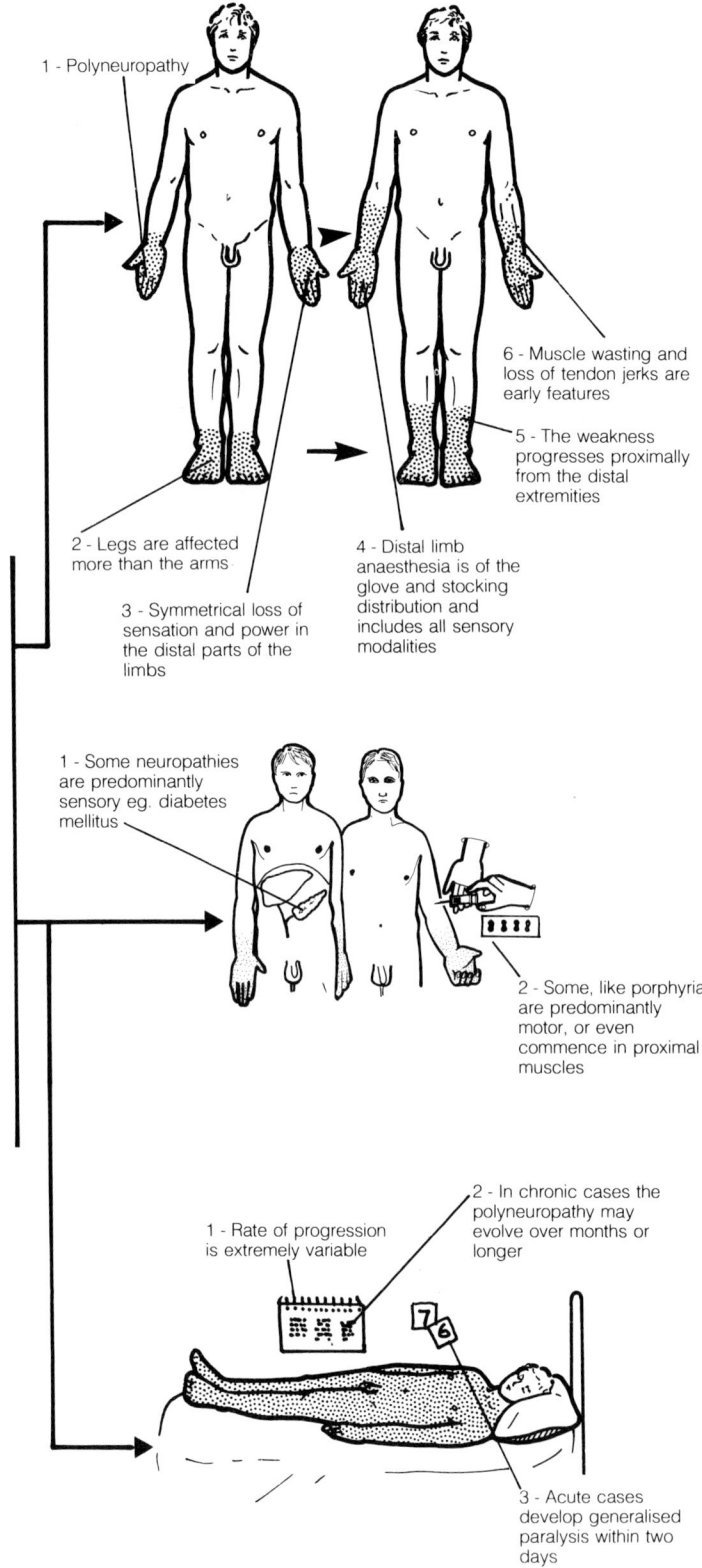

Polyneuropathy

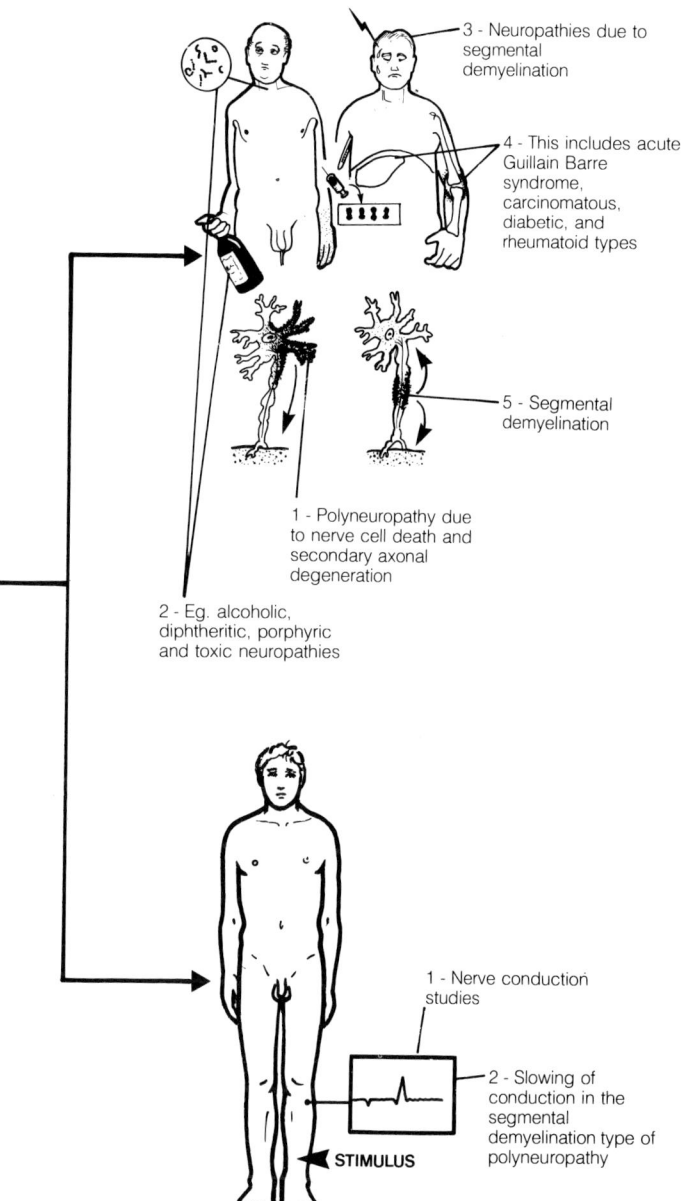

Pathologically, the polyneuropathy is either due to nerve cell death and secondary axonal degeneration (eg. alcoholic, diphtheritic, porphyric, and toxic neuropathies), or due to segmental demyelination of the peripheral nerve sheaths (eg. acute Guillain-Barré syndrome, carcinomatous, diabetic, rheumatoid polyneuropathies). Nerve conduction studies will show slowing of conduction in the segmental demyelination types of polyneuropathy, while with axonal degeneration the nerve conduction is either normal or absent.

In a few types of peripheral neuropathy, the affected nerves are palpably thickened. These conditions include leprosy (particularly thickening of the greater auricular nerve), amyloidosis and familial hypertrophic neuropathy.

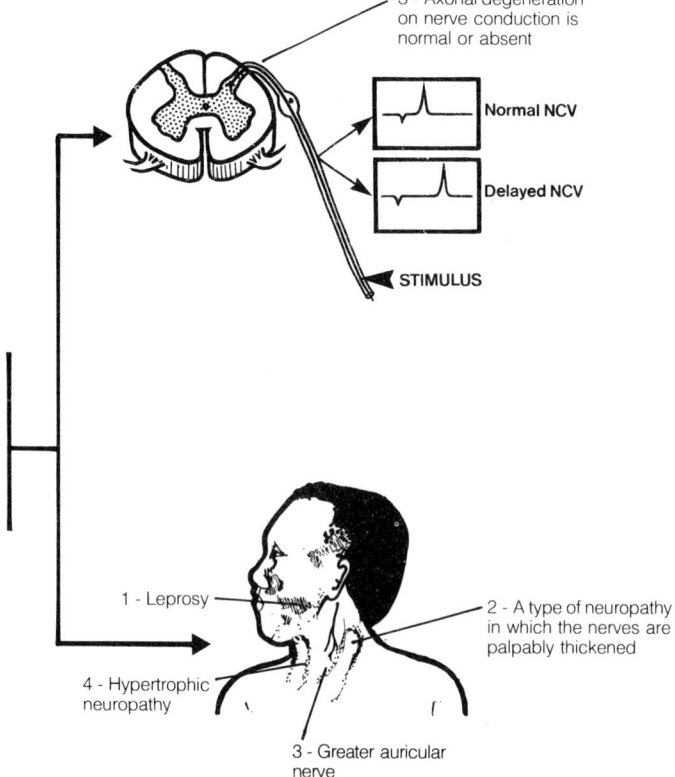

The commonest classification of polyneuropathy is by cause:-
Genetic – Peroneal muscular atrophy, Refsum's syndrome, hypertrophic neuropathy.

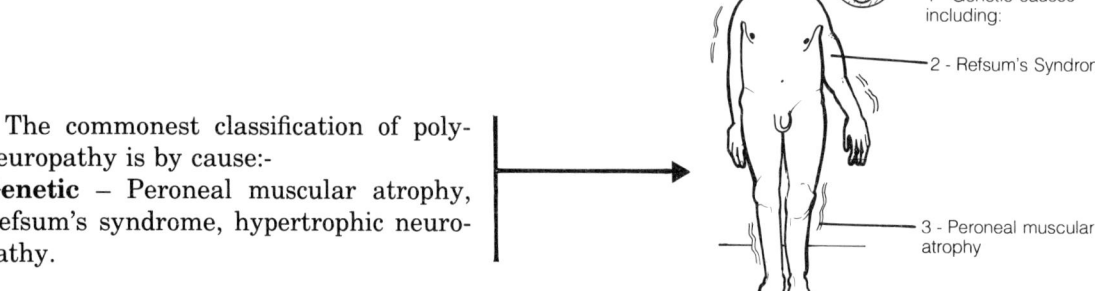

Polyneuropathy

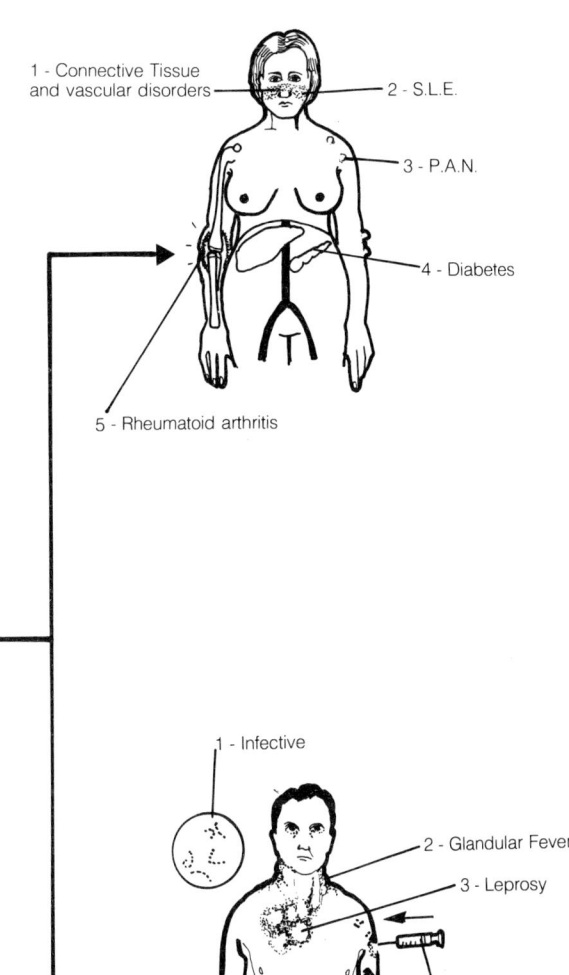

Connective Tisssue and Vascular Disorders – PAN, SLE, RA and diabetes (usually causing mononeuritis multiplex).
Infective – Diphtheria, leprosy, glandular fever, exanthematous disease, allergy from inoculations or Guillain-Barré syndrome.

Polyneuropathy

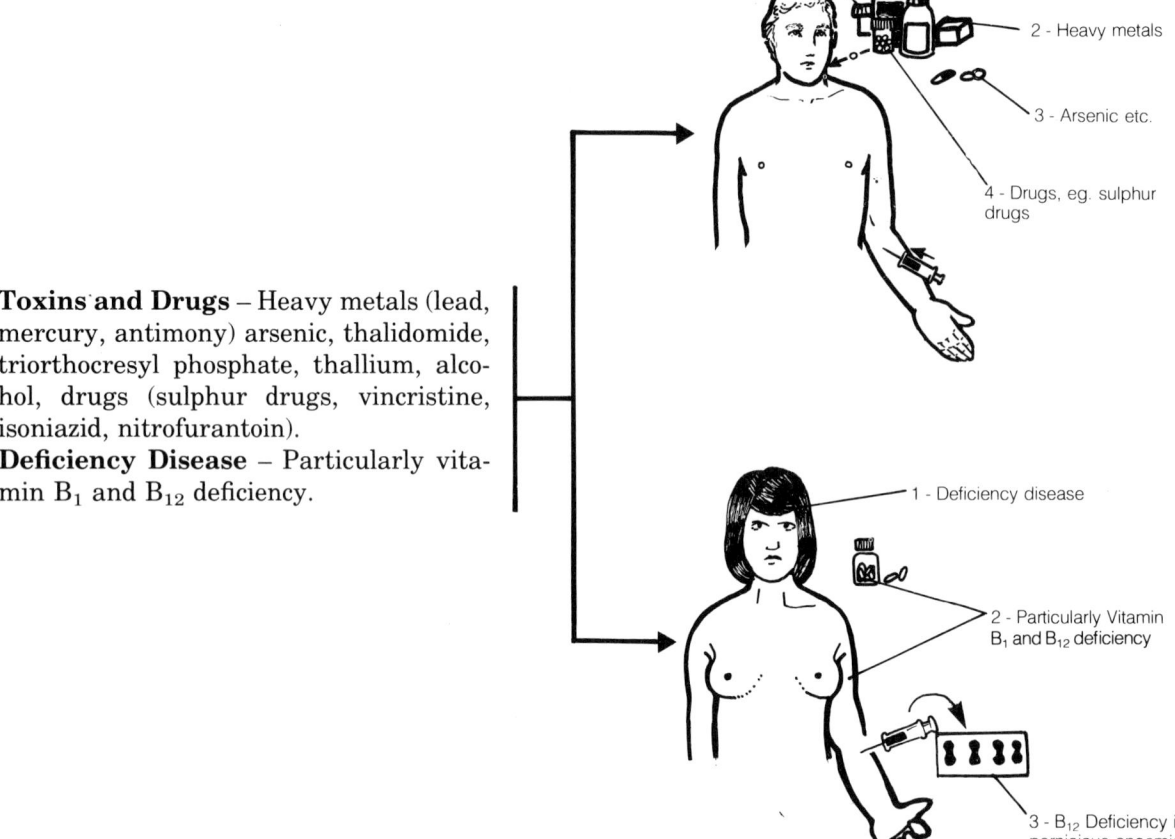

Toxins and Drugs – Heavy metals (lead, mercury, antimony) arsenic, thalidomide, triorthocresyl phosphate, thallium, alcohol, drugs (sulphur drugs, vincristine, isoniazid, nitrofurantoin).

Deficiency Disease – Particularly vitamin B_1 and B_{12} deficiency.

Metabolic – Diabetes, uraemia, porphyria, carcinoma, amyloidosis.

ACUTE INFECTIOUS POLYNEURITIS
(Guillain-Barré syndrome)

This unusual condition may abruptly follow an acute febrile illness (eg. upper respiratory tract infection, glandular fever, infectious hepatitis). There is headache, vomiting, and back pain prior to the onset of distal (or proximal) and symmetrical weakness, often in all four limbs. The condition may progress to affect the trunk musculature and cranial nerves and cause life-threatening paralysis within a few days of onset, requiring mechanical ventilation due to respiratory muscle paralysis.

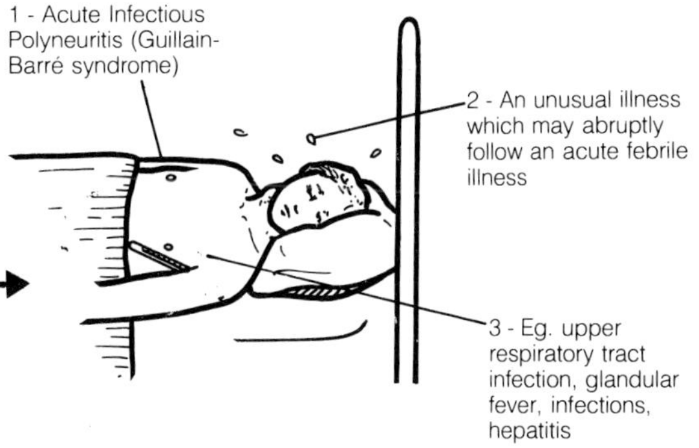

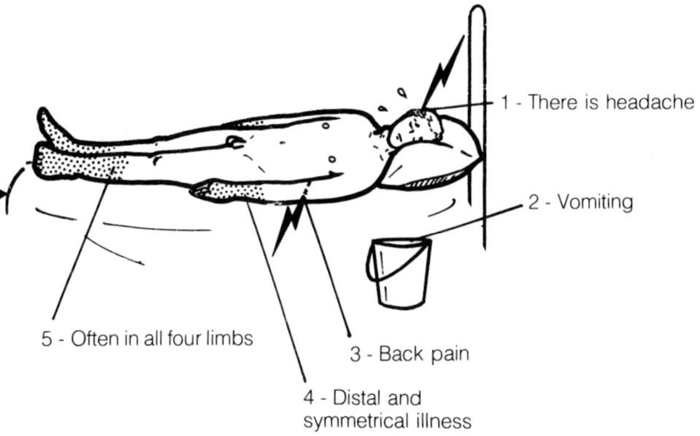

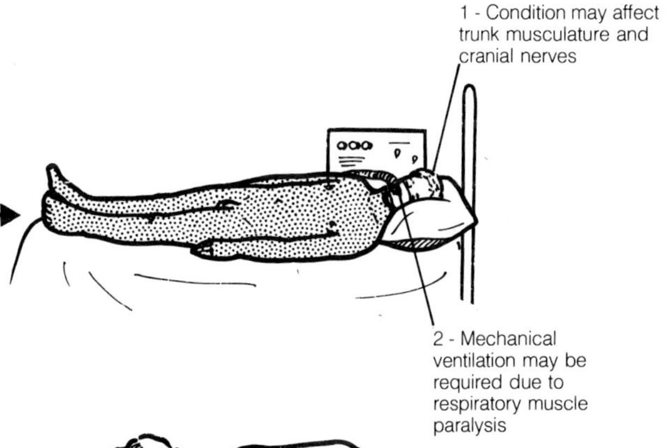

The nerve conduction studies confirm this demyelinating polyneuropathy and the CSF characteristically shows a high CSF protein with a normal cell count.

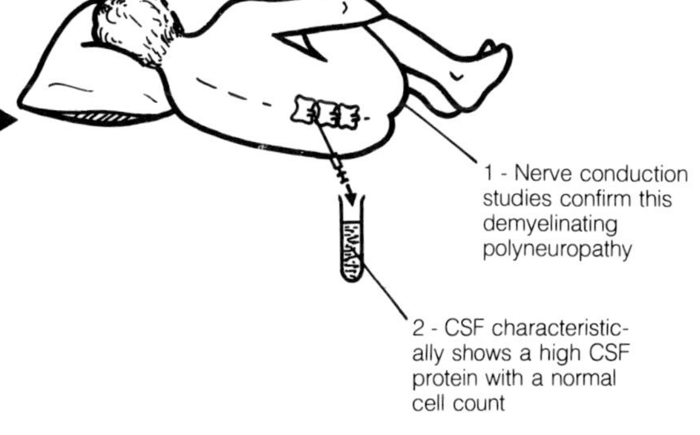

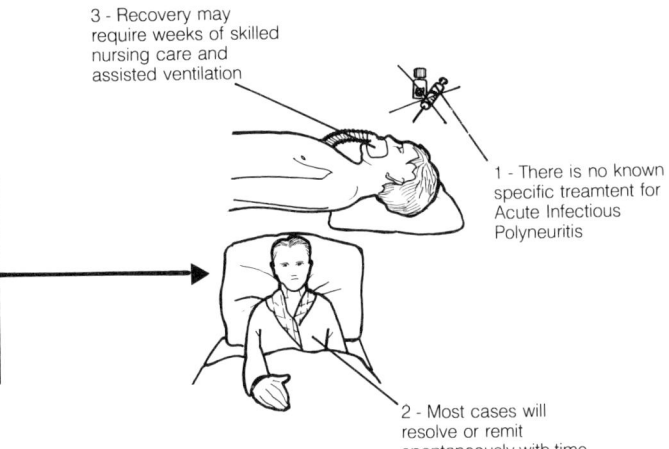

There is no known specific treatment for this condition but most cases will resolve or remit spontaneously with time, (and this may require weeks of assisted ventilation), such that skilled nursing care for as long as necessary will usually reap the rewards of recovery.

VITAMINS B_1 and B_{12} DEFICIENCY

Beriberi is a nutritional disorder relatively common in the Far East, in areas where polished rice is the staple diet; such a diet is deficient in thiamine (vitamin B_1). Beriberi presents with a painful peripheral neuritis – classic "glove and stocking" sensory loss with muscle weakness and wasting.

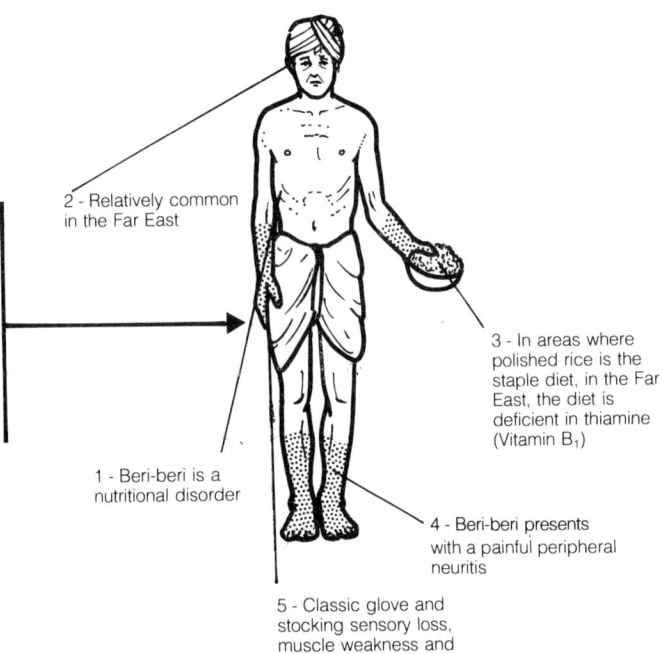

Vitamins B_1 and B_{12} Deficiency

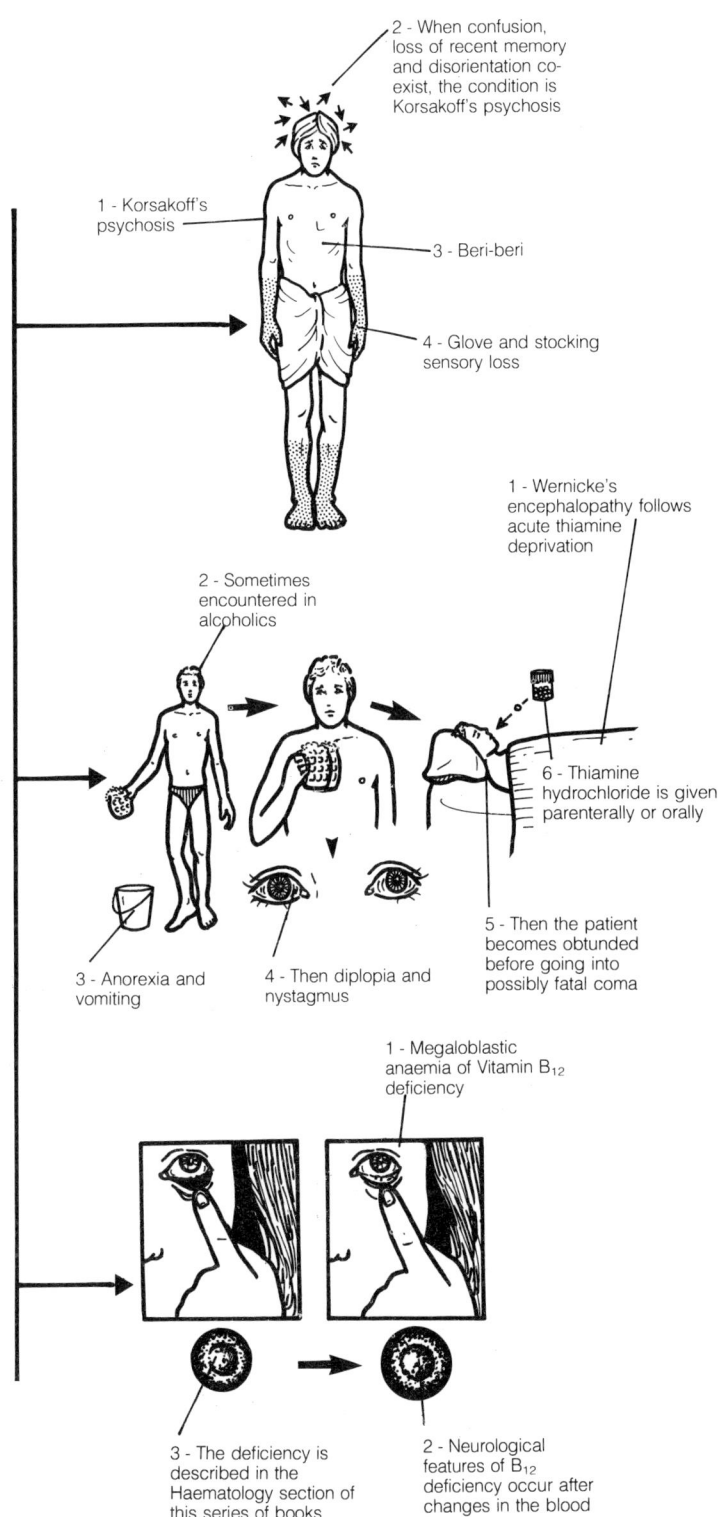

When confusion, loss of recent memory and disorientation co-exist, the condition is called **Korsakoff's psychosis.**

Wernicke's encephalopathy follows acute thiamine deprivation and is sometimes encountered in alcoholics. Anorexia and vomiting precede diplopia and nystagmus and then the patient becomes obtunded before slipping into a coma which may be fatal. Thiamine hydrochloride is given parenterally or orally as therapy.

The megaloblastic anaemia of vitamin B_{12} deficiency is well described elsewhere in this series of books and neurological features of B_{12} deficiency occur after changes in the blood picture.

Vitamins B_1 and B_{12} Deficiency

In **subacute combined degeneration** of the cord, there is degeneration of the dorsal columns of the spinal cord and then the lateral columns (including the pyramidal tracts) are afflicted; a polyneuritis is also part of the picture. The first symptom is usually paraesthesiae in the toes followed by numbness and weakness of the legs. The peripheral neuropathy leads to flaccid paralysis despite the pyramidal (UMN) lesion; nevertheless the Babinski response may be positive, confirming the pyramidal tract involvement. **Treatment** is with parenteral hydroxocobalamin, (see Pernicious Anaemia).

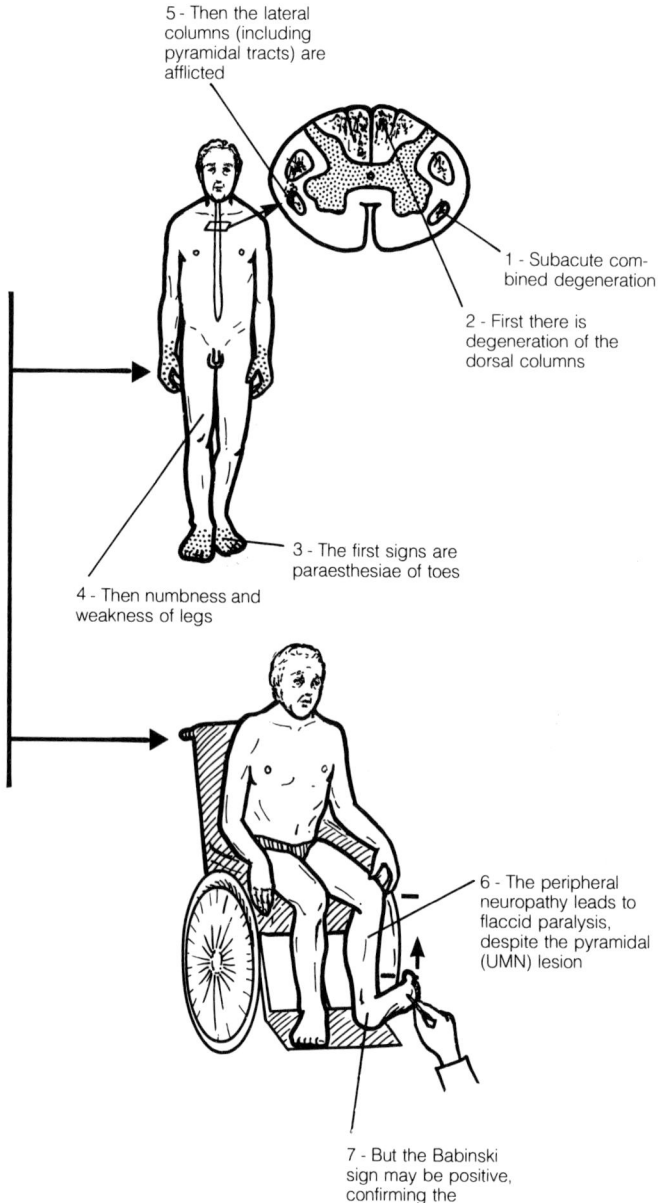

1 - Subacute combined degeneration
2 - First there is degeneration of the dorsal columns
3 - The first signs are paraesthesiae of toes
4 - Then numbness and weakness of legs
5 - Then the lateral columns (including pyramidal tracts) are afflicted
6 - The peripheral neuropathy leads to flaccid paralysis, despite the pyramidal (UMN) lesion
7 - But the Babinski sign may be positive, confirming the pyramidal tract involvement

MYASTHENIA GRAVIS

This disease is characterised by the abnormally rapid fatiguability of voluntary muscles during exercise due to impaired acetylcholine mediated transmission at the neuromuscular junctions. The presence of acetylcholine receptor autoantibody in the serum of some patients provides one causative mechanism of this transmission block. Indeed, a newborn child may demonstrate transient myasthenia gravis due to the transplacental passage of anti-body from a myasthenic mother. A **thymoma** is present in 15% of cases of myasthenia gravis and there is a higher incidence of thyroid disease and other auto-immune diseases, also in patients with myasthenia. The disease is more common in females and tends to present in the second or third decades of life (although patients with thymic tumours tend to present in later life).

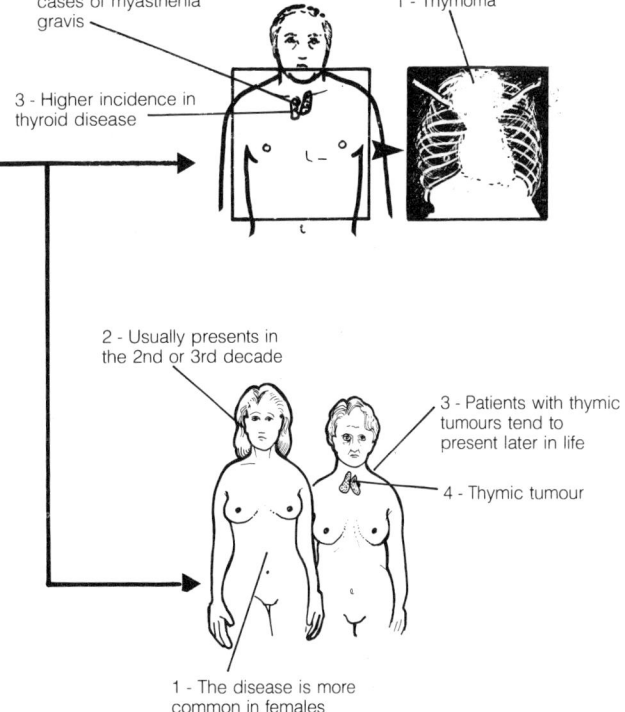

Myasthenia Gravis

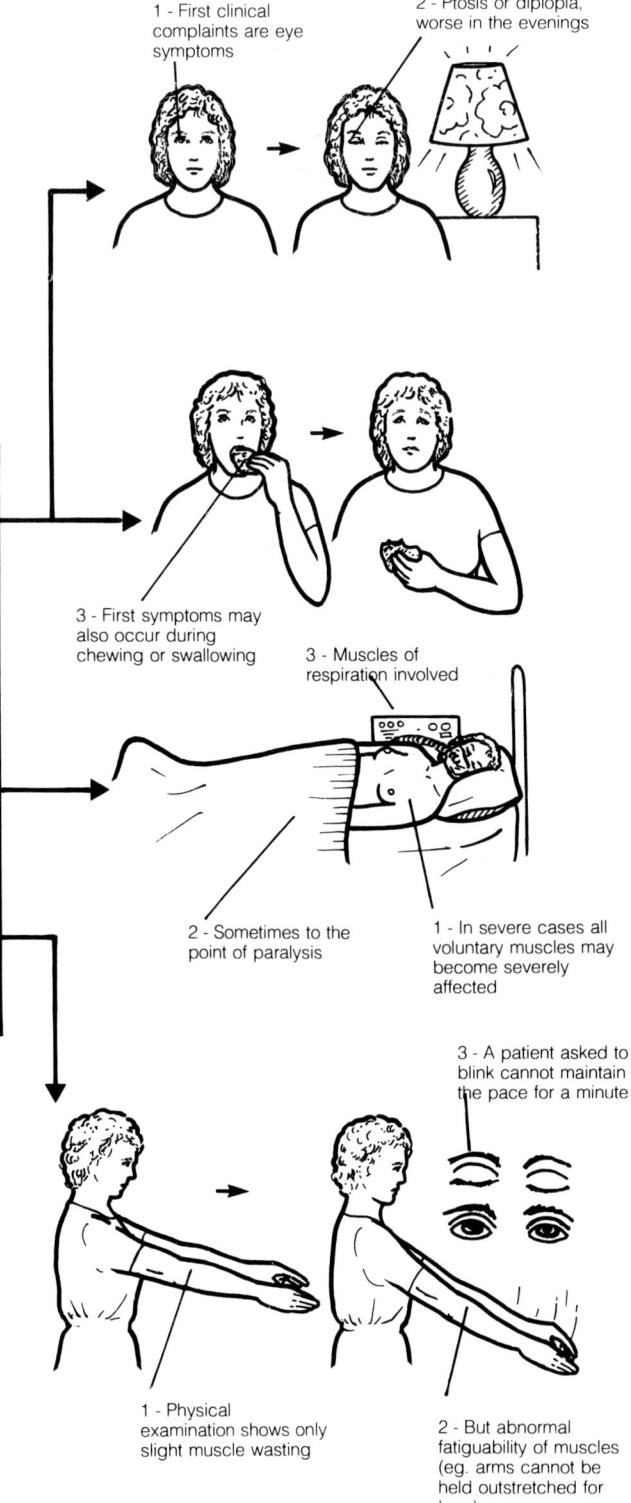

The first **clinical complaints** are commonly with eye symptoms (eg. ptosis, diplopia – worse in the evenings etc) or due to fatigue during chewing, swallowing (towards the end of a meal), or speaking (voice softens with use). In more severe cases, all voluntary muscles may become severely affected to the point of paralysis and when respiratory muscles become involved the disease becomes life-threatening. **Physical examination** often shows only slight muscle wasting but demonstrates abnormal fatiguability of muscles – (eg. if the patient tries to keep on blinking for one minute, there is deterioration in performance after a good initial performance, and the patient cannot keep the arms outstretched in front of him for long).

Although the fatiguability strongly suggests the diagnosis, there may be a differential diagnosis and with ocular signs this may be from IIIrd nerve palsy, or with other presentations from myopathies or motor neurone disease. There is a peculiar myasthenic syndrome, (the **Eaton-Lambert syndrome**) which occurs as a rare distant effect of carcinoma in which the patient complains of fatiguable weakness, often of the proximal limb muscles. Nerve conduction study results differ from myasthenia gravis and the condition is less responsive to therapy, although oral guanidine hydrochloride may be helpful.

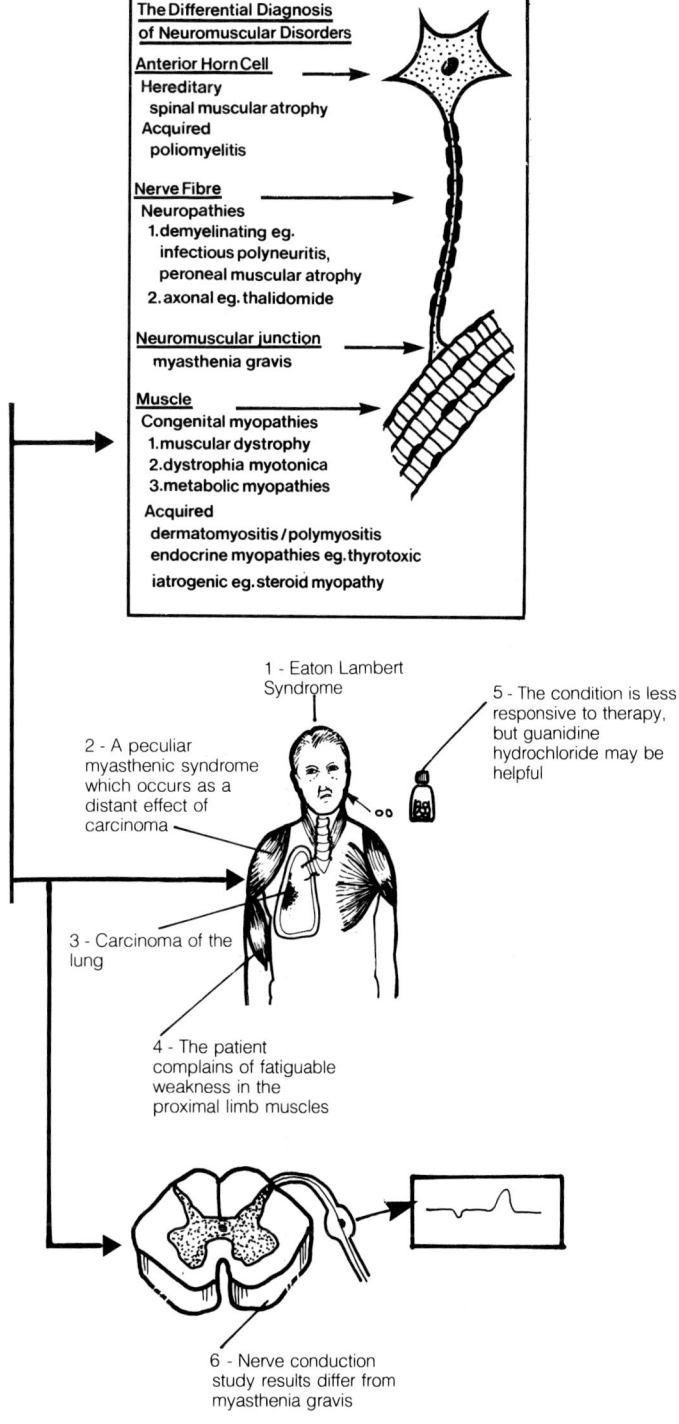

The **diagnosis** of myasthenia gravis is made by a therapeutic trial injection of the short acting anticholinesterase; edrophonium chloride (Tensilon) – 10mg i.v. stat. In myasthenia gravis, such an injection leads to marked and immediate improvement in the condition. In nerve conduction studies using repetitive nerve stimulation, muscle action potentials of progressively smaller amplitude are seen (c.f. larger amplitude in Eaton-Lambert syndrome). Skeletal muscle auto-antibodies may be circulating and a CXR may show a thymoma.

1 - Diagnosis of myasthenia gravis

2 - Diagnosis is made by the therapeutic trial injection of the short acting anticholinesterase; edrophonium chloride (tensilon) – 10mg i.v. stat

3 - In myasthenia gravis such an injection leads to a marked and immediate improvement in the condition

1 - Nerve conduction studies using repetitive nerve stimulation

2 - Muscle action potentials of progressively smaller amplitude are seen

Thymectomy may be dramatically effective therapy, particularly in young women and when performed early in their disease. However, thymectomy must be considered for all severe cases of myasthenia and the operation is not restricted to those with thymic tumours.

1 - Thymectomy may be dramatically effective

2 - Particularly in young women, when performed early in the disease

3 - Thymectomy must be considered for all severe cases of myasthenia

4 - The operation is not restricted to those with thymic tumours

Myasthenia Gravis

Medical treatment of myasthenia gravis comprises oral anticholinesterase therapy, (neostigmine 15mg q.d.s., or pyridostigmine 60mg q.d.s.). Muscarinic side effects may occur and if the dose of the anticholinesterase is increased too high, the muscle strength may actually become weaker due to the drug causing a 'depolarisating block'. The latter should be suspected if the pupils are constricted to smaller than 3mm, (suggesting high availability of acetylcholine at muscarinic receptors). With the presence of auto-antibodies and thymic involvement in disease causation, other therapies including corticosteroid and azathioprine therapies, thoracic duct drainage and plasmapheresis of auto-antibody have all been used as immunosuppressants in severe disease.

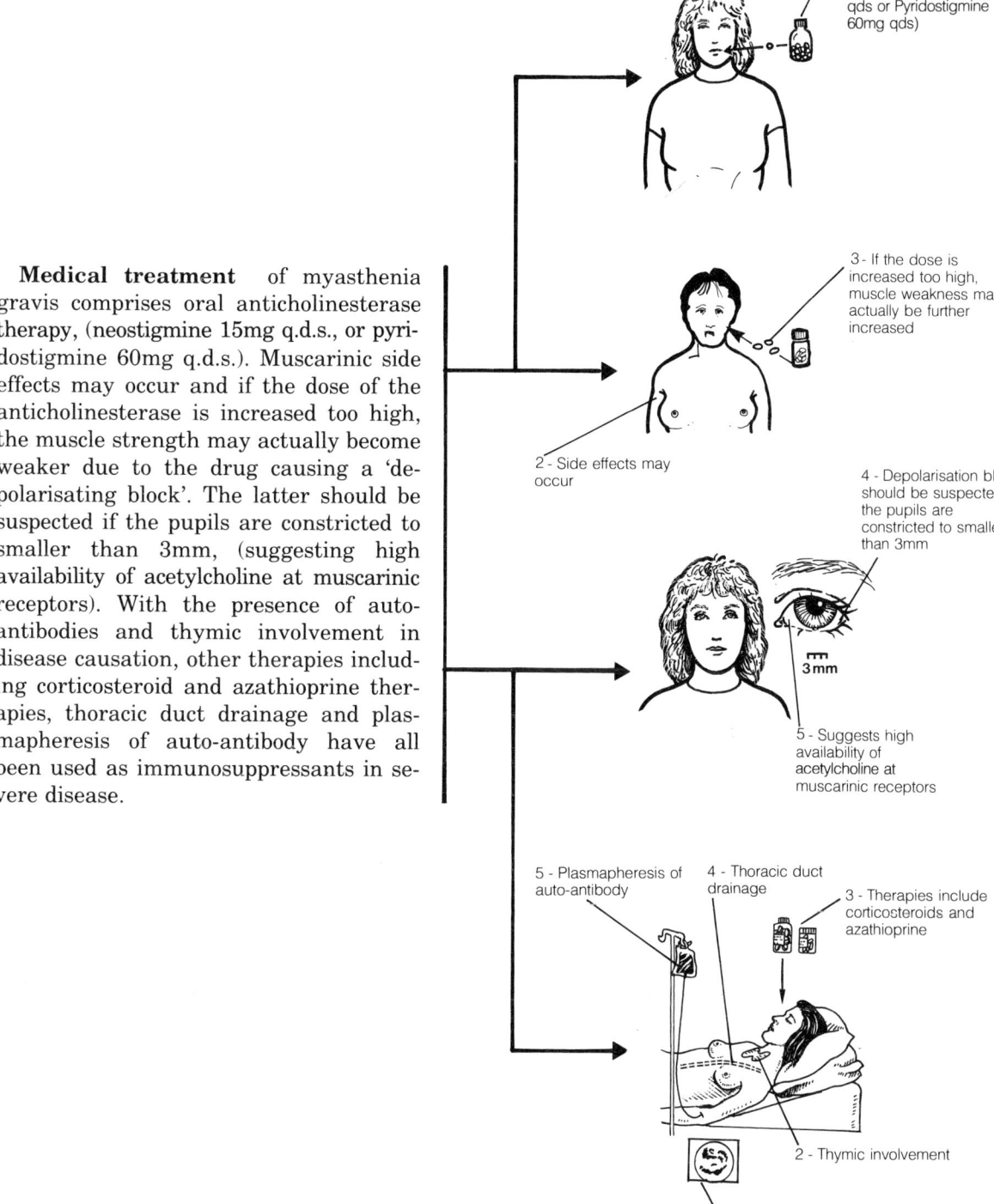

1 - Medical treatment comprises oral anti-cholinesterase therapy. (Neostigmine 15 mg qds or Pyridostigmine 60mg qds)

2 - Side effects may occur

3 - If the dose is increased too high, muscle weakness may actually be further increased

4 - Depolarisation block should be suspected if the pupils are constricted to smaller than 3mm

5 - Suggests high availability of acetylcholine at muscarinic receptors

5 - Plasmapheresis of auto-antibody

4 - Thoracic duct drainage

3 - Therapies include corticosteroids and azathioprine

2 - Thymic involvement

1 - Auto-antibodies

MYOPATHIES

Although the diagnosis of myopathy may often appear straightforward, there are several important, diagnostic tests which assist. The history is important, concentrating on the order of development of symptoms and the symmetry of weakness, and particularly the family history, as many myopathies are hereditary. The **physical examination** must concentrate on the pattern of weakness or wasting, (often proximal muscles rather than distal limb musculature). Of the ancillary tests, the serum aldolase and creatine phosphokinase (CPK) are often elevated in the presence of myopathy. The electomyogram (EMG) is often diagnostic in myopathy, distinguishing this from LMN lesions, myasthenia etc. The ultimate **diagnostic test** in suspected myopathy is the muscle biopsy for histological examination.

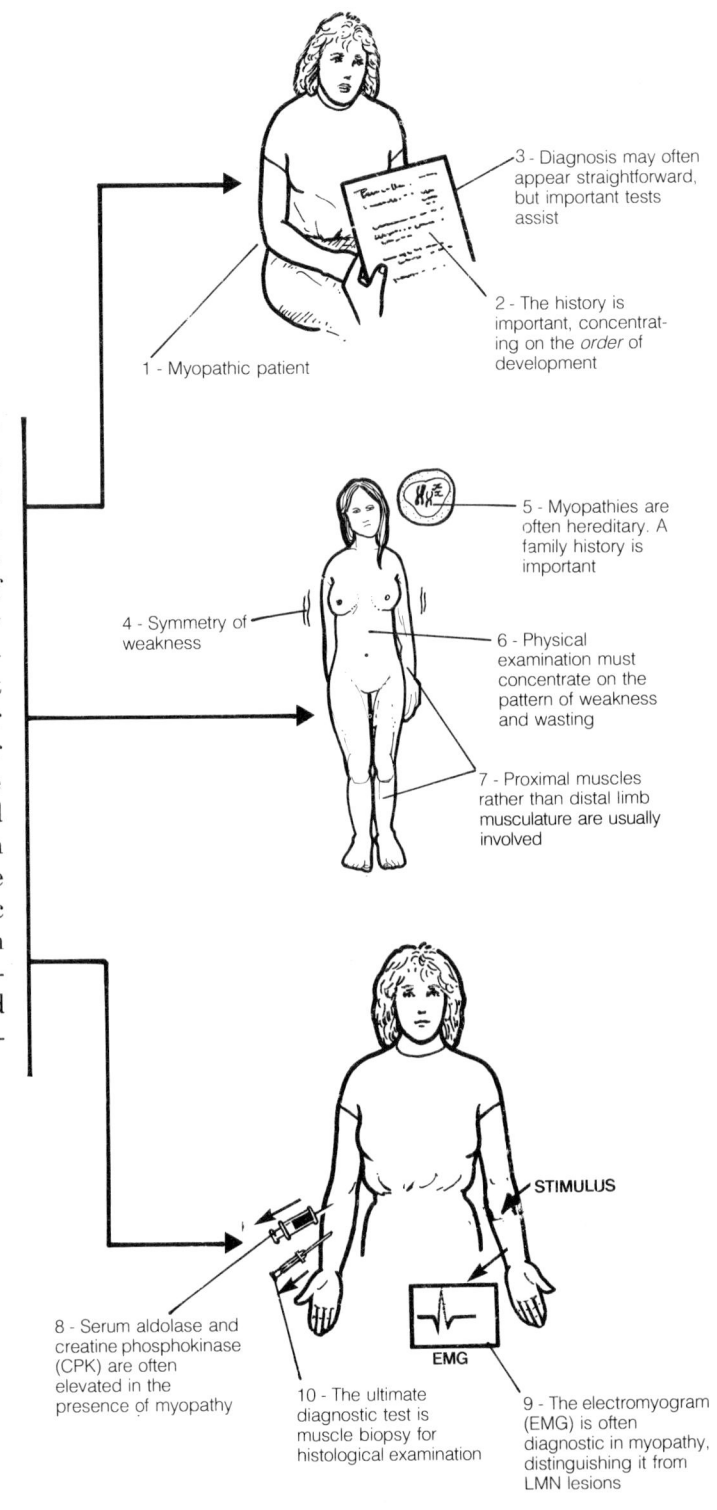

1 - Myopathic patient

2 - The history is important, concentrating on the *order* of development

3 - Diagnosis may often appear straightforward, but important tests assist

4 - Symmetry of weakness

5 - Myopathies are often hereditary. A family history is important

6 - Physical examination must concentrate on the pattern of weakness and wasting

7 - Proximal muscles rather than distal limb musculature are usually involved

8 - Serum aldolase and creatine phosphokinase (CPK) are often elevated in the presence of myopathy

9 - The electromyogram (EMG) is often diagnostic in myopathy, distinguishing it from LMN lesions

10 - The ultimate diagnostic test is muscle biopsy for histological examination

MUSCULAR DYSTROPHY

This is a group of hereditary disease of muscle that tends to afflict proximal limb muscles and leads to severe and symmetrical muscle wasting and weakness; there is no muscle fasciculation, the tendon reflexes are usually preserved until a very late point in the disease and LMN signs and sensory signs are absent.

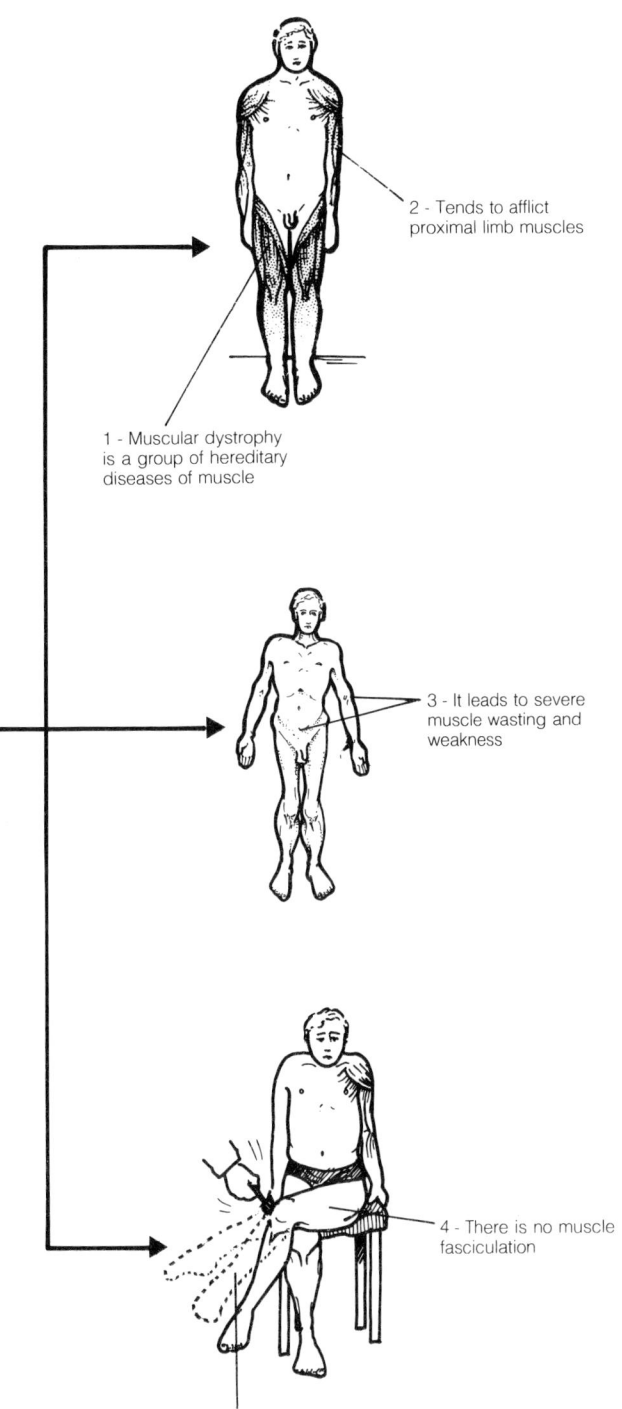

1 - Muscular dystrophy is a group of hereditary diseases of muscle

2 - Tends to afflict proximal limb muscles

3 - It leads to severe muscle wasting and weakness

4 - There is no muscle fasciculation

5 - Tendon reflexes are usually preserved until a very late stage in the disease

Pseudohypertrophic Muscular Dystrophy (Duchenne type)

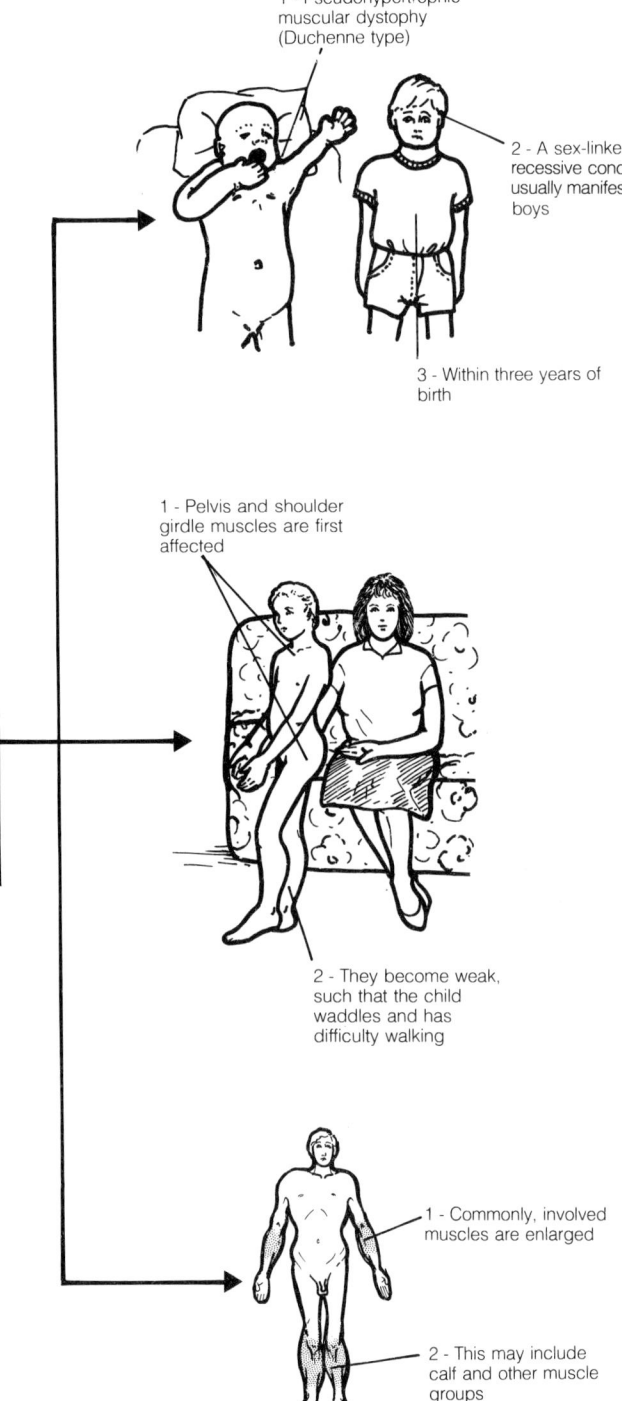

PSEUDOHYPERTROPHIC MUSCULAR DYSTROPHY (Duchenne type)

This sex-linked recessive condition usually manifests in boys within three years of birth. The pelvis and shoulder girdle muscles are first affected becoming weak, so that the child waddles and then has difficulty walking. Commonly, the involved muscles are enlarged and this may include the calf and other muscle

Pseudohypertrophic Muscular Dystrophy (Duchenne type)

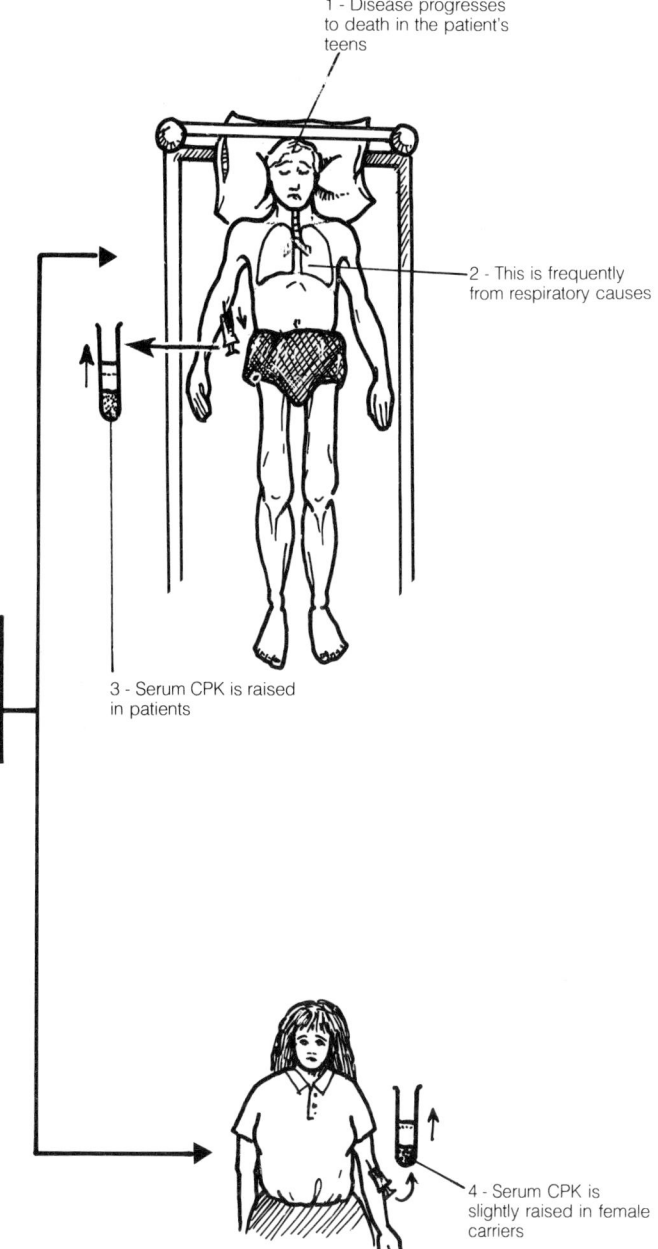

groups. The disease progresses to death usually in the teens, and frequently from respiratory causes. The serum CPK is raised in patients with this disease and slightly elevated in female carriers of the gene.

1 - Disease progresses to death in the patient's teens

2 - This is frequently from respiratory causes

3 - Serum CPK is raised in patients

4 - Serum CPK is slightly raised in female carriers

LIMB-GIRDLE MUSCULAR DYSTROPHY

This autosomal recessive condition usually has its clinical onset in the second to third decade with pelvic and shoulder girdle weakness which gradually (over perhaps many years) progress to death.

FACIO-SCAPULO – HUMERAL MUSCULAR DYSTROPHY

This autosomal dominant condition may manifest first at any age but the facial muscles, (particularly orbicularis oculi) may be afflicted. The limb girdles are also involved early and very insidiously the disease progresses. Although most patients will die from the disease, a longer life span is more likely than in the other muscular dystrophies. There is a separate form of ocular muscular dystrophy which does not progress beyond the ocular or facial muscles.

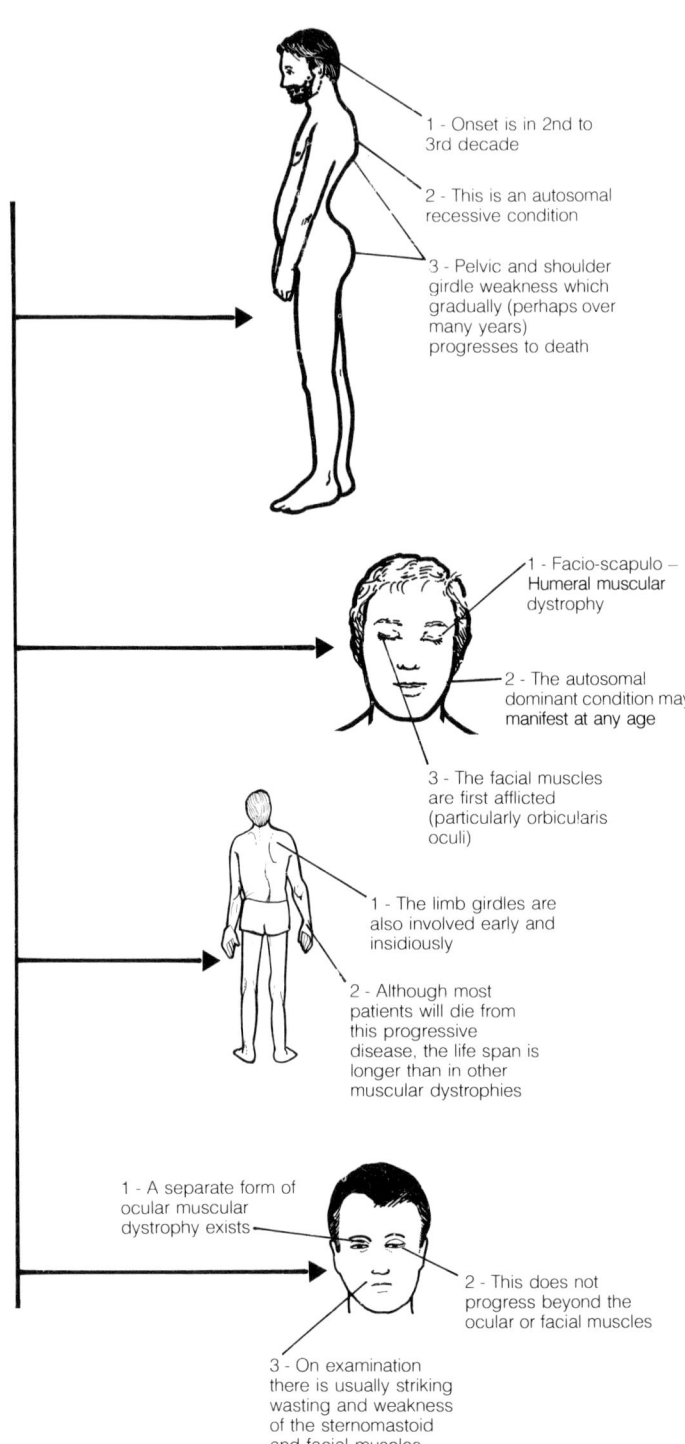

1 - Onset is in 2nd to 3rd decade

2 - This is an autosomal recessive condition

3 - Pelvic and shoulder girdle weakness which gradually (perhaps over many years) progresses to death

1 - Facio-scapulo – Humeral muscular dystrophy

2 - The autosomal dominant condition may manifest at any age

3 - The facial muscles are first afflicted (particularly orbicularis oculi)

1 - The limb girdles are also involved early and insidiously

2 - Although most patients will die from this progressive disease, the life span is longer than in other muscular dystrophies

1 - A separate form of ocular muscular dystrophy exists

2 - This does not progress beyond the ocular or facial muscles

3 - On examination there is usually striking wasting and weakness of the sternomastoid and facial muscles

MYOTONIC DYSTROPHY

This autosomal dominant condition usually has its clinical onset in the third decade of life, and myotonia, (the persistence of muscle contraction after voluntary contraction has finished) is the most characteristic feature. The early symptoms are often of difficulty in swallowing and later speaking or of generalised weakness. On examination there is usually striking wasting and weakness of sternomastoid muscles and facial muscles. Later, the limb girdle and other muscles become affected. All these muscles may demonstrate myotonia after voluntary contraction, and myotonia may be provoked in some muscles by tapping on the muscle — best demonstrated as "percussion myotonia" in the thenar muscles. The CPK is raised and the EMG shows myotonic discharges. Associated features in myotonic dystrophy include cataracts, baldness, gonadal atrophy and later dementia. The disease is progressive and fatal. Although guanine, procainamide and phenytoin may assist the myotonia they are not specific therapy.

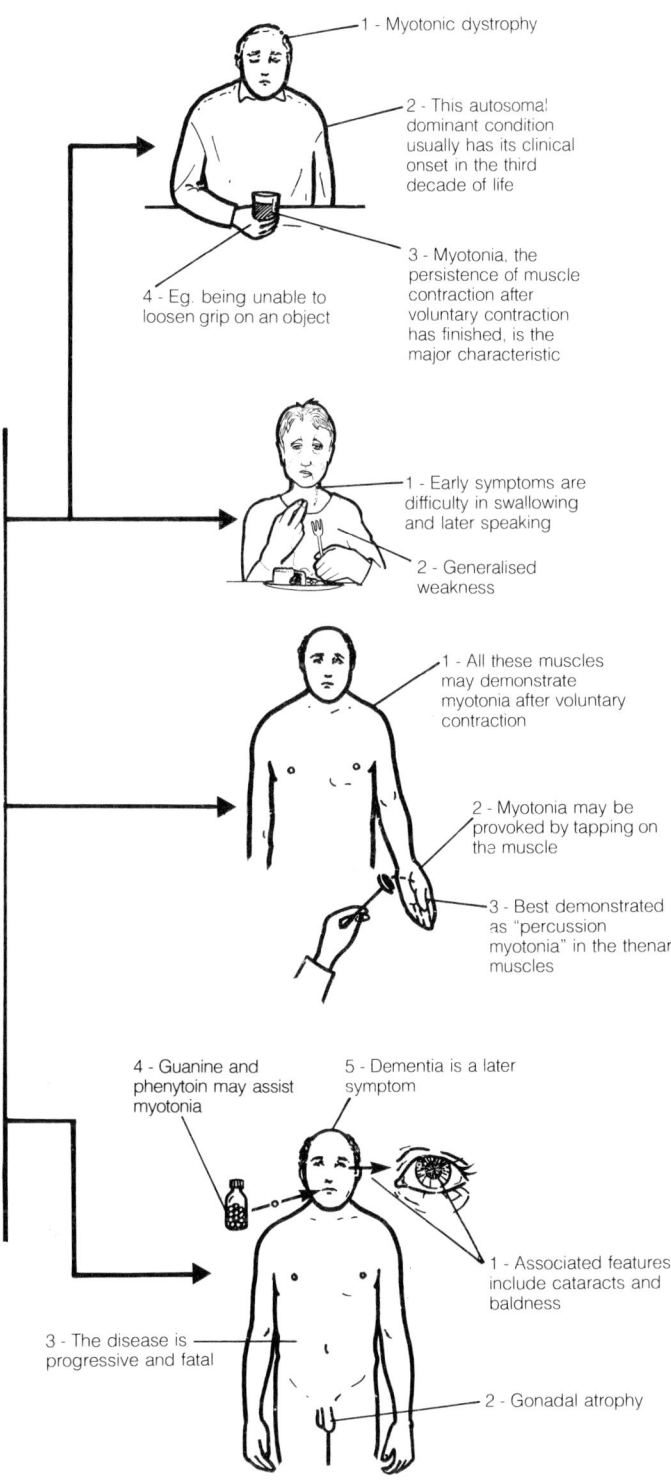

Myotonia congenita (Thomsen's disease) is a rare mendelian dominant condition that manifests first in childhood with myotonia and often hypertrophic muscles. Although the course of the disease is indolent, it may ultimately prove fatal.

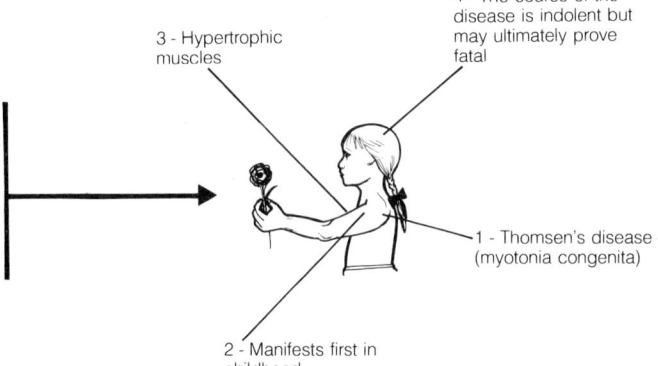

ACQUIRED MYOPATHIES

There are certain well recognised myopathies associated with endocrine and metabolic diseases, and, like most typical muscle diseases, proximal limb (or limb girdle) muscles are worst affected. Thus, in Cushing's syndrome or thyrotoxicosis, (or indeed in diabetic amyotrophy), there is proximal limb muscle weakness with the patient having difficulty in standing up from a low chair, (he tends to

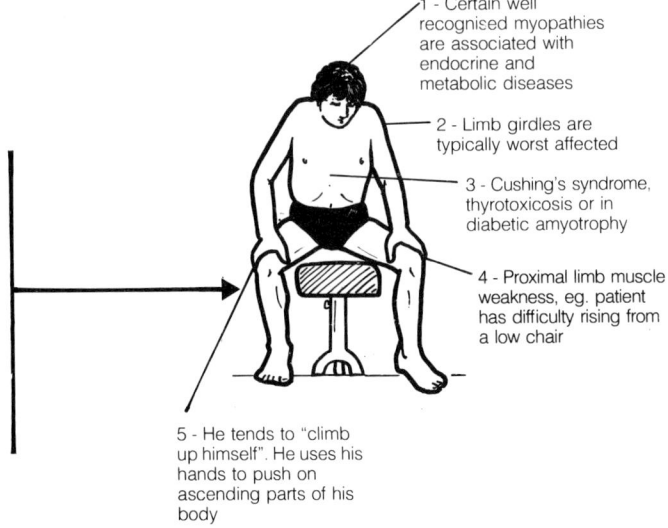

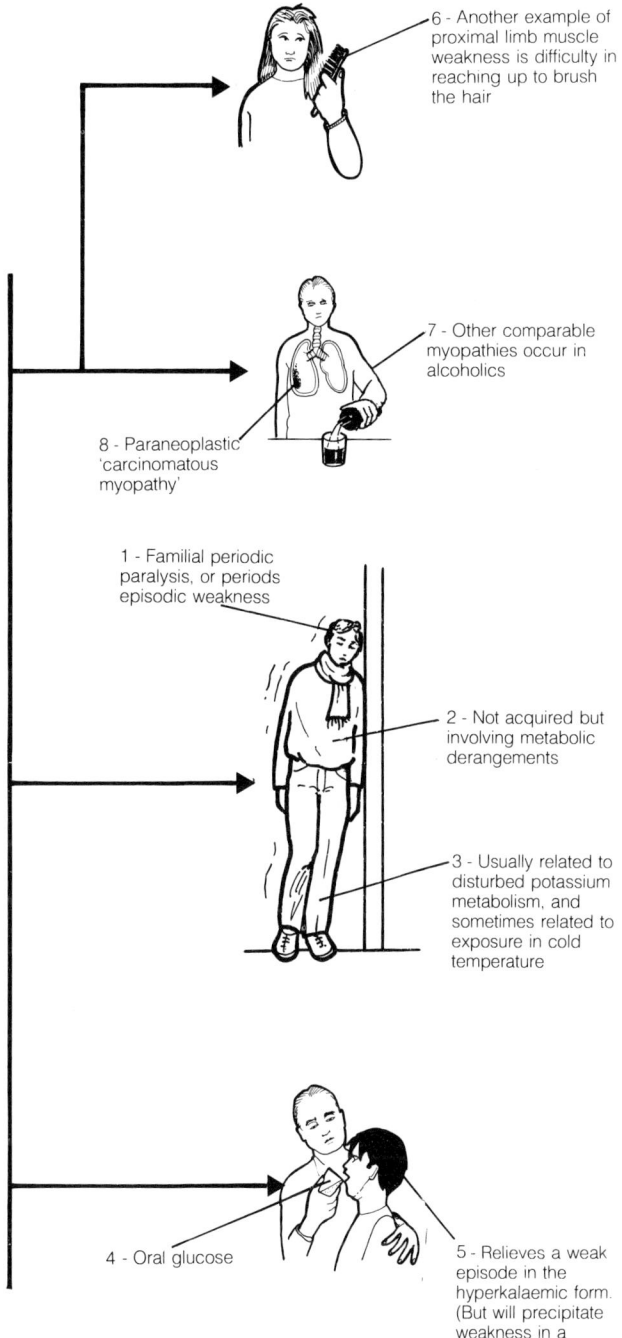

"climb up himself" using his hands to push up on ascending parts of his body in order to stand erect), or having difficulty in reaching up to brush his hair. Other comparable myopathies may occur in alcoholism, McArdle's disease and the paraneoplastic 'carcinomatous myopathy', (where myopathy occurs as a distant effect from a tumour).

Not acquired, but involving metabolic derangements are the group of **'familial periodic paralyses'** with periods of episodic weakness, usually related to disturbed potassium metabolism and sometimes related to exposure to cold temperature. Oral glucose will precipitate a weak episode in the hypokalaemic variety and relieve a weak episode in the hyperkalaemic form.

POLYMYOSITIS

Polymyositis refers to an inflammatory condition of muscles which differs from the true myopathies in that the damage to the muscles is due to inflammatory destruction of the fibres rather than a primary muscle disease. The onset is commonly in middle age and there are associations with connective tissue (autoimmune) disorders. Polymyositis may also occur as a distant effect of a carcinoma (eg. lung cancer); indeed, the diagnosis of polymyositis in an adult should be followed by a careful screen for cancer. The condition dermatomyositis embraces the co-existence of a pathognomonic facial skin rash and polymyositis.

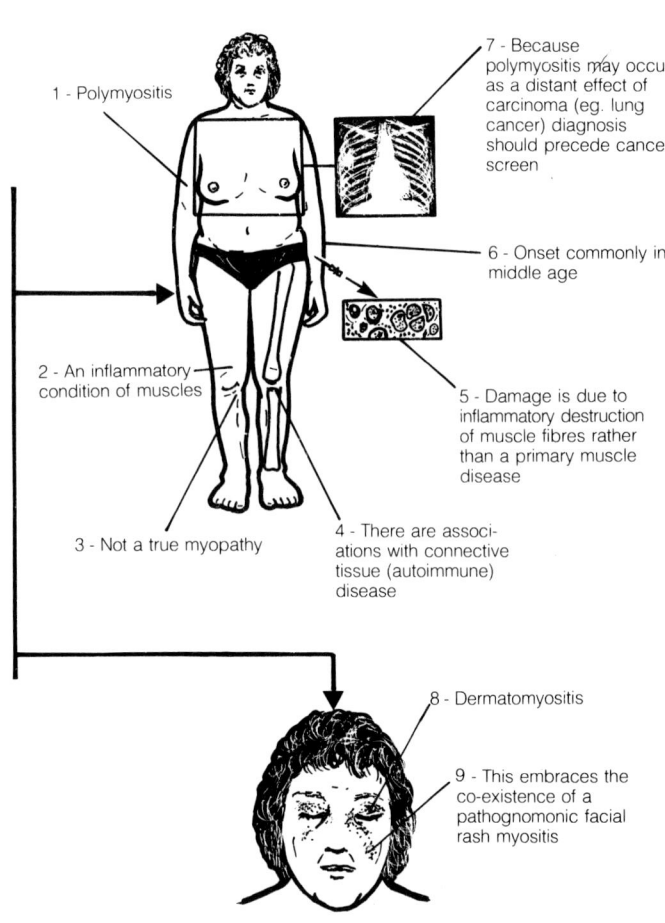

Clinically, polymyositis usually causes weakness and wasting of proximal muscles; the neck extensors are commonly affected and the head may droop forwards. In the more acute cases, a fever, polymorphonuclear leucocytosis, high ESR and raised CPK are present and the muscles may become tender and swollen,

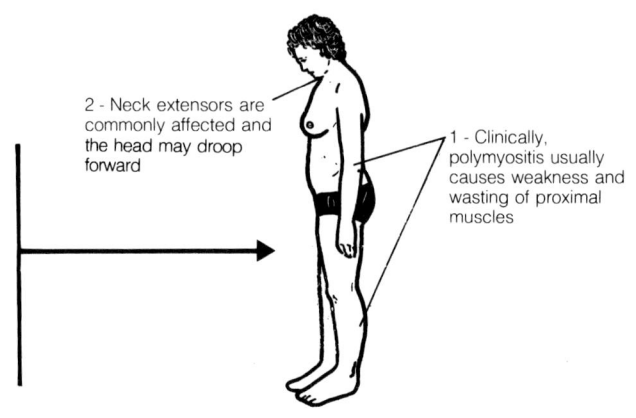

(rare in the other myopathies). In the more chronic cases, slowly progressive muscle weakness and wasting are the dominant clinical features. The EMG findings are quite distinct from both LMN lesions and from true myopathies, notably the presence of fibrillation in the EMG of polymyositis. The other disorders from which polymyositis must be distinguished include polymyalgia rheumatica (where "muscle stiffness" is the dominant symptom) and some unusual infestation of muscle (eg. trichinosis, toxoplasmosis).

Treatment of polymyositis is by prednisolone, (20mg tds reducing to a low maintenance dose when the condition remits), and treatment of any underlying neoplasm.

Psychiatry

A **psychiatric illness** may be defined as a clinical condition in which the patient's behaviour or experiences and thoughts are qualitatively and quantitatively beyond the socially accepted range.

There is one apparently fundamental division in psychiatry with: 1) The **neuroses**, (psychiatric illnesses where the patient has insight into his problems), and 2) the **psychoses**, (illnesses where the patient has no insight). Thus, a patient with an obsessional neurosis who is compelled to wash his face one hundred times a day, realises (even though compelled by anxiety to repeat the act over and over again), that this is absurd. Conversely, a psychotic may perform dangerous, criminal, anti-social or purely bizarre acts with no realisation of their absurdity or consequence. The neuroses are intriguing in that most are clinical syndromes only because they are (just) beyond the extremes of normal feelings or behaviour. Thus, every normal person has experienced depression and anxiety but in normal people these feelings do not become overwhelmingly powerful, preventing other feelings or destroying life's normal pattern.

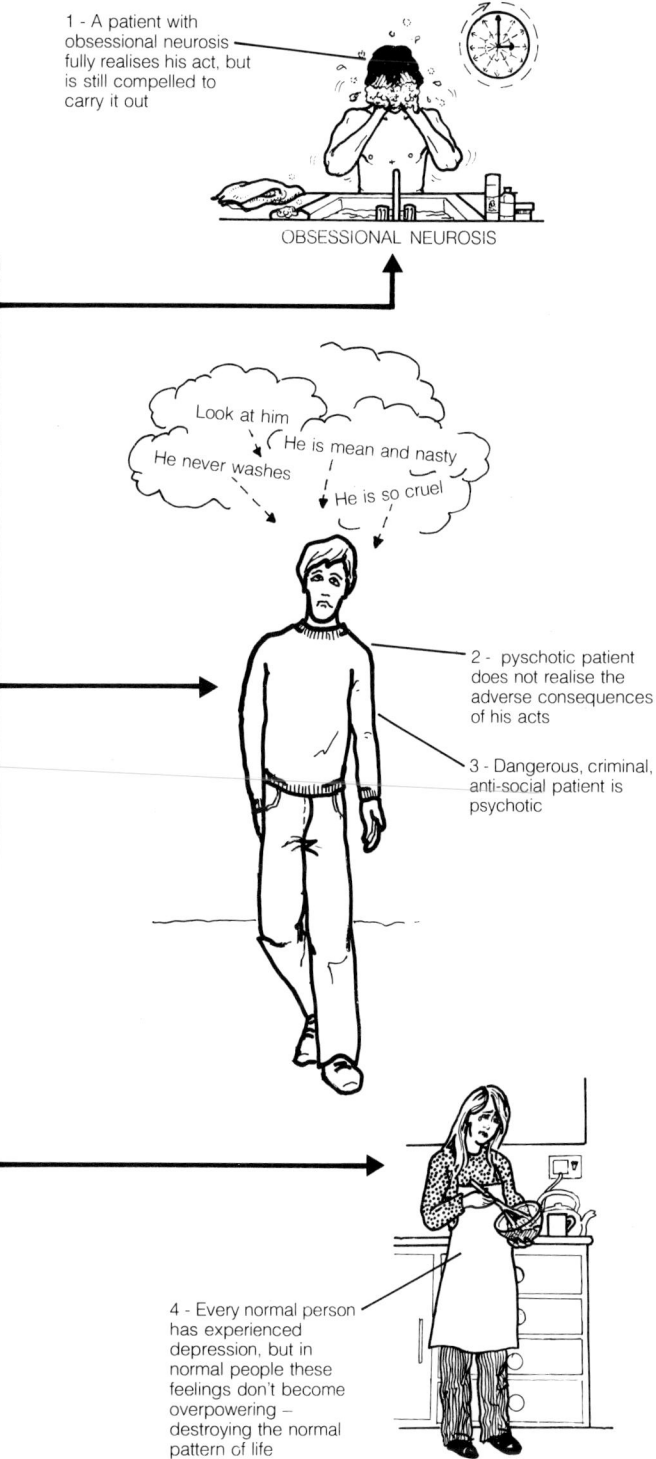

1 - A patient with obsessional neurosis fully realises his act, but is still compelled to carry it out

OBSESSIONAL NEUROSIS

2 - pyschotic patient does not realise the adverse consequences of his acts

3 - Dangerous, criminal, anti-social patient is psychotic

4 - Every normal person has experienced depression, but in normal people these feelings don't become overpowering – destroying the normal pattern of life

CLASSIFICATION OF PSYCHIATRIC DISORDERS

This easy, perhaps old-fashioned, classification has the great virtue of simplicity and this has great merit in such a complex subject.

The disadvantages of this classification will be alluded to in the later text, and as all classifications are imperfect, it is suggested that this serves as the introduction:–

0. Mental defect/subnormality

1. The **neuroses**
   i) anxiety states
   ii) hysterical conversion states/hysteria
   iii) reactive depression (neurotic depression)
   vi) obsessional neurosis

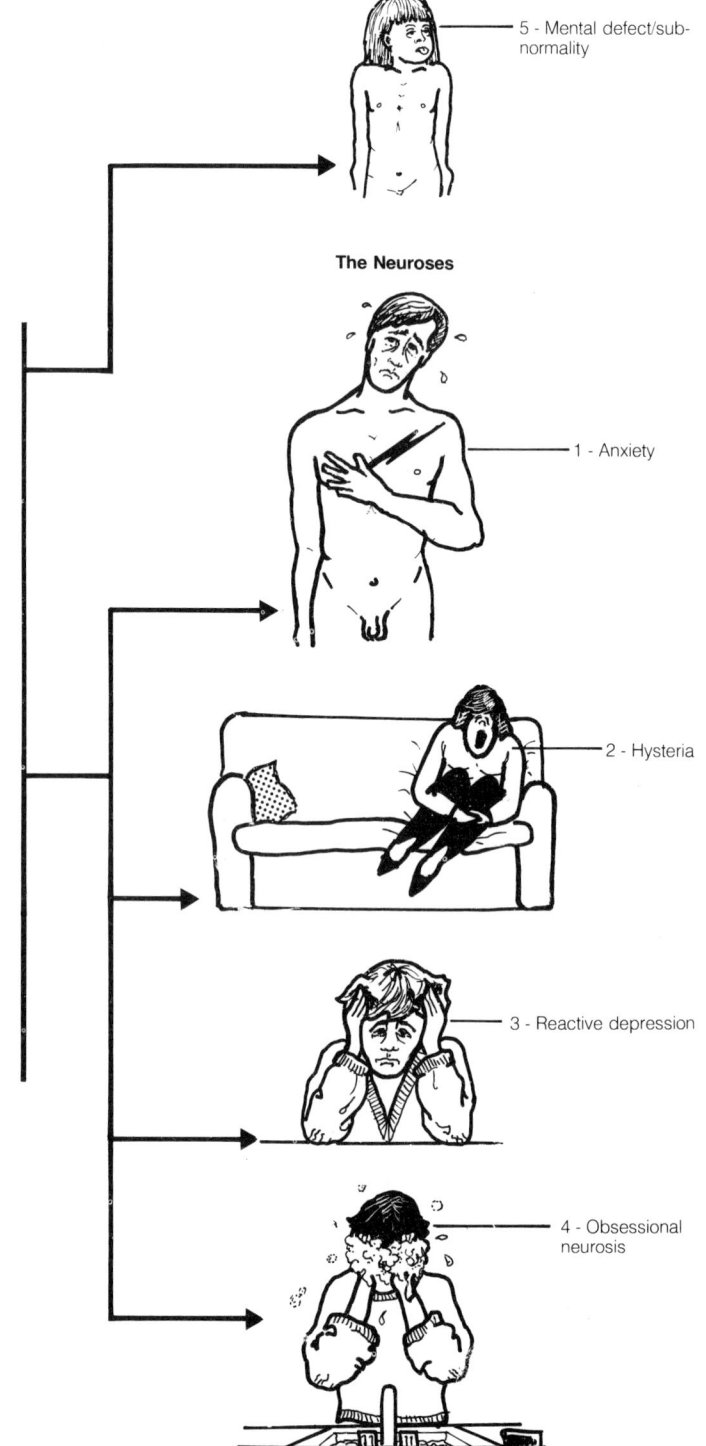

Classification of Psychiatric Disorders

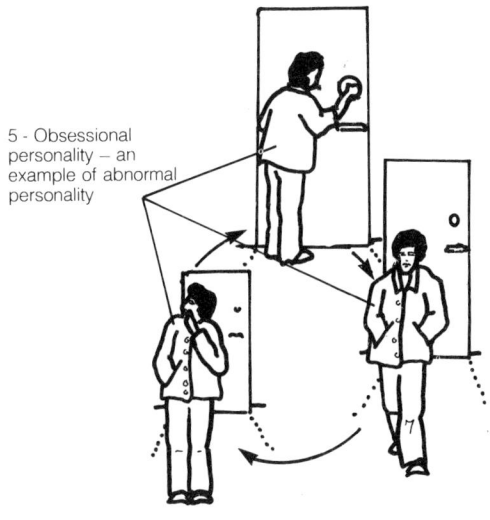

5 - Obsessional personality – an example of abnormal personality

2. Abnormal personalities

3. The psychoses
i) Functional psychoses – in which, so far, there is no evidence of a specific CNS lesion
  a) Manic depressive psychosis
  b) Schizophrenia

ii) Organic psychoses – in which the psychiatric disease is related to physical disease.

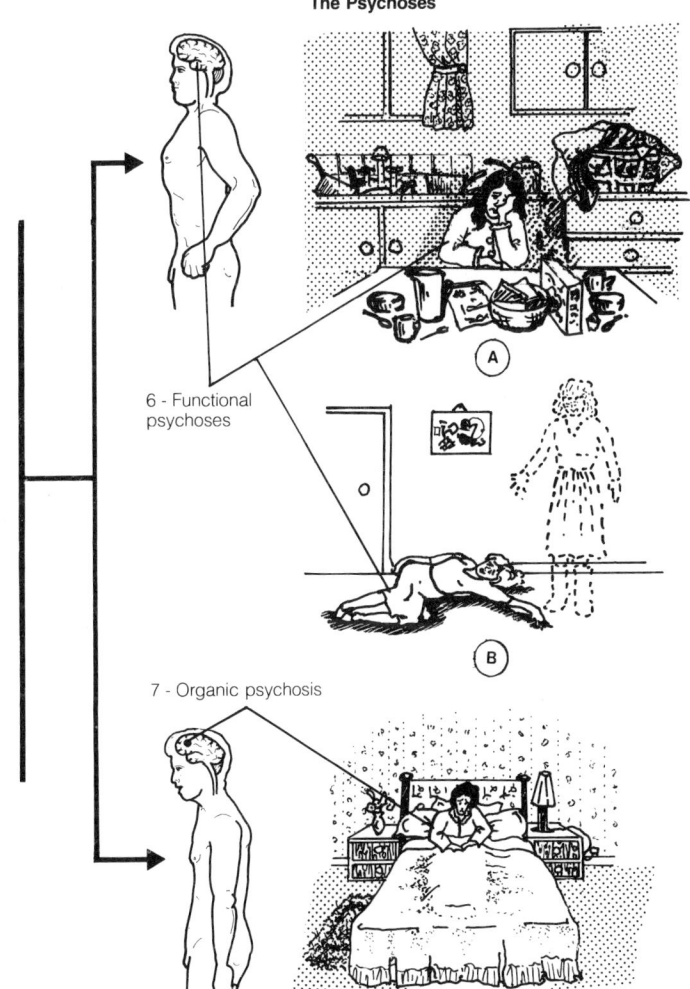

The Psychoses

6 - Functional psychoses

7 - Organic psychosis

201

THE PSYCHIATRIC HISTORY AND EXAMINATION

The clinician's purpose is to first understand the patient's problem and this is achieved by a lengthy dialogue/interview with the patient; both history taking and the psychiatric examination take place side by side as the experienced psychiatrist records and unravels the patient's history and psyche.

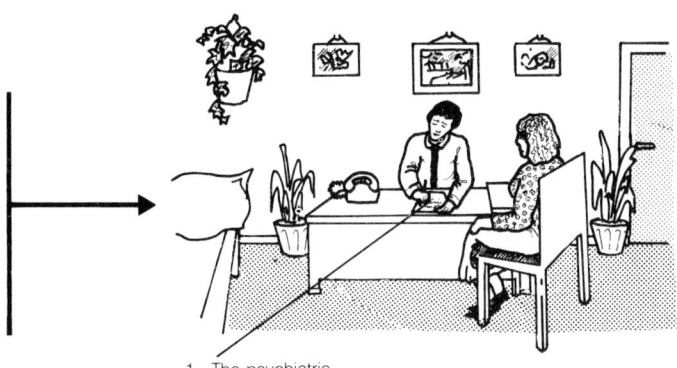

1 - The psychiatric history to assess the time of onset, length exacerbating factors, physical accompaniments

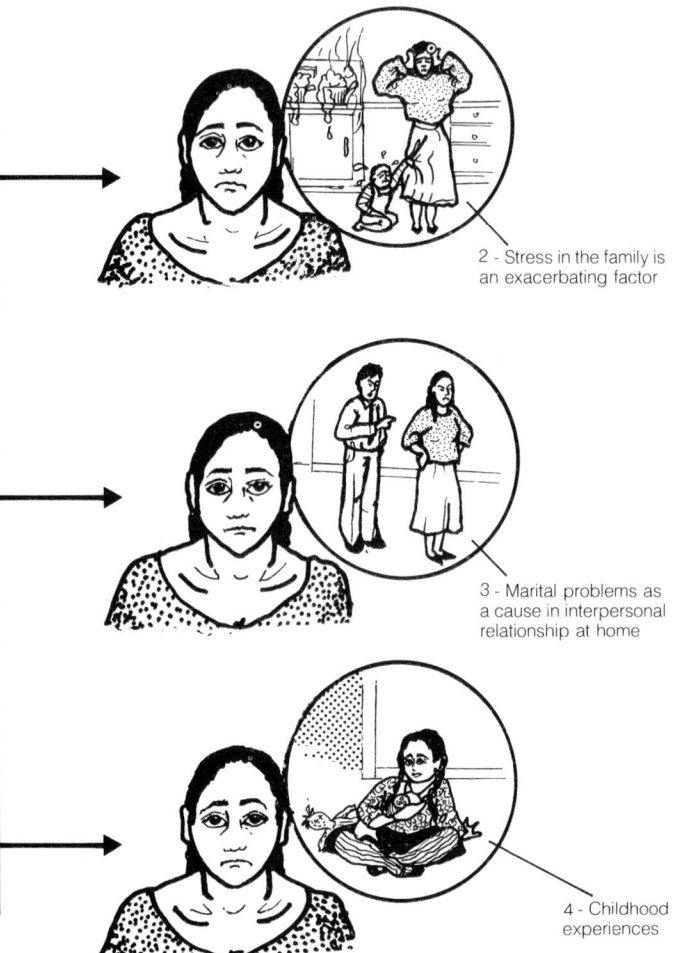

2 - Stress in the family is an exacerbating factor

3 - Marital problems as a cause in interpersonal relationship at home

4 - Childhood experiences

As in any speciality of medicine, the **history taking** commences with a record of the symptoms that have brought the patient to medical attention and then a full enquiry as to onset, length, exacerbating factors, physical accompaniments etc. Particular attention is paid to possible precipitants and stresses that might provoke the symptoms. The rest of the history includes everything that a good medical history contains but pays particular attention to family and social factors – interpersonal relationships at home and work. The clinician will enquire to a greater depth into the patient's personal history, from childhood experiences through to future aspirations. Never must these questions be phrased in a way to offend the patient but rather to set him talking about aspects of his life that may have contributed to the presenting state of mental conflict. Frequently, guilt, shame or inhibitions underly the patient's problems and it is only by gentle persuasion that these will be revealed.

The Psychiatric History and Examination

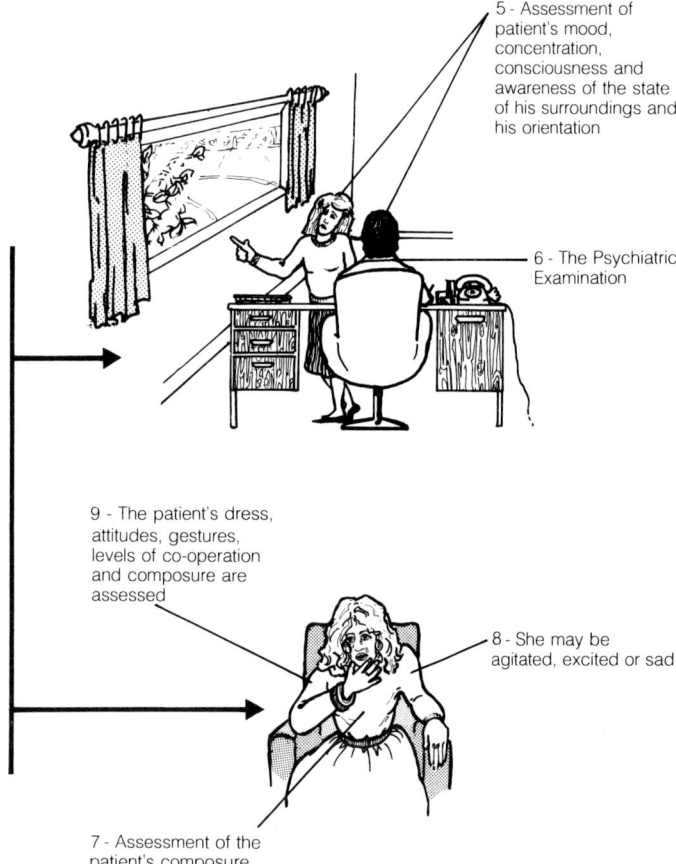

5 - Assessment of patient's mood, concentration, consciousness and awareness of the state of his surroundings and his orientation

6 - The Psychiatric Examination

9 - The patient's dress, attitudes, gestures, levels of co-operation and composure are assessed

8 - She may be agitated, excited or sad

7 - Assessment of the patient's composure

The **psychiatric examination** commences with the assessment of behaviour and then mood. An important initial evaluation is the level of consciousness and the degree of orientation or awareness the patient has with his surroundings; these two will govern the rapport that can be struck up in the consultation. The patient's dress, attitudes, gestures and general levels of activity cooperation and composure are all assessed during the conversation. The patient may be noted to be agitated or widely excited, to be "beyond contact", to be profoundly sad. All these observations are recorded. Similarly observations on mood and emotional display are noted.

The Psychiatric History and Examination

The patient's conversation ("talk") and thoughts are next assessed. For the conversation that commences at the outset of the consultation it will soon be obvious whether the patient is thinking fast and fluently or whether thoughts are slow, interrupted, not easily formulated, bizarre in content or logic etc. In general, thoughts are accelerated in agitation and anxiety and retarded in depression. Recurring topics of conversation (eg. suicide) should be carefully documented. Thought disorders will be more completely discussed later and any evidence of specific disorders of thought (eg. thought blocking, thought broadcasting, delusions etc.) should be carefully described in the psychiatric notes. The degree of insight must also be assessed.

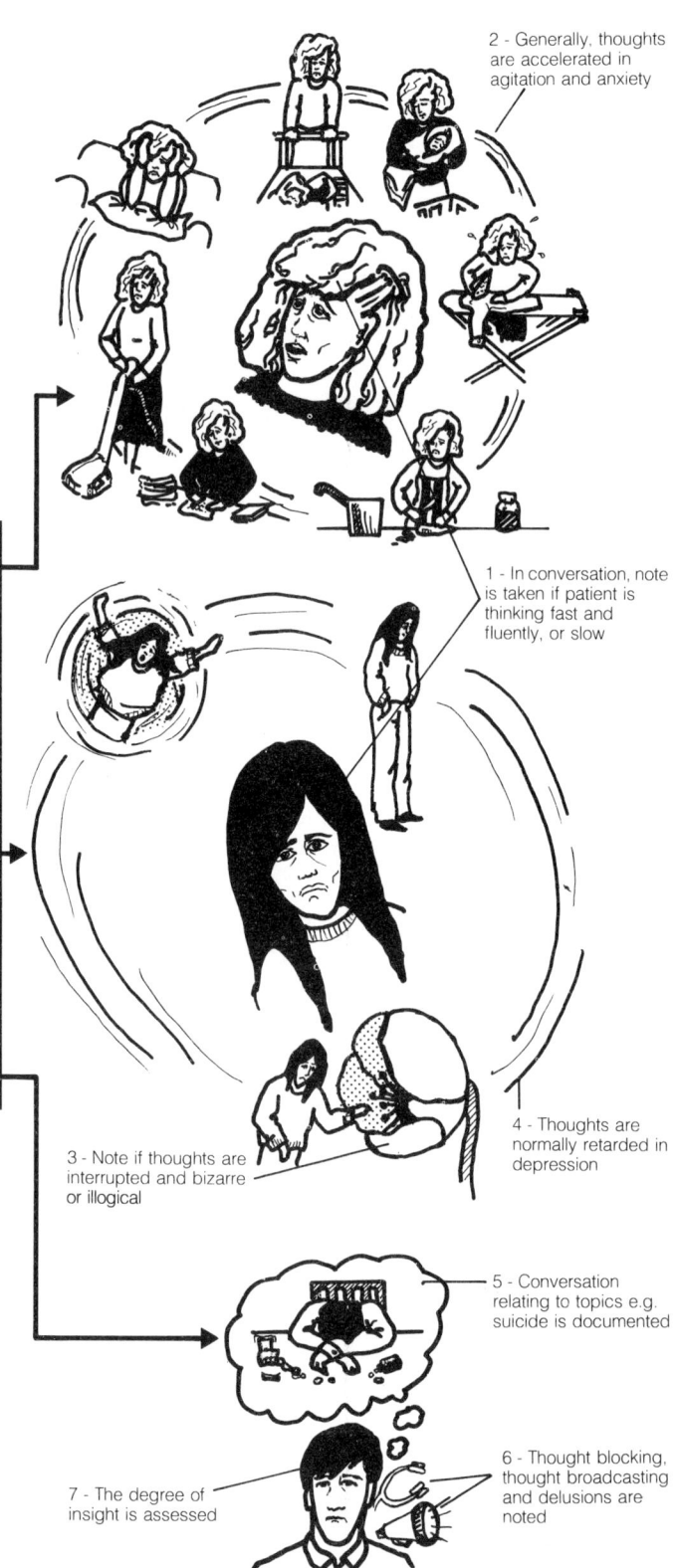

2 - Generally, thoughts are accelerated in agitation and anxiety

1 - In conversation, note is taken if patient is thinking fast and fluently, or slow

3 - Note if thoughts are interrupted and bizarre or illogical

4 - Thoughts are normally retarded in depression

5 - Conversation relating to topics e.g. suicide is documented

6 - Thought blocking, thought broadcasting and delusions are noted

7 - The degree of insight is assessed

Perceptual disturbances are sought throughout the interview. Illusions are perceptual misinterpretations and are most commonly encountered in the organic psychoses (eg. delirium), whilst hallucinations are false perceptions occurring in the absence of stimuli (eg. voices speaking "within the patient's head"). Although they may rarely be induced in normal people, hallucinations strongly imply a psychosis.

8 - In illusions, there is a misinterpretation of an object such that an omelette may be considered as a chocolate bar! Delirium tremens of alcoholism is a common cause

ILLUSION

9 - In hallucinations, a patient perceives an object or objects where in fact none exists

HALLUCINATION

10 - Cognitive functions such as memory concentration and intellect are tested

In the assessment of cognitive functions, memory, concentration, intellect and level of general knowledge for current events are all either formally tested or else they are assessed from the patient's performance at interview.

11 - Level of general knowledge for current events are also tested from patient's performance at interview

THE NEUROSES

Although there is frequently considerable overlap, it is helpful to distinguish anxiety states, hysteria and obsessional neurosis as three sub-types of neurosis.

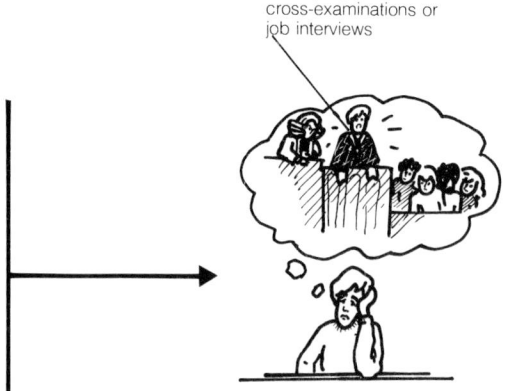

1 - "Normal" or healthy anxiety e.g. courtroom cross-examinations or job interviews

Anxiety – Everybody has experienced anxiety – a feeling of fear and apprehension. "Healthy anxiety" is experienced by most people under conditions of unaccustomed stress, (eg. interviews for jobs, court room cross examinations etc.)

Such anxiety is a normal response of the body to unaccustomed stress and is accompanied by extra-activity within the sympathetic nervous system leading to: tachycardia (perhaps with palpitations) and raised blood pressure, dry mouth, diarrhoea, frequency of micturition, sweating, headache, dilated pupils. This generalised adrenergic response to stress– this "flight and fright" response is an adaptive response seen throughout mammals and assists the body to counter stresses, (physical and mental).

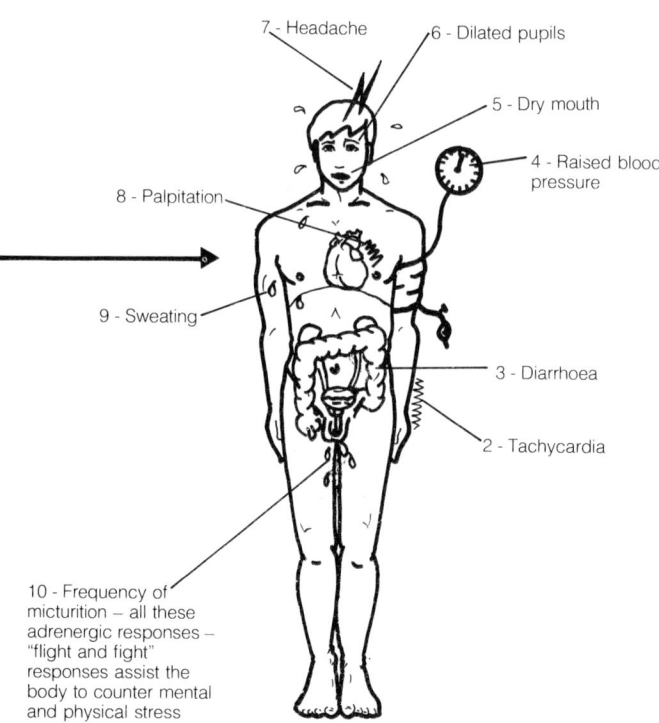

7 - Headache
6 - Dilated pupils
5 - Dry mouth
4 - Raised blood pressure
8 - Palpitation
9 - Sweating
3 - Diarrhoea
2 - Tachycardia
10 - Frequency of micturition – all these adrenergic responses – "flight and fight" responses assist the body to counter mental and physical stress

The Neuroses

However, **morbid anxiety** is quite different, continuing without a stress stimulus, pervading the entire mental life of the patient and detracting from the body's performance against stress. The patient is well aware that his anxiety is unfounded, but he cannot shrug it off.

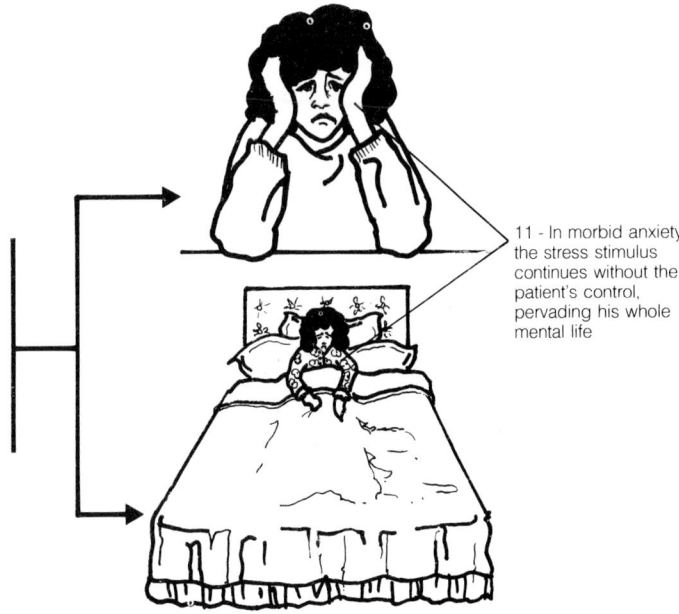

11 - In morbid anxiety the stress stimulus continues without the patient's control, pervading his whole mental life

The clinical presentation of the patient with morbid anxiety may be with the symptoms of continuous apprehension and the systemic concomitants described above. However, equally likely are complaints of "tremors", "butterflies in the stomach", "dyspepsia", "being constantly strung up", irritability or tension headaches.

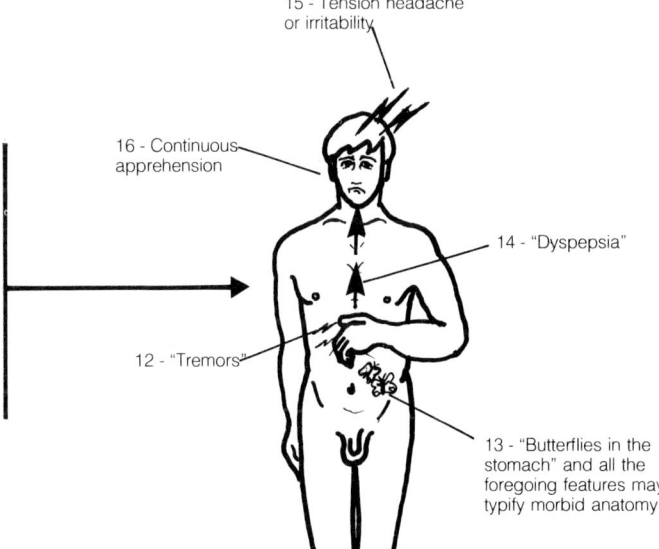

15 - Tension headache or irritability
16 - Continuous apprehension
14 - "Dyspepsia"
12 - "Tremors"
13 - "Butterflies in the stomach" and all the foregoing features may typify morbid anatomy

The Neuroses

There are many other symptoms in anxiety states. Anxiety tends to increase the tone in the voluntary muscles and this increased muscular tension in the muscles of the head, (particularly frontalis muscle), causes frontal headaches. Sleeping is typically poor in patients with anxiety states – both the getting off to sleep and broken sleep during the night.

Once healthy anxiety has been excluded, organic causes of anxiety states which include thyrotoxicosis, phaeochromocytomas, hypoglycaemic episodes, and even temporal lobe epilepsy – should also be considered in the differential diagnosis. Further, anxiety states may complicate predominantly depressive or even schizophrenic illness.

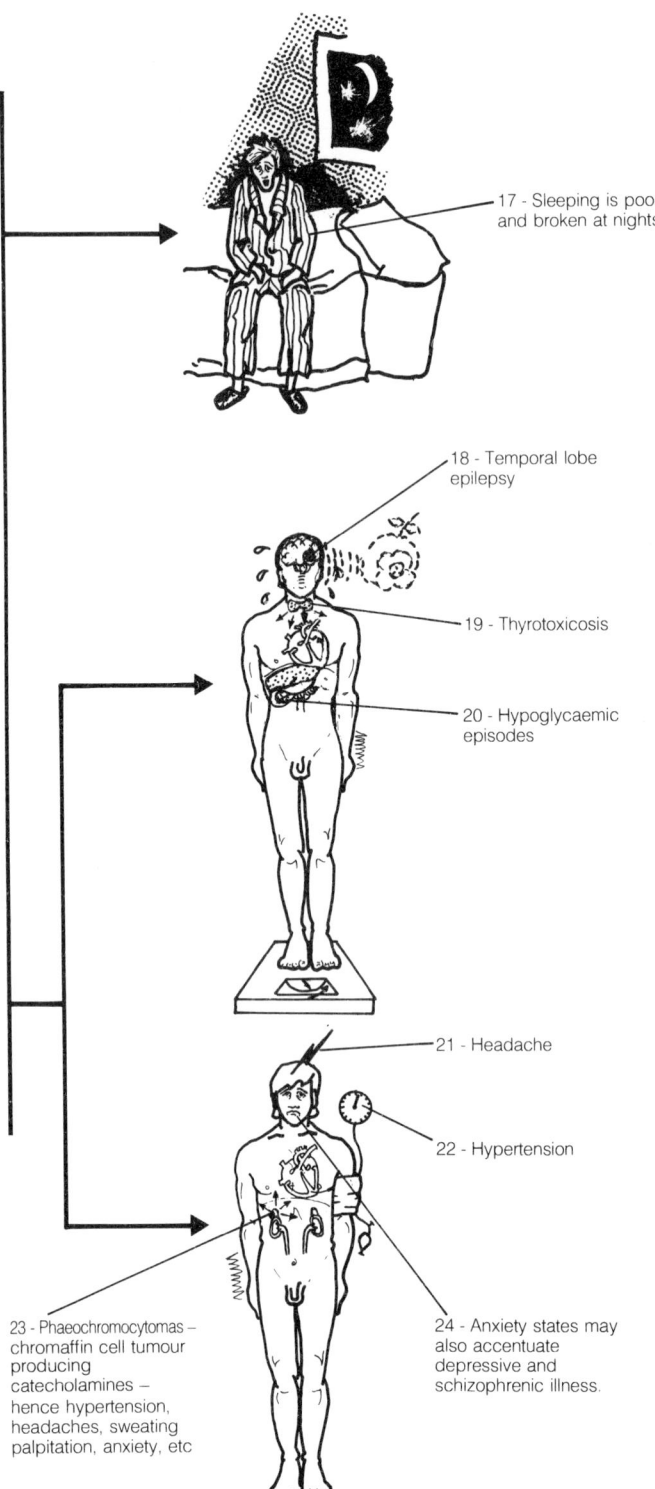

17 - Sleeping is poor and broken at nights

18 - Temporal lobe epilepsy

19 - Thyrotoxicosis

20 - Hypoglycaemic episodes

21 - Headache

22 - Hypertension

23 - Phaeochromocytomas – chromaffin cell tumour producing catecholamines – hence hypertension, headaches, sweating palpitation, anxiety, etc

24 - Anxiety states may also accentuate depressive and schizophrenic illness.

The Neuroses

Anxiolytic drugs (notably the benzodiazepine group eg. diazepam 10 mg tds) are useful in the management of acute anxiety states but psychotherapy is the mainstay of management for chronic cases.

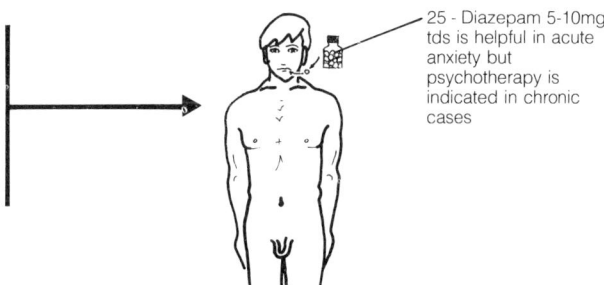

25 - Diazepam 5-10mg tds is helpful in acute anxiety but psychotherapy is indicated in chronic cases

Phobias – Agoraphobia (fear of open spaces) is perhaps the commonest severe phobic anxiety state and tends to occur in young adult women. Thus a newly married woman becomes housebound for fear of travelling in the big outside world. Such a phobia may often have a hysterical basis and can be incapacitating.

Another variety of severe phobia has an underlying obsessional basis – for example, the fear of being unclean or contaminated that results in over-elaborate exercises in hygiene. Much more mild and common are specific phobias – for example, fear of spiders, fear of the dark etc.

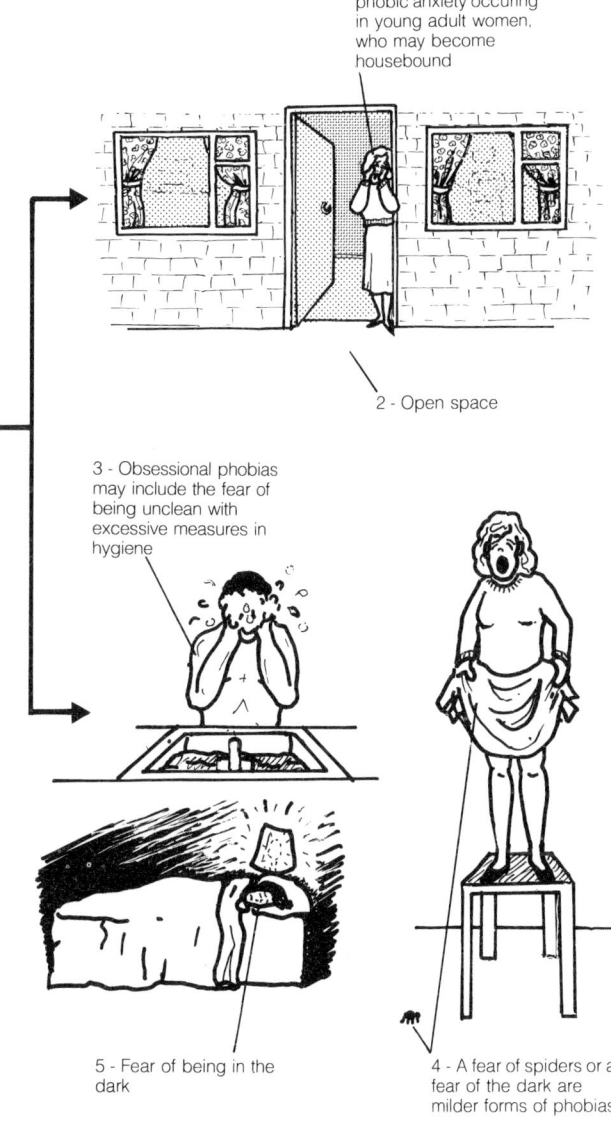

1 - Agoraphobia (fear of open spaces) is a phobic anxiety occuring in young adult women, who may become housebound

2 - Open space

3 - Obsessional phobias may include the fear of being unclean with excessive measures in hygiene

5 - Fear of being in the dark

4 - A fear of spiders or a fear of the dark are milder forms of phobias

The optimum therapy for phobic anxiety states usually includes behavioural therapy and anxiolytic drugs (eg. diazepam 10 mg tds).

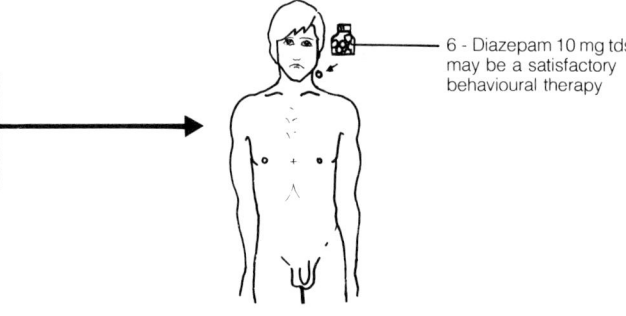

6 - Diazepam 10 mg tds may be a satisfactory behavioural therapy

Hysteria – In hysteria, mental or physical symptoms are developed by the patient as an attempted solution to a conflict or plight. The distinction of hysteria from malingering is that the malingerer consciously contrives his symptoms whereas the symptoms are at least partly subconsciously developed in hysteria.

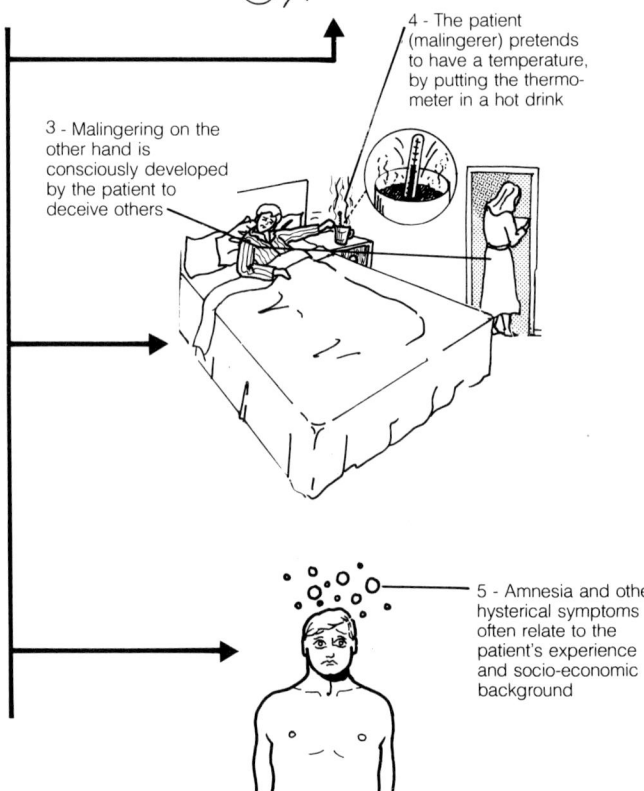

1 - In hysteria, the patient develops mental and physical symptoms (often subconsciously developed) to solve his/her conflict or plight

2 - Hysterical aphonia or inability to produce speech sounds from the larynx, not due to organic disease

3 - Malingering on the other hand is consciously developed by the patient to deceive others

4 - The patient (malingerer) pretends to have a temperature, by putting the thermometer in a hot drink

The type of symptom developed by the hysteric depends largely on his experience and socio-cultural background and may well relate to the precipitating conflict or stress – eg. hysterical amnesia etc.

5 - Amnesia and other hysterical symptoms often relate to the patient's experience and socio-economic background

The Neuroses

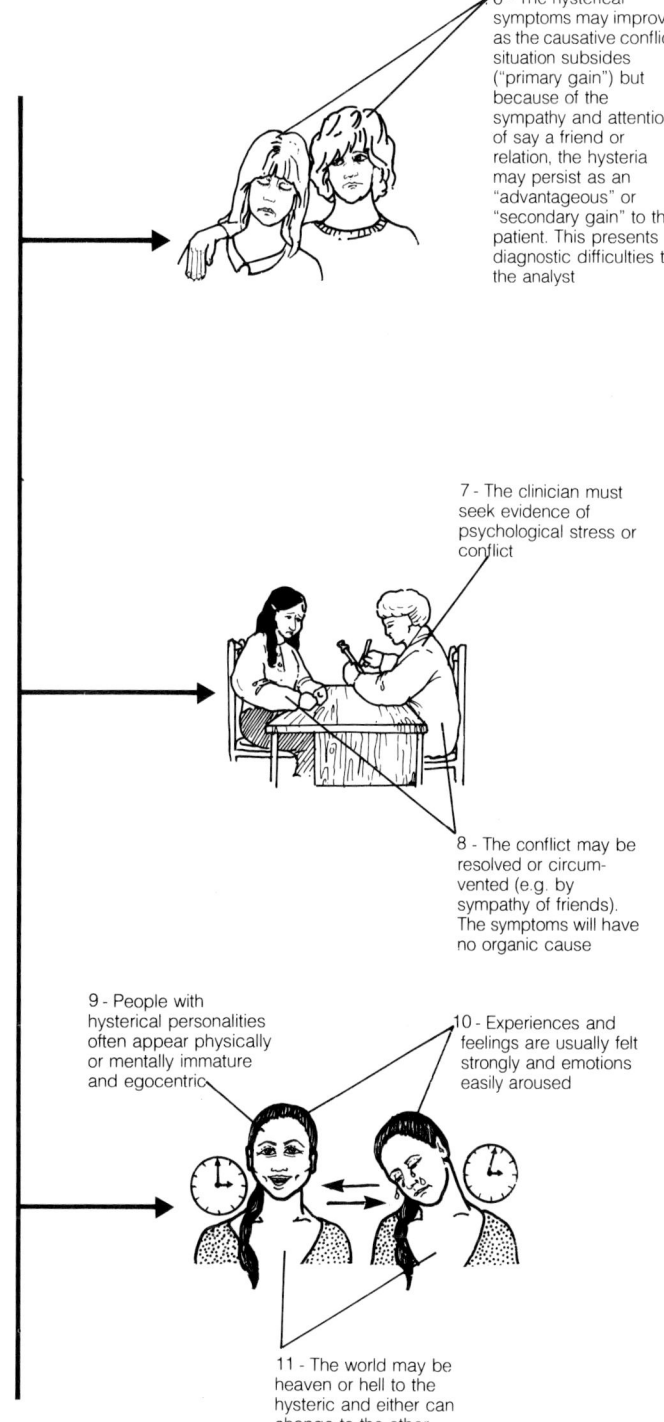

The hysterical symptoms may circumvent the conflict situation ("primary gain") but because of extra sympathy, attention and modifications in life style and pressures, the hysterical symptom may persist because it remains advantageous ("secondary gain"). The precipitating cause of the hysterical symptoms may then be difficult for the analyst to discover.

Hysteria must be a **positive diagnosis**. The clinician must seek evidence of a psychological stress or conflict which is partly resolved or circumvented by the development of physical symptoms for which there is no organic cause.

Hysteria is more common but by no means inevitable in people with hysterical personalities. People with such personalities often appear immature, (mentally and perhaps physically also), and egocentric. Experiences and feelings are usually felt strongly and emotions easily aroused. Interpersonal relationships are rarely deep or maintained. To the person with a hysterical personality the world is either "heaven" or "hell", and can quickly change from one to the other!

The Neuroses

The **treatment** of hysteria requires the removal of the source of conflict, the reduction or elimination of any "secondary gain" and assistance in bringing the patient to a more rational solution to stress by social readjustments. The skilled psychotherapist will not confront the patient with a direct attack on the conversation symptom but initially seek to circumvent the symptom. The acute hysteria reaction is treated by heavy sedation, (eg. chlorpromazine intramuscularly 50 mg 4-6 hourly).

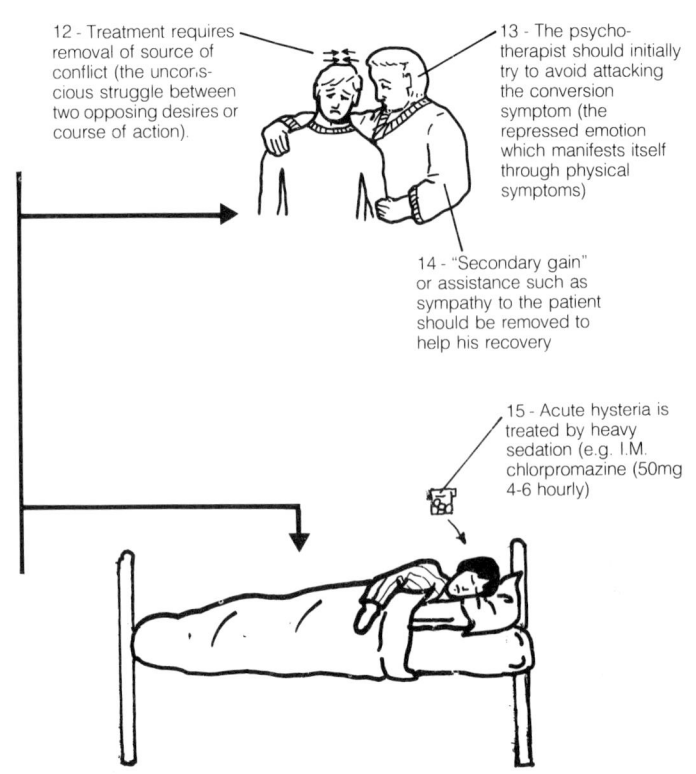

12 - Treatment requires removal of source of conflict (the unconscious struggle between two opposing desires or course of action).

13 - The psychotherapist should initially try to avoid attacking the conversion symptom (the repressed emotion which manifests itself through physical symptoms)

14 - "Secondary gain" or assistance such as sympathy to the patient should be removed to help his recovery

15 - Acute hysteria is treated by heavy sedation (e.g. I.M. chlorpromazine (50mg 4-6 hourly)

Anorexia Nervosa – This condition usually afflicts adolescent or young adult females and manifests as a failure to eat, or more accurately : "food rebuttal". Food rebuttal is the more accurate term as the anorectic may appear to have a normal appetite at table, yet by hiding or discarding food or even by self-induced emesis, the food is not digested. Weight loss is invariable and secondary amenorrhoea common; a growth of lanugo hair particularly on the back is also common.

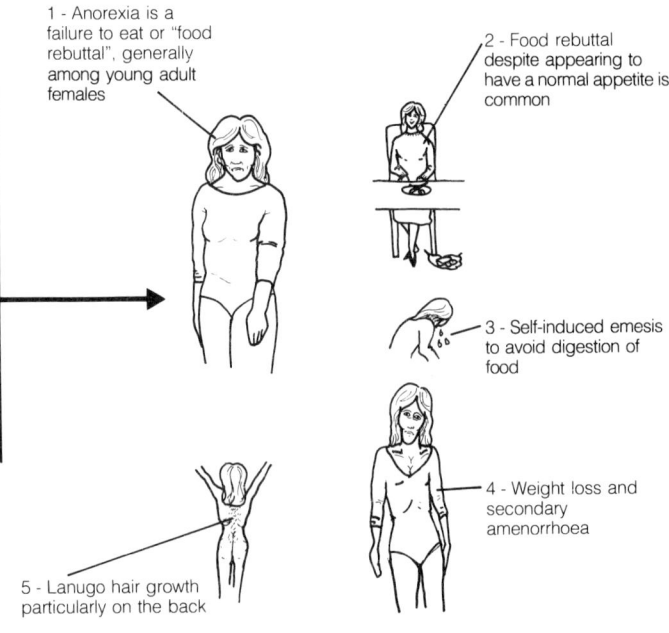

1 - Anorexia is a failure to eat or "food rebuttal", generally among young adult females

2 - Food rebuttal despite appearing to have a normal appetite is common

3 - Self-induced emesis to avoid digestion of food

4 - Weight loss and secondary amenorrhoea

5 - Lanugo hair growth particularly on the back

The Neuroses

The underlying stresses that induce anorexia are usually those of maturation from a girl to womanhood, particularly where there is family conflict together with an intolerable self-image of being overweight.

6 - A concomitant family conflict may add to the causes

7 - The causes of anorexia may be those of maturation from a girl to womanhood

8 - An intolerable self image of being overweight is another cause

10 - Psychotropic drugs, e.g. chlorpromazine may help reduce tension

9 - Treatment includes supervised feeding in a pleasant surrounding and a support for the psyche

Treatment involves supervised feeding in congenial surroundings and well-maintained support for the psyche. Psychotropic drugs (eg. chlorpromazine) may reduce tension and help the patient.

11 - Forced nasogastic feeding may be necessary to avoid starvation

12 - A few patients may recover but the prognosis is always uncertain

13 - Supportive care e.g. I.V. feeding

The Neuroses

In severe cases, nasogastric tube feeding is essential as a few cases will otherwise starve to death. The prognosis for less severe cases is never certain. Some continue in a chronic anorexic state whereas others recover.

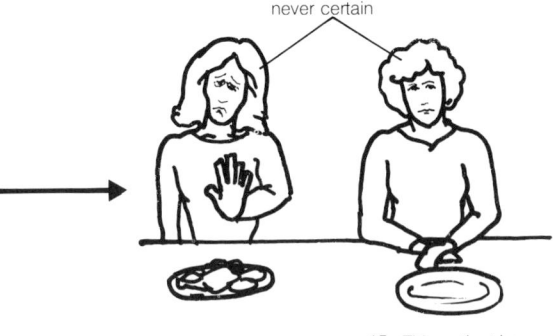

14 - The prognosis for less severe cases is never certain

15 - This patient has fully recovered from her anorexic state

Obsessional Neurosis – An obsession is a persistent thought or compulsion to action which the patient cannot rid from his mind, although he realises that this is senseless. A cardinal feature of these thoughts is that they occur against the patient's will and dominate the patient even though he may try to put them out of his mind. Thus a patient may feel compelled to wash his hands over and over and over again, or dress and redress many times in an elaborate ritual with a specific order for each detail. After some period of time, the patient presents to medical attention, when the symptom "has got out of control". Depression frequently accompanies the obsessional neurosis.

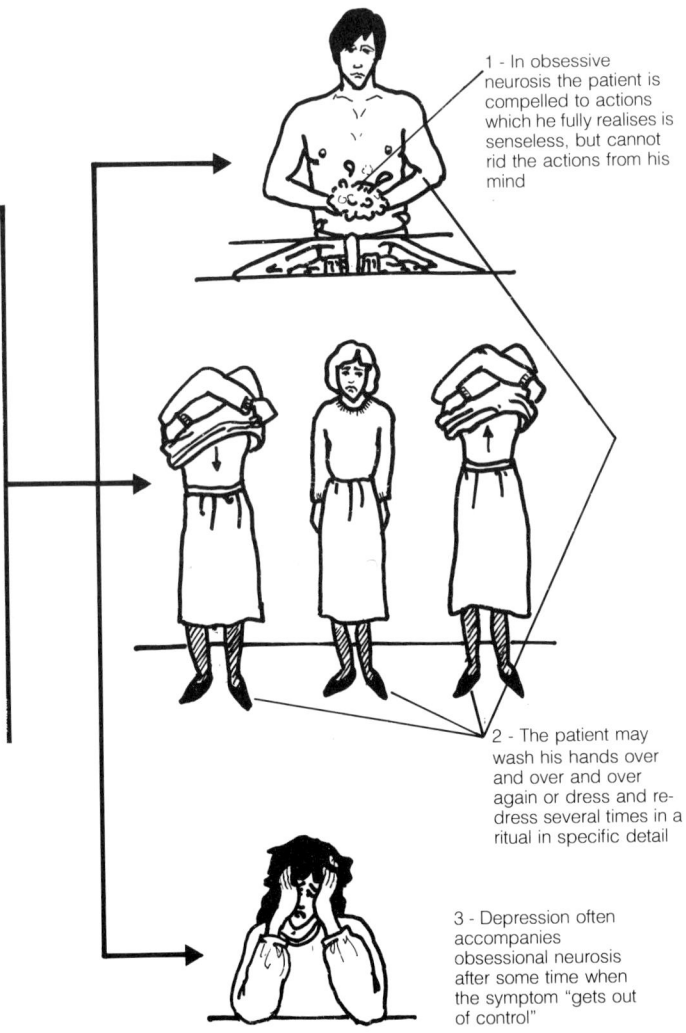

1 - In obsessive neurosis the patient is compelled to actions which he fully realises is senseless, but cannot rid the actions from his mind

2 - The patient may wash his hands over and over and over again or dress and redress several times in a ritual in specific detail

3 - Depression often accompanies obsessional neurosis after some time when the symptom "gets out of control"

The Neuroses

Obsessional neurosis is more common in brain damaged patients and is also more commonly seen in those people with obsessional personalities, although the personality may never give rise to the neurosis. People with obsessional personalities are from an early age pedantic, neat, punctilious and meticulous with an excessive concern for order and the need for re-checking that things have been done. Many of these people are tense and anxious and easily upset by disturbances in their otherwise ordered lives. Depression and obsessional neurosis may sometimes follow.

Treatment of obsessional neurosis is often different with supportive care being most important. Anxiolytic or antidepressive drugs may be appropriate in some individuals, in general, psychotherapy is not successful. Spontaneous remissions are common and the long term prognosis is often good.

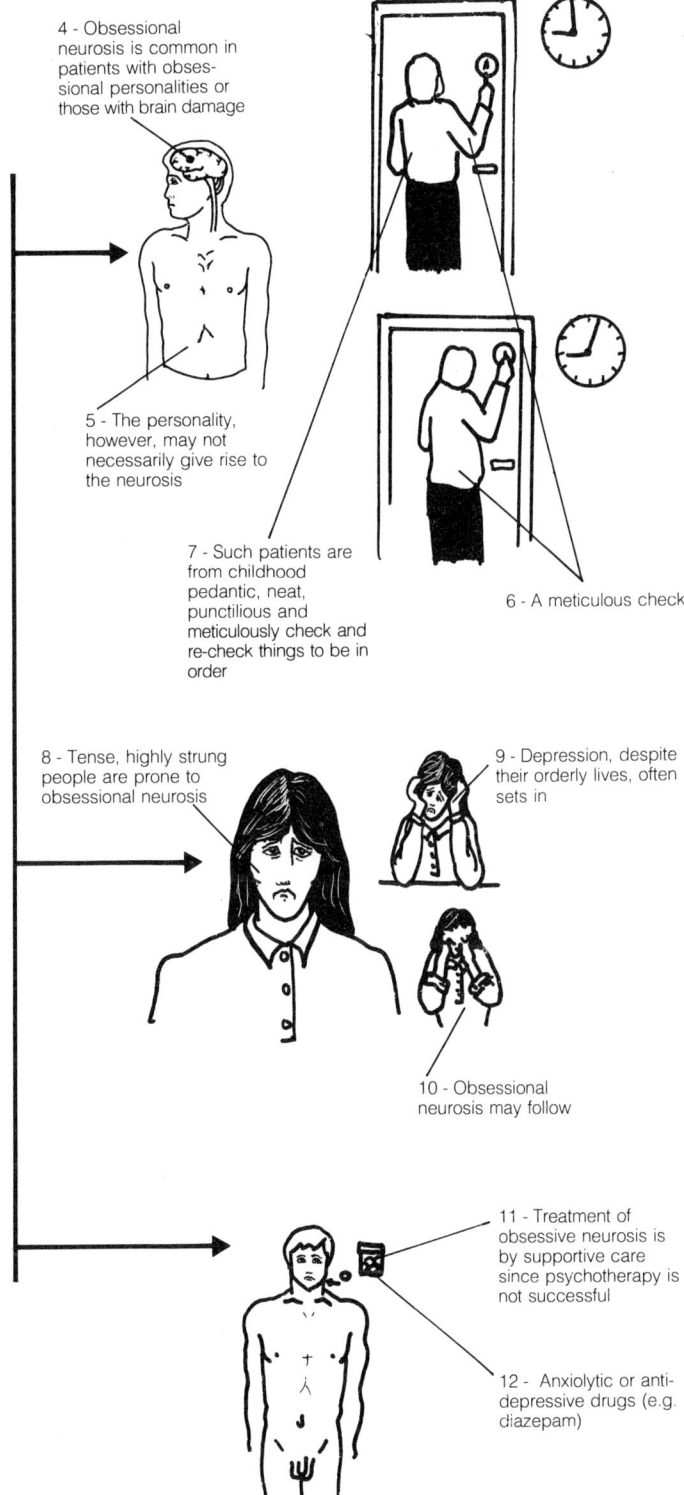

4 - Obsessional neurosis is common in patients with obsessional personalities or those with brain damage

5 - The personality, however, may not necessarily give rise to the neurosis

6 - A meticulous check

7 - Such patients are from childhood pedantic, neat, punctilious and meticulously check and re-check things to be in order

8 - Tense, highly strung people are prone to obsessional neurosis

9 - Depression, despite their orderly lives, often sets in

10 - Obsessional neurosis may follow

11 - Treatment of obsessive neurosis is by supportive care since psychotherapy is not successful

12 - Anxiolytic or antidepressive drugs (e.g. diazepam)

THE CLASSIFICATION OF DEPRESSIVE STATES AND REACTIVE DEPRESSION

Traditionally, two divisions of depressive state have been recognised:-

i) **Endogenous Depression** – A depression that arises and develops in the absence of any apparent precipitating enviromental cause; (see manic-depressive psychosis).

ii) **Reactive Depression** – In this state, the depression results from a reaction to environmental stress.

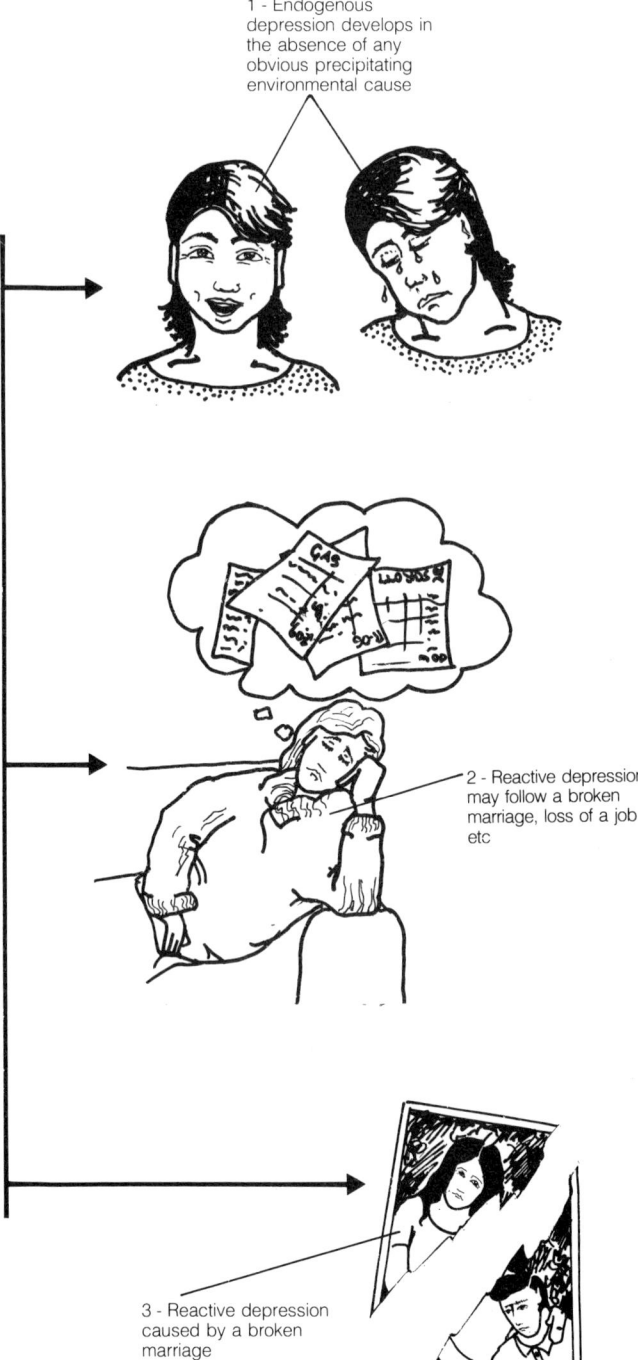

1 - Endogenous depression develops in the absence of any obvious precipitating environmental cause

2 - Reactive depression, may follow a broken marriage, loss of a job etc

3 - Reactive depression caused by a broken marriage

The Classification of Depressive States and Reactive Depression

Reactive Depression – Although a broken marriage or loss of occupation will lead to "gloom" or a depressed mood in most people for a time, this depression is amplified in those with a hypersensitive personality, to whom the event may only confirm an inner feeling of inadequacy. Such a person is often pre-conditioned for this reaction by his life pattern and inward expection of failure. Thus, such people have often timid or anxiety-prone and withdrawn personalities.

The **symptoms of depression** (see endogenous depression) are characterised by their tendency to "wax and wane" in response to environmental changes. There is usually difficulty in getting off to sleep, the patient lying awake pondering all the problems and stresses. The depressive mood is usually less severe than in endogenous depression and suicide attempts are usually "cries for help". The mood is responsive to environmental changes and psychotherapy and herein lies the key to reversal of this neurosis. Antidepressant therapy is sometimes appropriate.

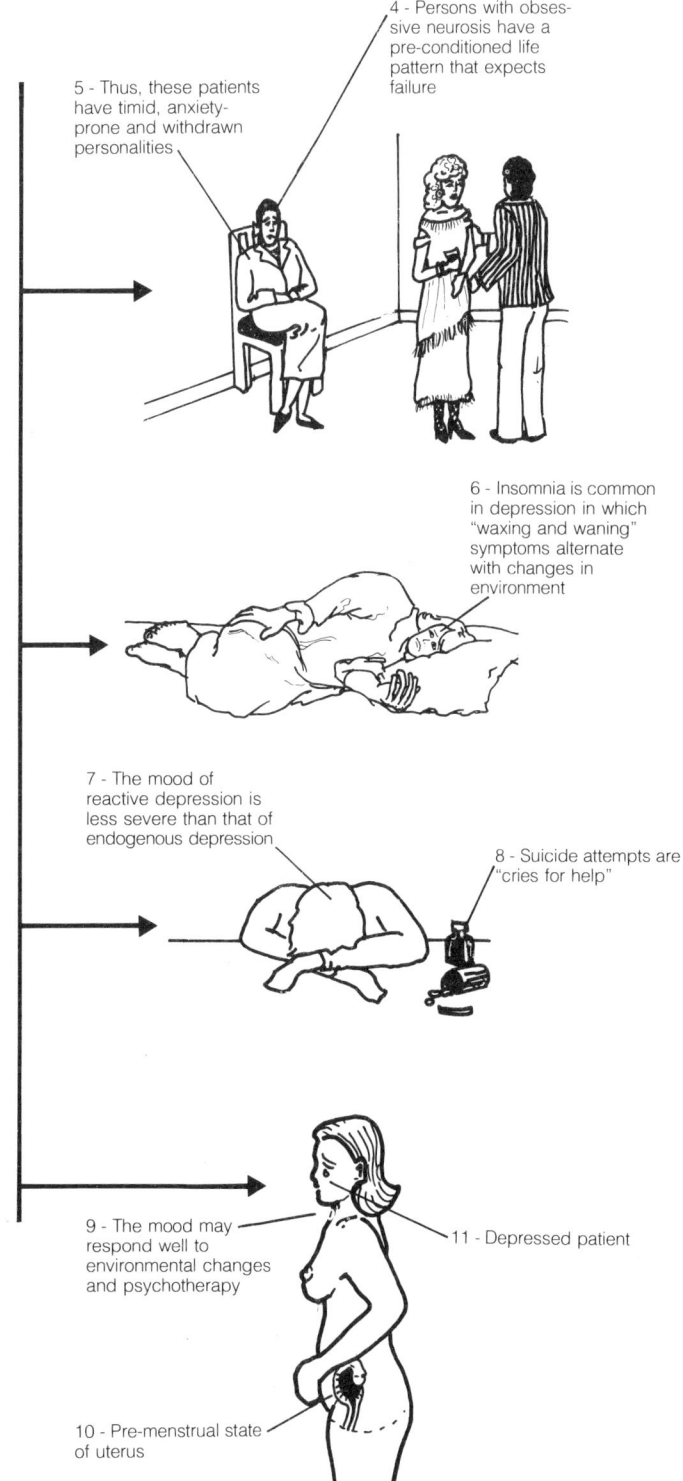

The Classification of Depressive States and Reactive Depression

Particular forms of depressive reactions are recognised in association with endocrinological changes, notably:– premenstrual depression, post-partum depression and involutional (peri-climacteric or menopausal) depression. Specific organic illnesses are well-recognised precipitants of depression, (eg. jaundice, chronic painful illness). Depressive states caused by these physical illnesses or states may be as profound and insoluble as endogenous depression and it is for this reason that many experts prefer to classify all the depressive states together under the affective disorders.

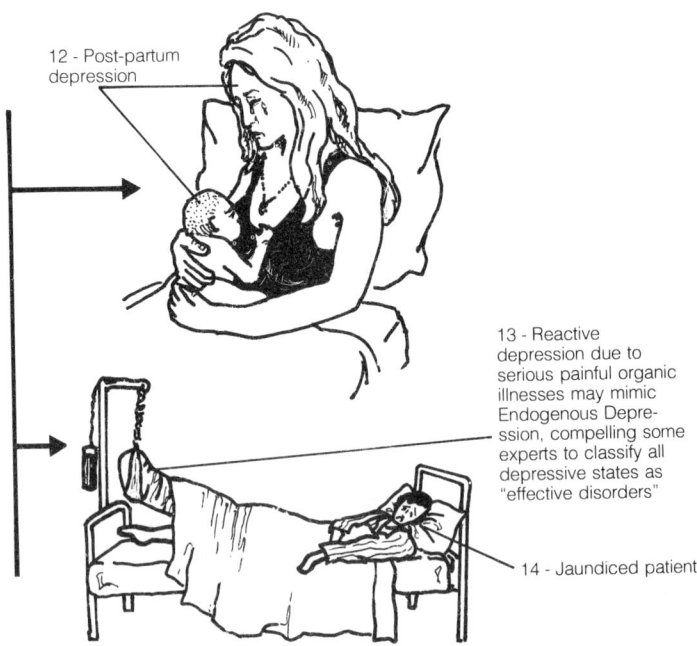

12 - Post-partum depression

13 - Reactive depression due to serious painful organic illnesses may mimic Endogenous Depression, compelling some experts to classify all depressive states as "effective disorders"

14 - Jaundiced patient

Abnormal Personalities The personality of a person is the distinctive individual character of that person and comprises a unique blend of affect/mood, intellect, desires, emotions and even physique. The personality is a relatively unchanging property of each person. The "abnormal personality" is an important concept in psychiatry as it underlies many psychiatric illnesses. In the U.K., the term "psychopath" is used for people with personalities leading to anti-social conduct, but abnormal personalities extend far beyond this limited definition. In most people, the variations in personality are within an accepted spectrum and "personality disorders" tend to be mild – perhaps at or only just beyond the extreme of normal. Personalities can be subgrouped, at least to some degree:-

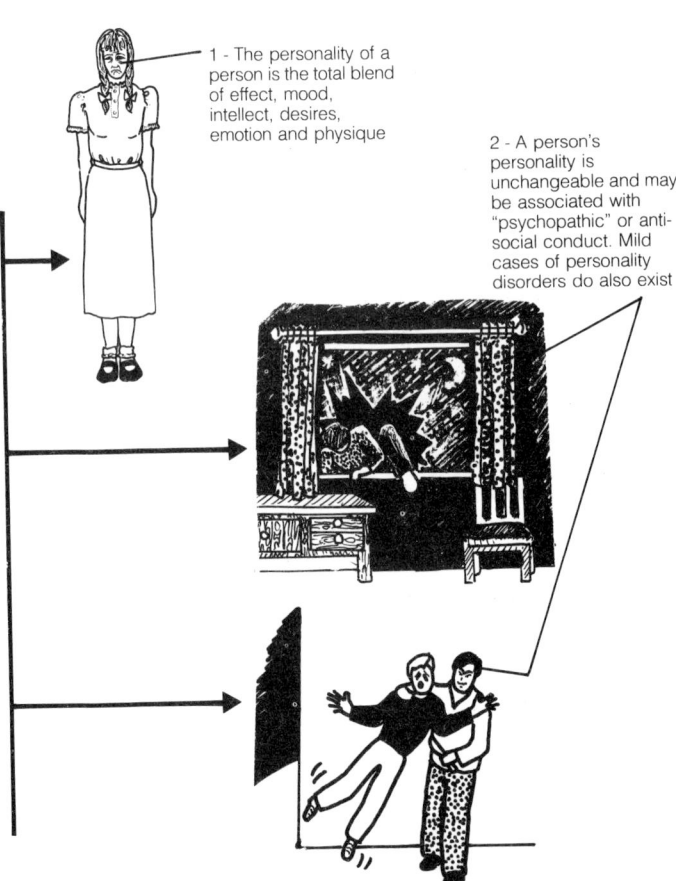

1 - The personality of a person is the total blend of effect, mood, intellect, desires, emotion and physique

2 - A person's personality is unchangeable and may be associated with "psychopathic" or anti-social conduct. Mild cases of personality disorders do also exist

The hysterical personality has already been described above with the adjectives and phrases: egocentric, emotionally labile, experiences felt strongly and shallow interpersonal relationships. The **obsessional personality** has also been described above and using the adjectives and phrases: pedantic, neat, puctilious, meticulous, excessive concern for order and the need for re-checking that things have been done. People with marked hysterical or obsessional personalities have some problems with integration into society and hysteria and obsessional neurosis, respectively, may develop.

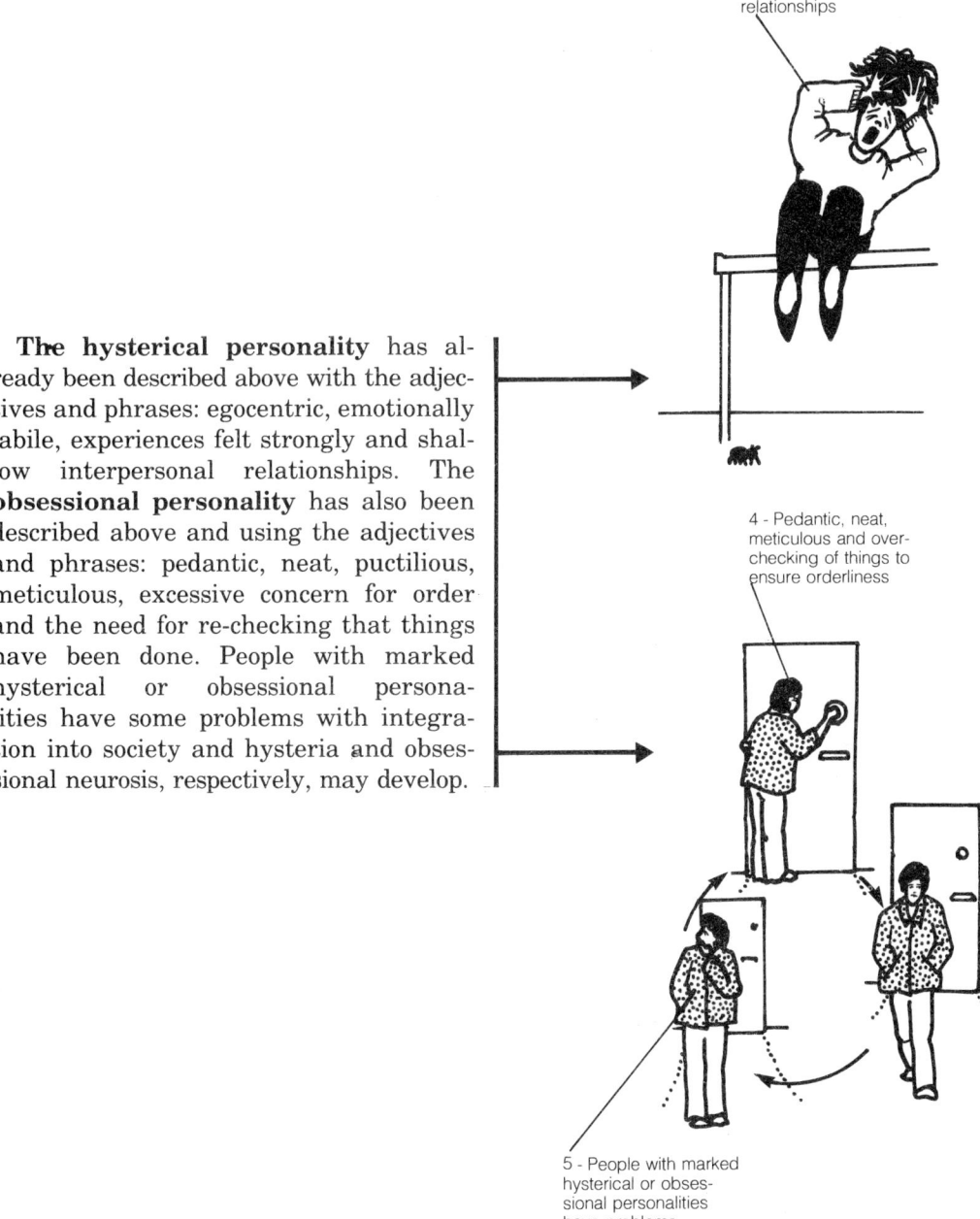

3 - Hysterical personality with emotionally labile and shallow inter-personal relationships

4 - Pedantic, neat, meticulous and over-checking of things to ensure orderliness

5 - People with marked hysterical or obsessional personalities have problems integrating in society

The schizoid personality describes a character who is shy, quiet and withdrawn; but, more than just this, he appears withdrawn in himself, an introvert. Such a person relates poorly with others and this makes his detachment from society more permanent. Emotions rarely surface and marriages are often unsuccessful.

If the person is of sufficient intellect, the schizoid trait may be advantageous to, (or even the cause of!) an academic life, where the person gains the respect of society by his works and by being aloof and seclusive.

Less socially acceptable is the person whose introversion demonstrates fanatical traits. Perhaps 50% of schizophrenics have this pre-morbid personality. **The paranoid personality** describes a suspicious and extremely sensitive character who over-reacts to even mild criticism. People with paranoid personalities may fanatically adhere to or propagate a religion, a political creed, "a cause" etc. Criticism of their following may lead to fury and violence.

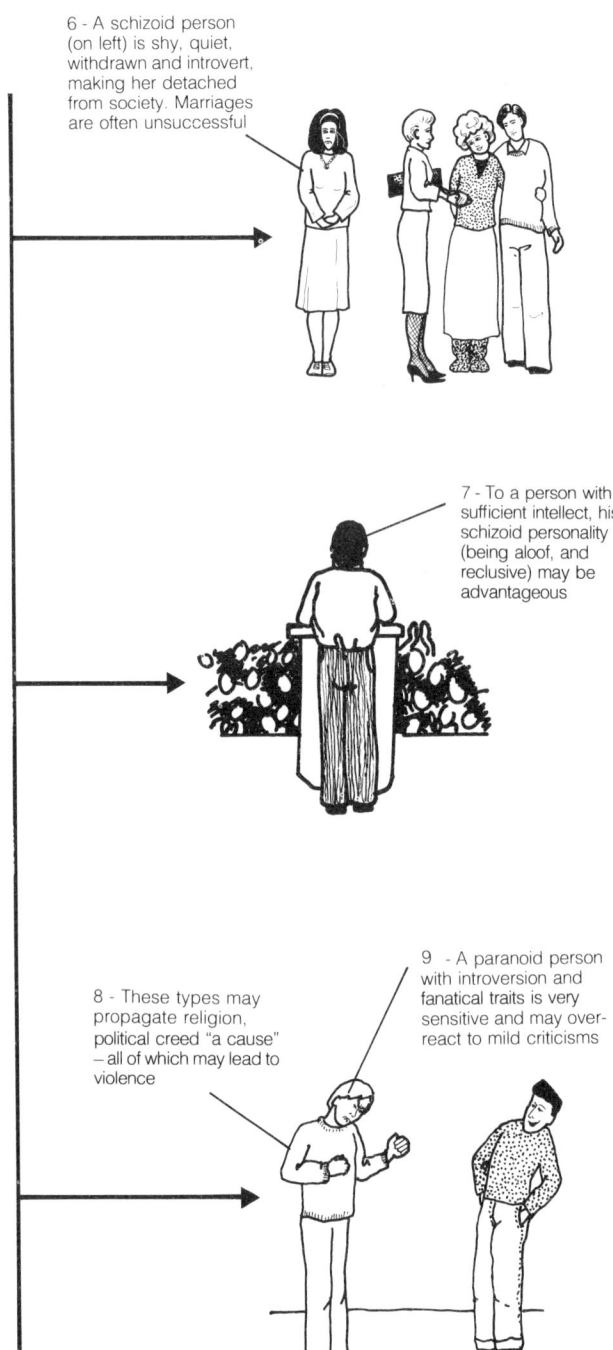

6 - A schizoid person (on left) is shy, quiet, withdrawn and introvert, making her detached from society. Marriages are often unsuccessful

7 - To a person with sufficient intellect, his schizoid personality (being aloof, and reclusive) may be advantageous

8 - These types may propagate religion, political creed "a cause" – all of which may lead to violence

9 - A paranoid person with introversion and fanatical traits is very sensitive and may over-react to mild criticisms

The Classification of Depressive States and Reactive Depression

The antisocial personality (psychopath) is perhaps the most important problem to society as these people are basically unable to control their impulses or emotions and are lacking in foresight. The antisocial personality may be a product of a neglected childhood environment and the most worrying parts of the personality differ between individuals, (eg. sadism, uncontrollable rages etc.). The true psychopath is unreliable, immoral by usual standards, untruthful and with criminal tendencies.

Bearing in mind the introductory remarks on personalities, it should be remembered that the antisocial personality may only be at one end of the normal spectrum and it is not an illness per se. However, immorality and criminal tendencies, (with an ambivalent disregard for morals and laws) may lead to legal and medical intervention. At this time, group psychotherapy may help patients to become more aware of the repercussions of their acts on others, and some improvement.

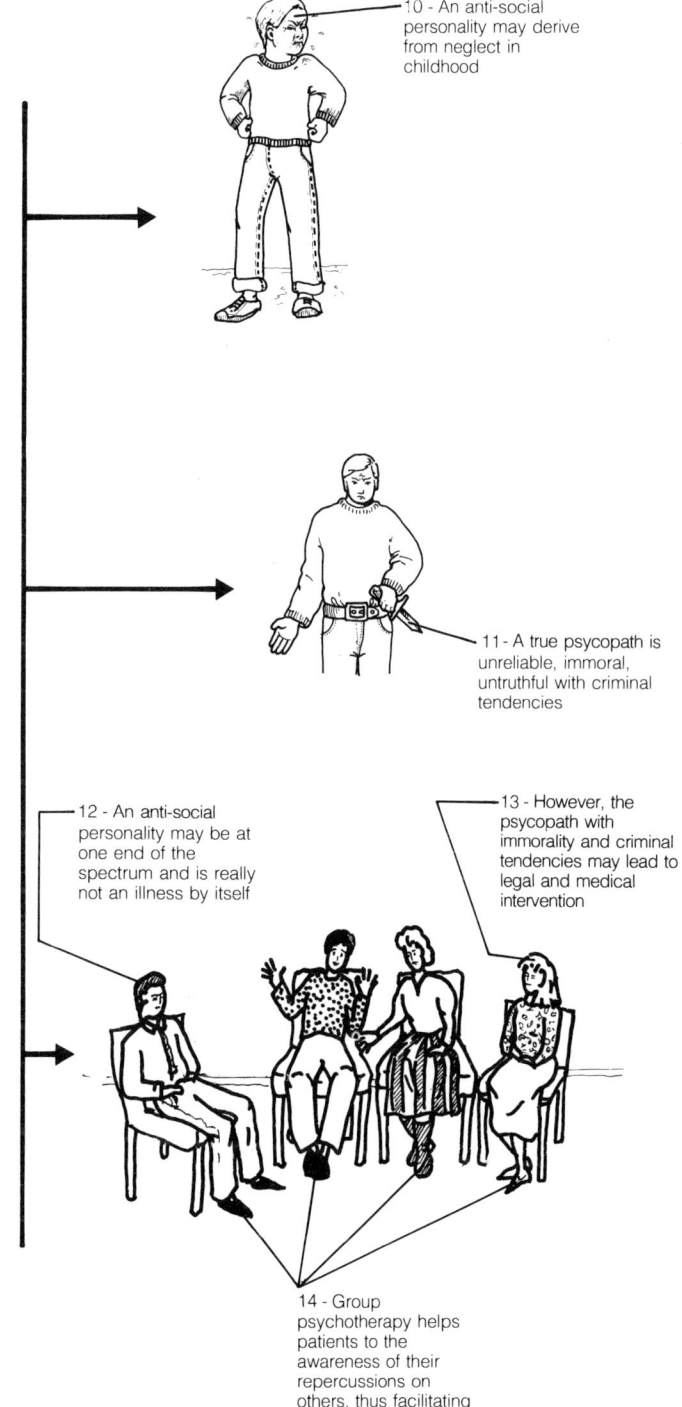

10 - An anti-social personality may derive from neglect in childhood

11 - A true psycopath is unreliable, immoral, untruthful with criminal tendencies

12 - An anti-social personality may be at one end of the spectrum and is really not an illness by itself

13 - However, the psycopath with immorality and criminal tendencies may lead to legal and medical intervention

14 - Group psychotherapy helps patients to the awareness of their repercussions on others, thus facilitating an improvement

Functional Psychoses

Lastly, the person with an **inadequate personality** is a negative thinker, being easily led and deceived, submitting easily to pressures. These are usually unsuccessful people whose lives are studded with failures and mistakes. Other personality types will be mentioned in the chapter.

FUNCTIONAL PSYCHOSES
Manic depressive illness – This term has been used to describe the range or "swing" of a severe affective disorder from endogenous depression with delusion through to mania, this afflicts perhaps 2% of the population. The two ends of this spectrum will be discussed separately:

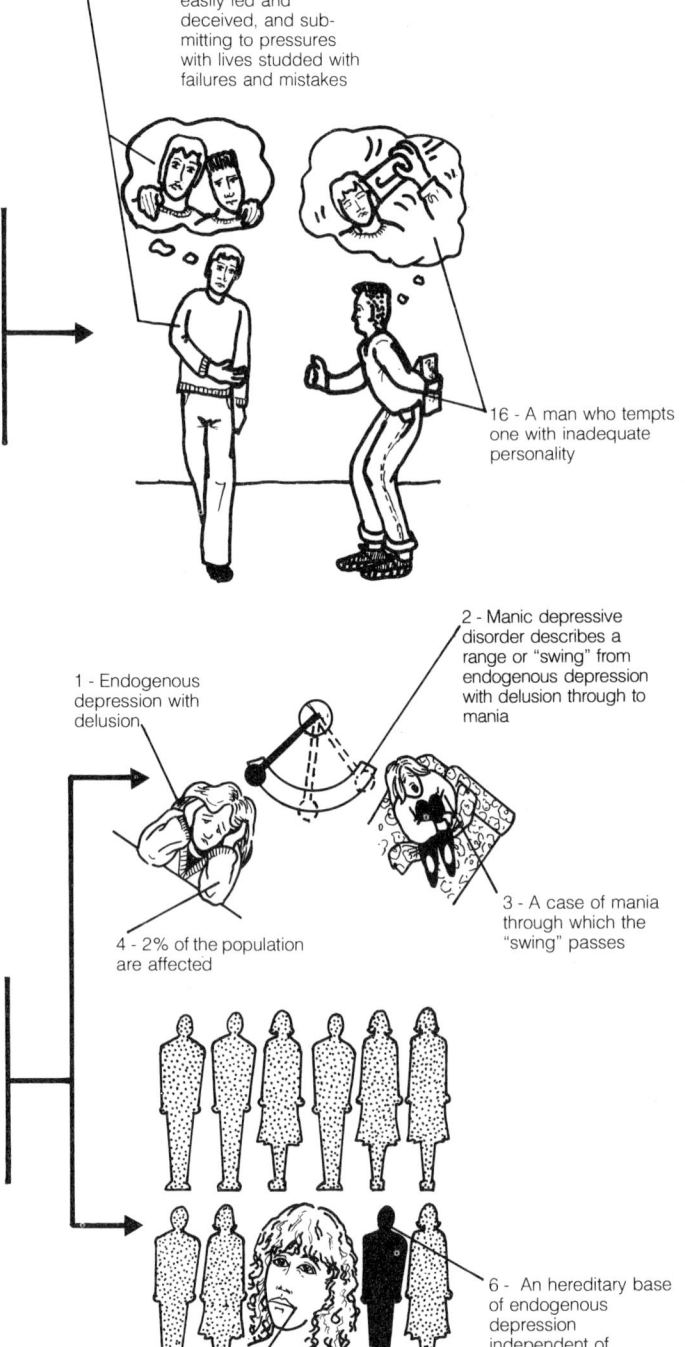

Endogenous Depression – In depression, there is a sustained and unrelenting mood of sadness and misery. There is no definable precipitating cause and a changing environment does not alleviate the condition. There is a hereditary basis to the development of endogenous depression – quite apart form any environmental factors affecting the family; at least 10% of relatives suffer endogenous depression.

Endogenous depression has been described as occurring typically in those people of a cyclothymic personality, (a personality with large mood swings from extreme cheerfulness and jollity to gloom and despair), and with a "pyknic" build (truncal obesity). However, an obsessional personality is also associated with endogenous depression.

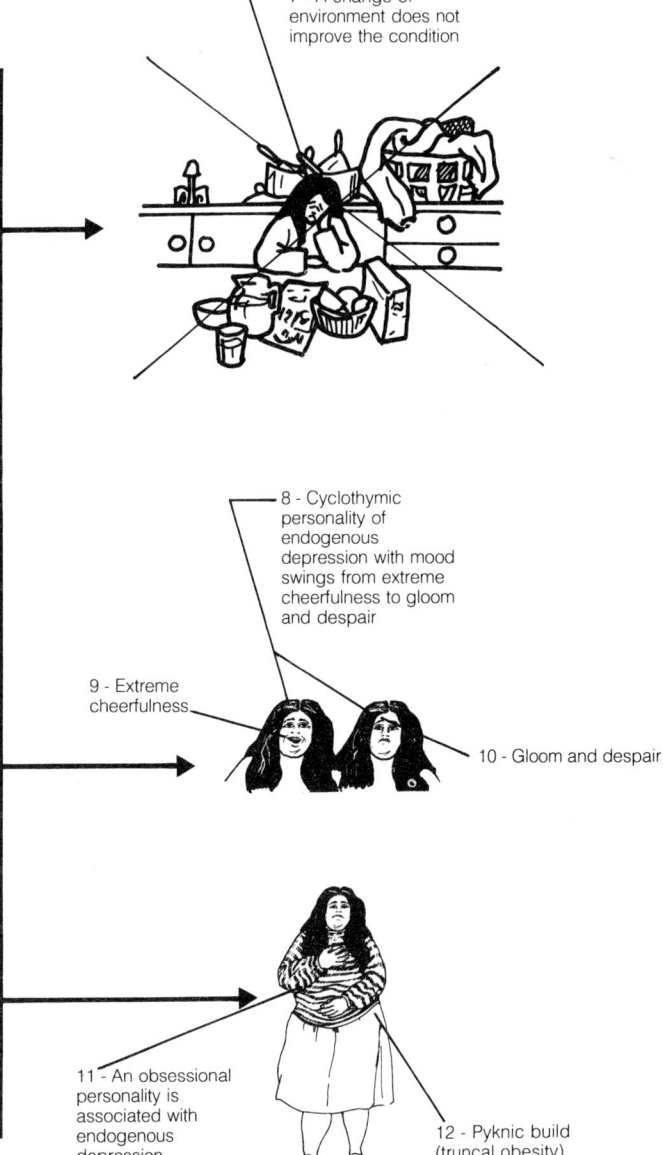

Functional Psychoses

The **clinical presentation** may be: "poor work performance", "no energy", "excessive tiredness" or other epiphenomena of depression. History taking will always disclose a mood disturbance with perpetual inner misery and expectations of a bleak future. The patient dwells on minor problems to an extreme length. A varying degree of anxiety is commonly present. Psychomotor activities are retarded such that thought and concentration, talk, intellectual activities, even movements are slow and laboured – facts about which the patient is well aware and about which he may bitterly complain.

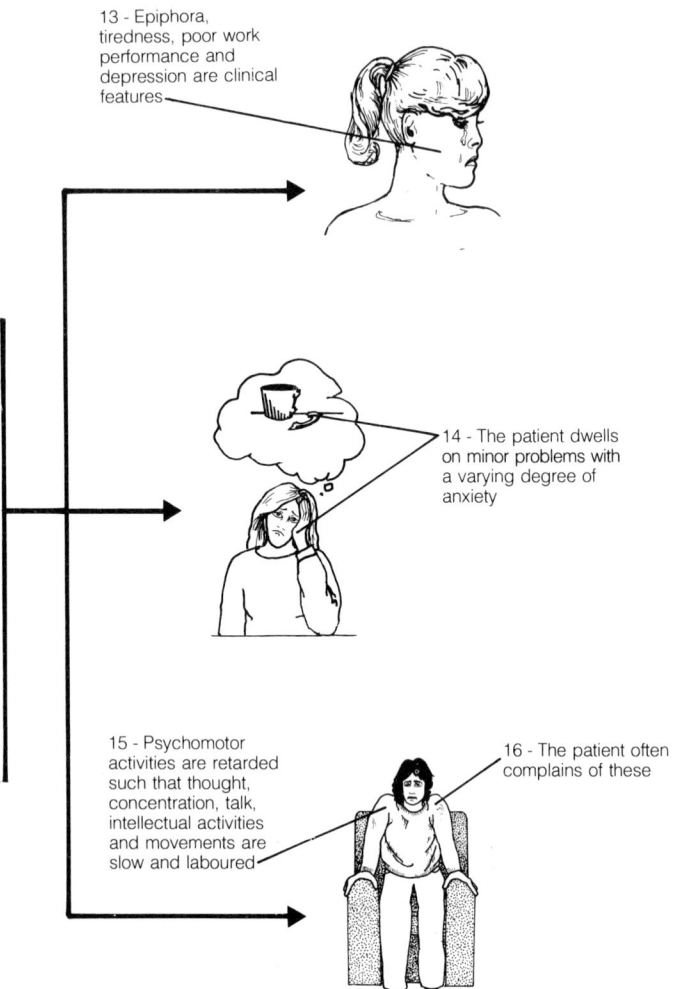

13 - Epiphora, tiredness, poor work performance and depression are clinical features

14 - The patient dwells on minor problems with a varying degree of anxiety

15 - Psychomotor activities are retarded such that thought, concentration, talk, intellectual activities and movements are slow and laboured

16 - The patient often complains of these

Functional Psychoses

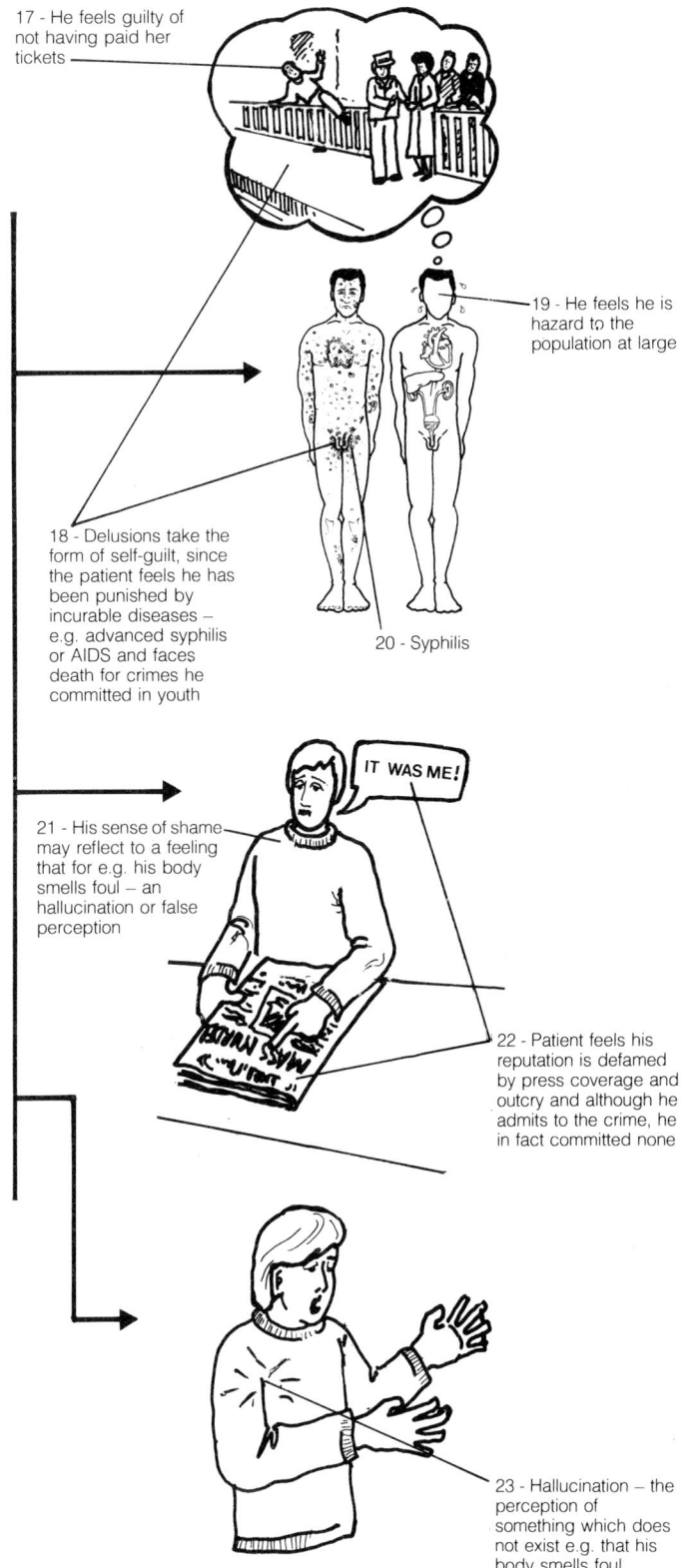

17 - He feels guilty of not having paid her tickets

19 - He feels he is hazard to the population at large

18 - Delusions take the form of self-guilt, since the patient feels he has been punished by incurable diseases – e.g. advanced syphilis or AIDS and faces death for crimes he committed in youth

20 - Syphilis

21 - His sense of shame may reflect to a feeling that for e.g. his body smells foul – an hallucination or false perception

22 - Patient feels his reputation is defamed by press coverage and outcry and although he admits to the crime, he in fact committed none

23 - Hallucination – the perception of something which does not exist e.g. that his body smells foul

Delusions are not uncommon and frequently take the form of self-guilt to be punished by damnation, poverty or incurable disease. Thus a severely depressed man who had consistently evaded paying for train tickets in his youth, much later became convinced that retribution had come upon him with the acquisition of advanced syphilis which would lead to his death and before that prove a health hazard to the population at large.

Other examples include depressives who confess to crimes that have received press coverage and public outcry. Hallucinations may occur and once again tend to relate to the patient's sense of shame – eg. That his body smells foul.

Functional Psychoses

The physical accompaniments of depression begin with apathy and easy exhaustion. Thus, minor work loads become impossible to perform even over an extended time period, or even impossible to contemplate. Loss of appetite and weight loss are common and hypochondriasis frequently relates to "constipation". Insomnia is very frequent, most characteristically with early morning wakening – being unable to get back to sleep and lying awake pondering about the gloomy present and future. There is commonly absent libido and consequently impotence. Weight loss is common.

Anxiety is present to some degree in every depressive, and is commonly manifest in the elderly depressive with constant fretting over minor matters and physical manifestations eg. hand wringing.

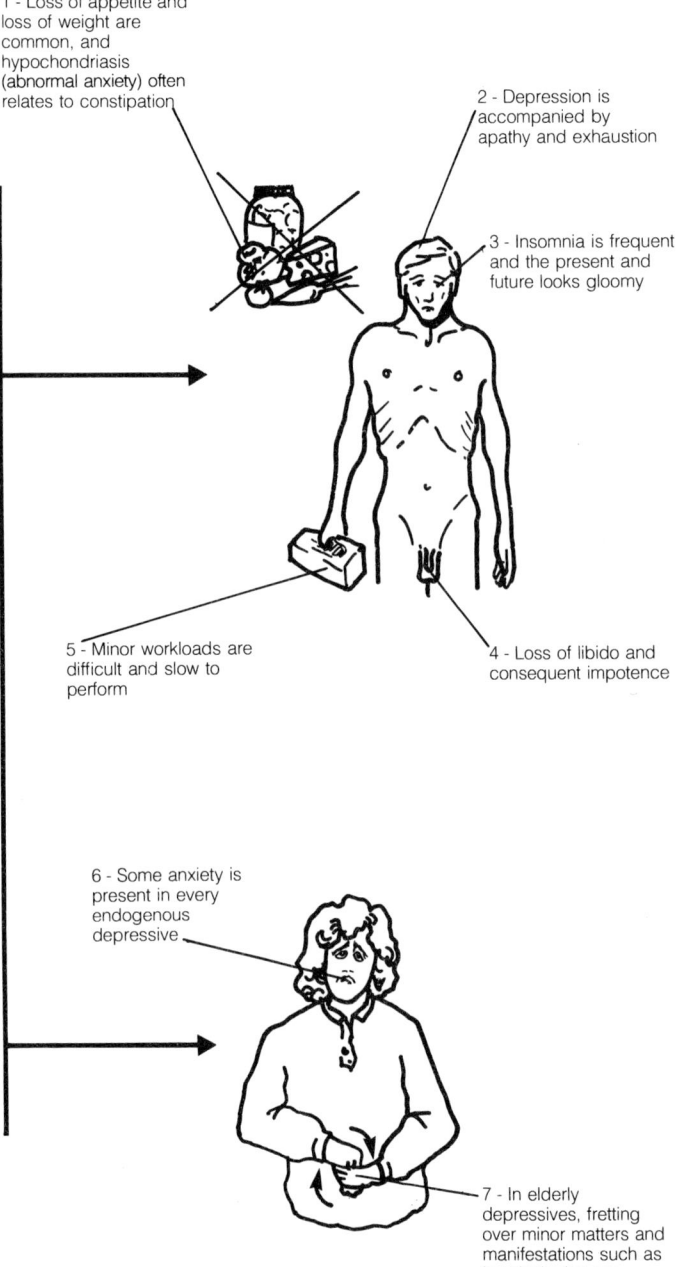

1 - Loss of appetite and loss of weight are common, and hypochondriasis (abnormal anxiety) often relates to constipation

2 - Depression is accompanied by apathy and exhaustion

3 - Insomnia is frequent and the present and future looks gloomy

4 - Loss of libido and consequent impotence

5 - Minor workloads are difficult and slow to perform

6 - Some anxiety is present in every endogenous depressive

7 - In elderly depressives, fretting over minor matters and manifestations such as handwringing are common

Functional Psychoses

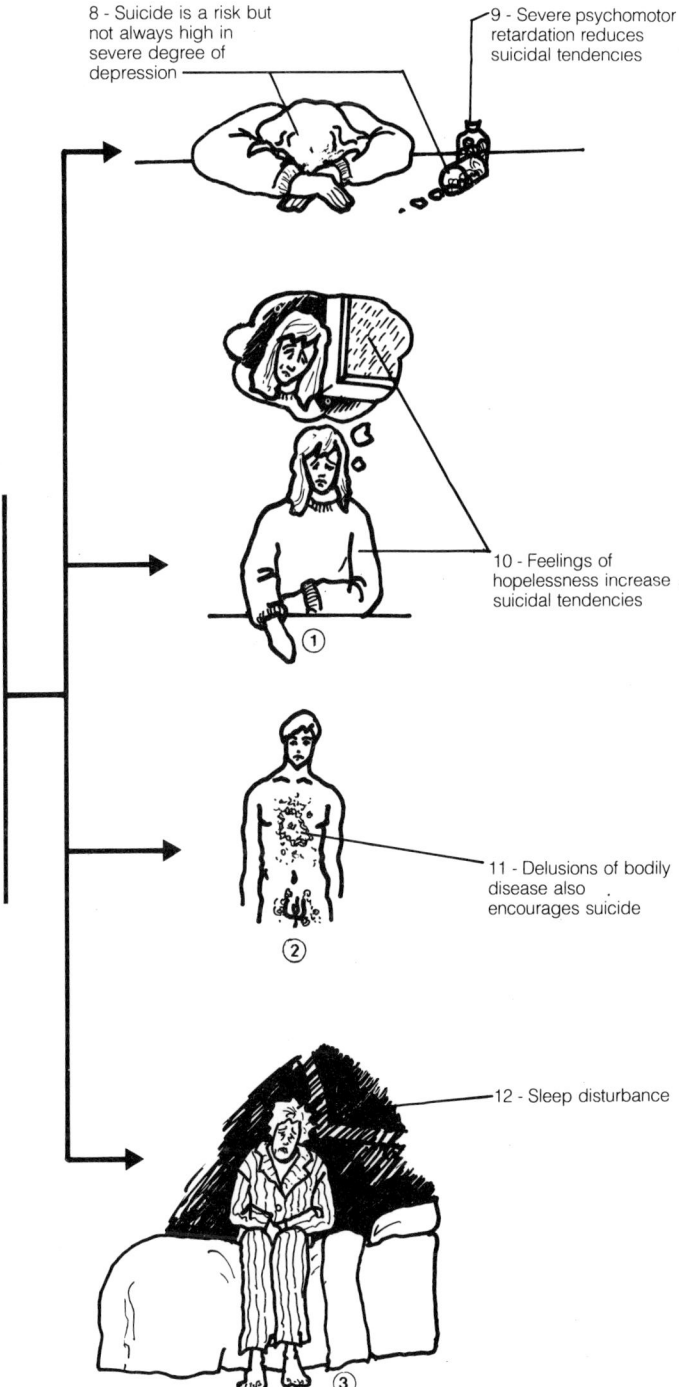

Suicide and attempted suicide is always a risk in endogenous depression and the risk is not always proportionate to the degree of depression; indeed, severe psychomotor retardation leads to a lesser likelihood of attempted suicide. Although it is difficult to accurately ear-mark high risk cases, several features of a depressive illness are recognised as being associated with suicide attempts:– 1) Feelings of hopelessness concerning the future; 2) delusions of guilt, unworthiness or bodily disease; 3) severe sleep disturbance;

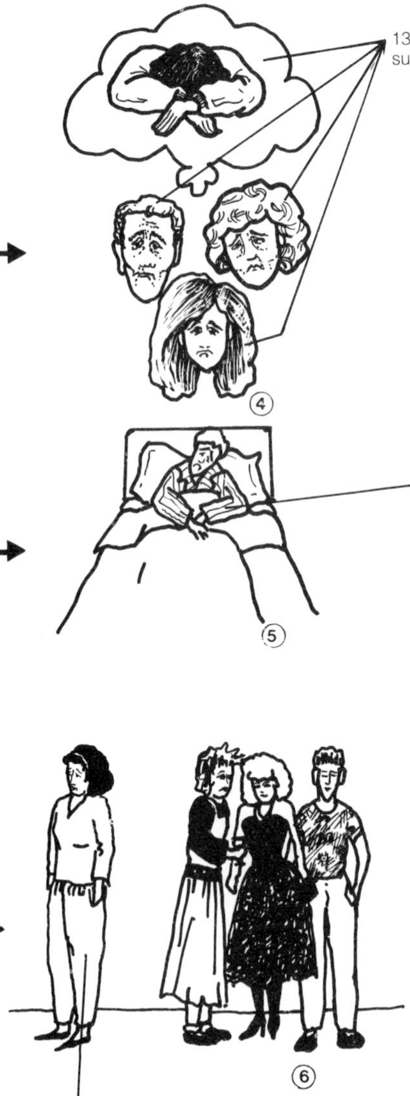

4) a family history of suicide, pre-occupation with suicide and a past history of suicide attempts; 5) associated physical illness; 6) social isolation.

13 - Family history of suicide

14 - Associated physical illness

15 - Social isolation

Elderly patients suffering a recent bereavement or chronic illness are particularly at a risk of suicide, especially where they live alone. Management involves: anticipation, social rehabilitation and specific treatment.

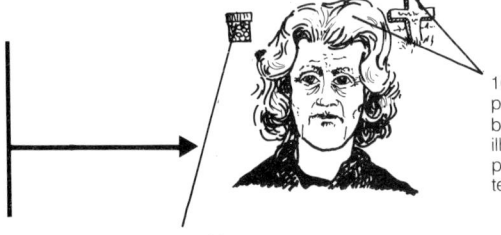

16 - Depressed elderly patients, following bereavement or chronic illness, living alone are prone to suicidal tendencies

17 - Management includes anticipation, social rehabilitation and specific treatment

Functional Psychoses

Differential Diagnosis – Various organic brain diseases may cause depression. Thus pre-senile or senile (eg. arteriosclerotic) dementias may be associated with depression and so may Parkinsonism. Tumours of the limbic system or patients with limbic lobe epilepsy may also suffer depression. Drugs (eg. corticosteroids, propranolol methyl dopa, the contraceptive pill) may cause depression. Organic visceral disease (eg. pancreatic carcinoma) may cause depression as may other illnesses, e.g. influenza or glandular fever. Depression may accompany myxoedema.

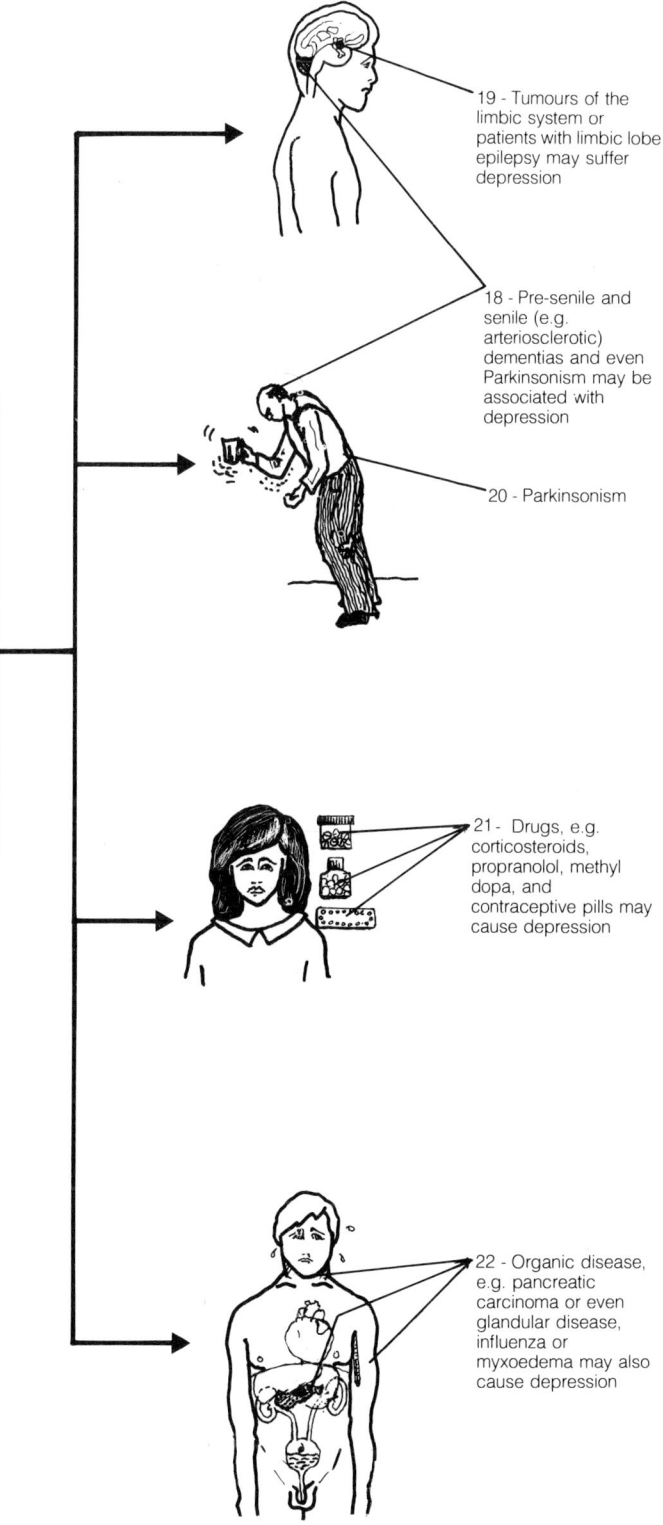

19 - Tumours of the limbic system or patients with limbic lobe epilepsy may suffer depression

18 - Pre-senile and senile (e.g. arteriosclerotic) dementias and even Parkinsonism may be associated with depression

20 - Parkinsonism

21 - Drugs, e.g. corticosteroids, propranolol, methyl dopa, and contraceptive pills may cause depression

22 - Organic disease, e.g. pancreatic carcinoma or even glandular disease, influenza or myxoedema may also cause depression

Functional Psychoses

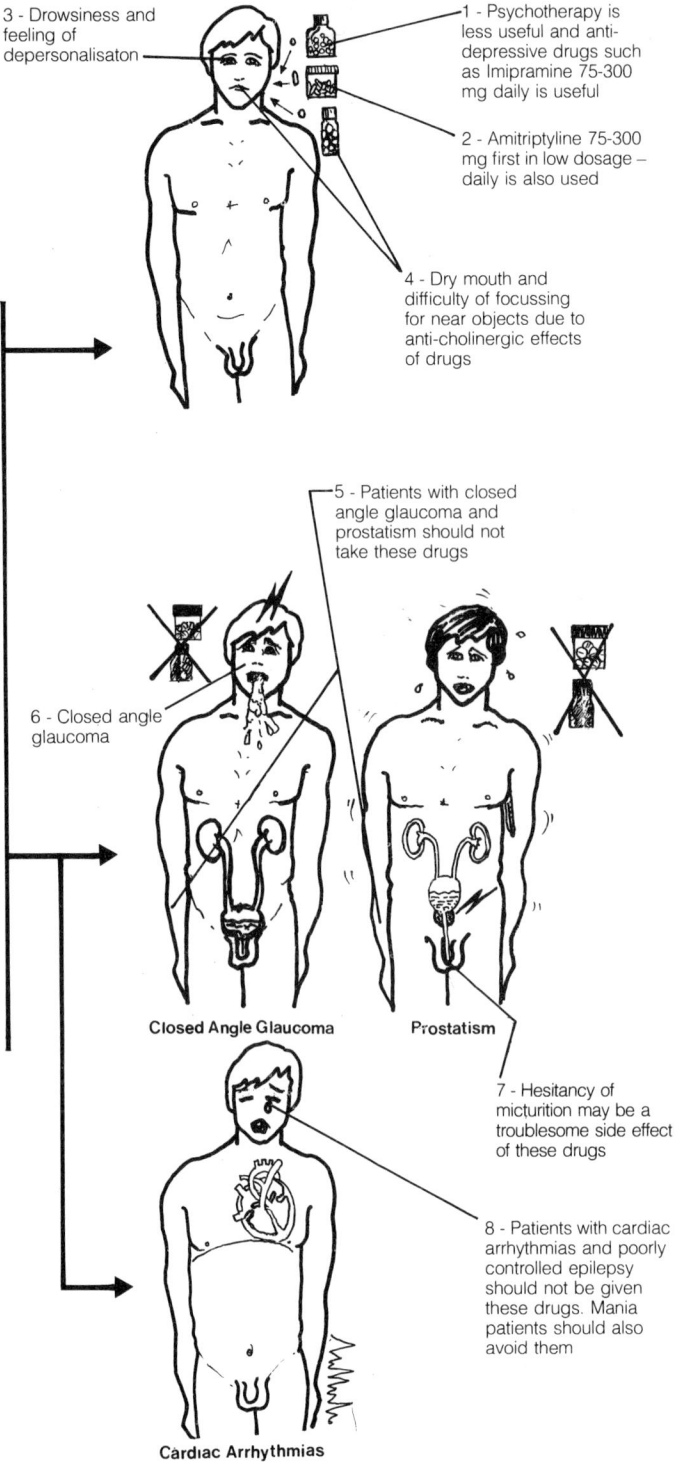

Treatment – In general, psychotherapy is less useful in endogenous than reactive depression and treatment is usually with drugs. The tricyclic antidepressants are usually the most effective group of drugs. The relief of symptoms may take a couple of weeks of administration. Imipramine (75-300 mg daily) and amitriptyline (75-300 mg) daily are the most commonly prescribed drugs and are prescribed initially in the lower dosage; amitriptyline is more sedative than imipramine. Drowsiness and feelings of depersonalisation may occur and anticholinergic effects (dry mouth, difficulty in focussing for near objects, hesitancy of micturition), all may produce troublesome side effects. Patients with closed angle glaucoma or prostatism should not be prescribed these drugs. Cardiac arrhythmias are a relative contraindication as is poorly controlled epilepsy. None of the antidepressants should be prescribed in mania.

Contraindications to tricyclic antideprressants

Functional Psychoses

Mianserin is a tetracyclic antidepressant with only minor inhibitory effects on removal re-uptake of noradrenaline and serotonin; its mode of action in depression may be the promotion of noradrenaline release. Mianserin has fewer anticholinergic effects and less cardiotoxicity but is probably also a less potent antidepressant than the tricyclics.

The monoamine oxidase inhibitors (eg. iproniazid and tranylcypromine) have undoubted activity in endogenous depression but are not recommended before a trial of tricyclic antidepressants. There are a large number of drug interactions with monoamine oxidase inhibitors, (eg. with methyl dopa, with alcohol etc.) and, further, tyramine or dopa containing foods (eg. cheeses, broad beans), that are consumed during the period of drug administration can lead to dangerous hypertensive crisis. The use of these drugs is thus more restricted.

Although not first choice in therapy, electro-convulsive therapy (ECT) is the most effective form of treatment currently available for endogenous depression and is safe if carried out on a carefully selected population and by experts. Psychosurgery is now used uncommonly.

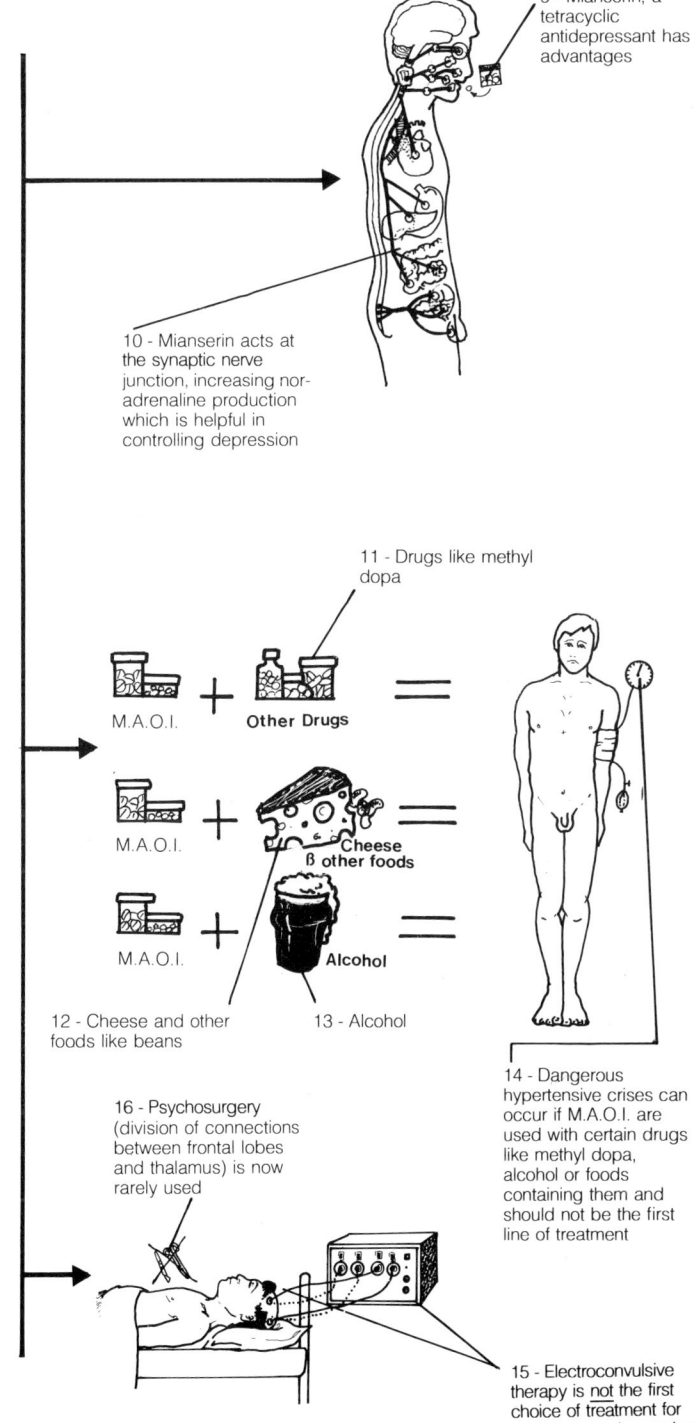

9 - Mianserin, a tetracyclic antidepressant has advantages

10 - Mianserin acts at the synaptic nerve junction, increasing noradrenaline production which is helpful in controlling depression

11 - Drugs like methyl dopa

12 - Cheese and other foods like beans

13 - Alcohol

14 - Dangerous hypertensive crises can occur if M.A.O.I. are used with certain drugs like methyl dopa, alcohol or foods containing them and should not be the first line of treatment

16 - Psychosurgery (division of connections between frontal lobes and thalamus) is now rarely used

15 - Electroconvulsive therapy is not the first choice of treatment for endogenous depression

Hypomania and Mania

Less common than depression, these conditions usually arise in patients with cyclothymic personalities, (having large mood swings from abnormal jollity to **deep gloom**), or in those with hypomanic personalities, (being excessively energetic and cheerful). In mania, there is uncontrollable excitement. In hypomania the level of activity is excessive, (even by the standards of the pre-morbid hypomanic personality), particularly in incessant talk and restlessness, but the condition stops just short of mania.

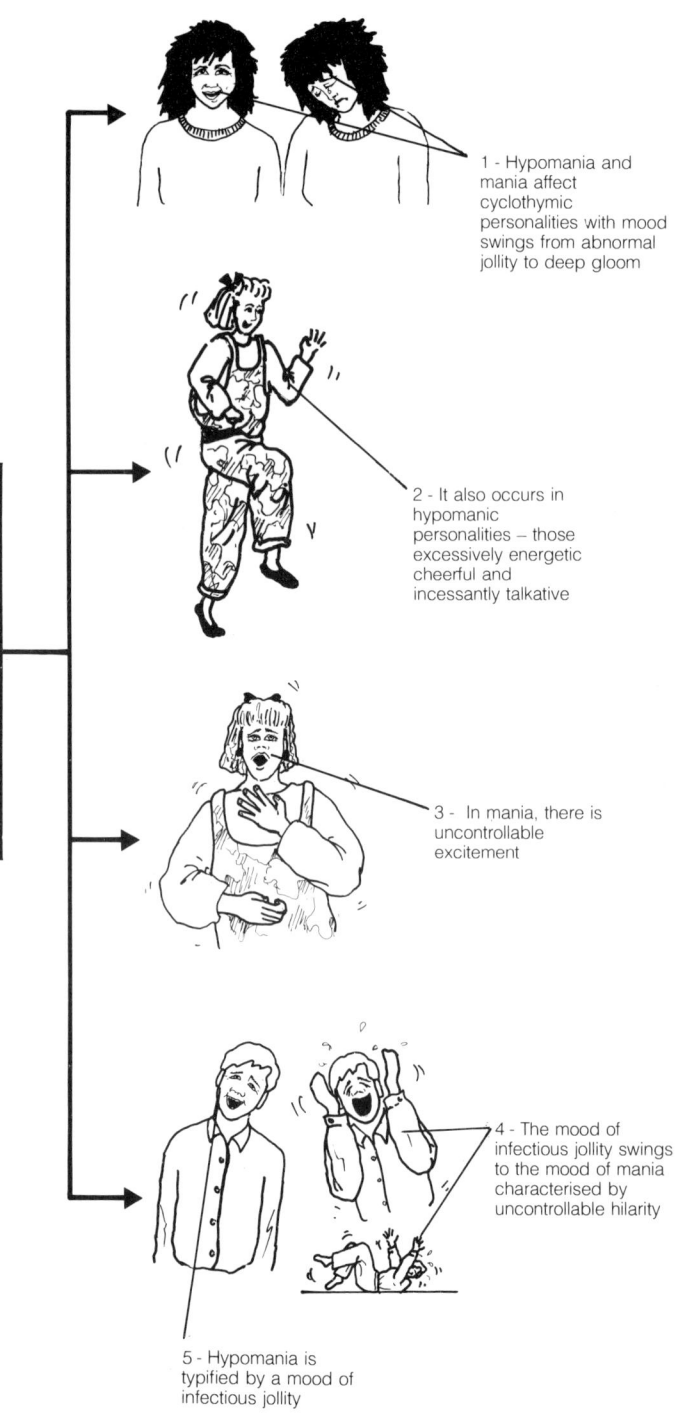

1 - Hypomania and mania affect cyclothymic personalities with mood swings from abnormal jollity to deep gloom

2 - It also occurs in hypomanic personalities – those excessively energetic cheerful and incessantly talkative

3 - In mania, there is uncontrollable excitement

4 - The mood of infectious jollity swings to the mood of mania characterised by uncontrollable hilarity

5 - Hypomania is typified by a mood of infectious jollity

Functional Psychoses

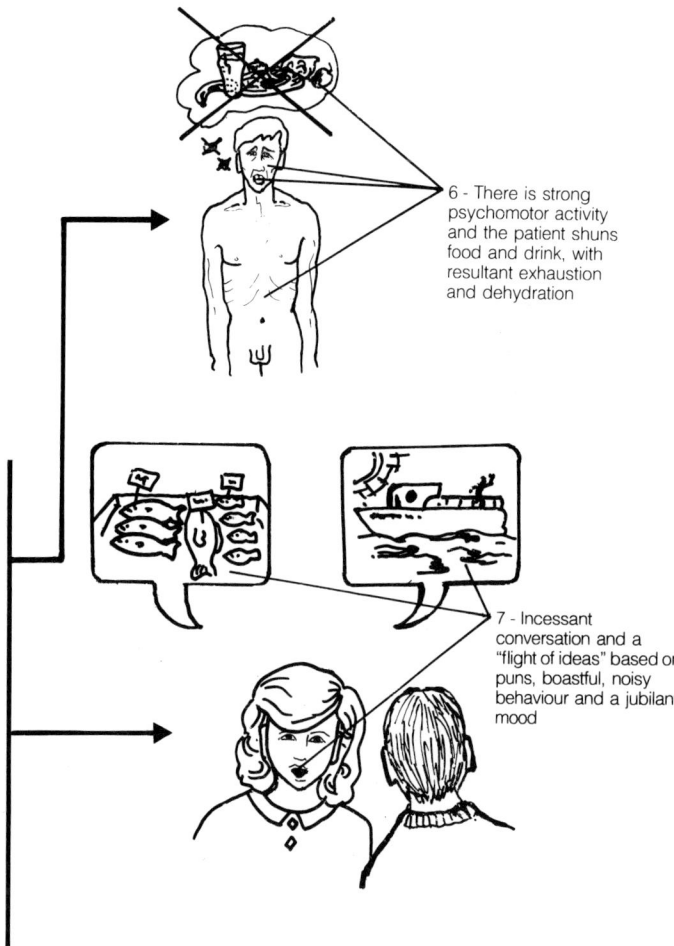

6 - There is strong psychomotor activity and the patient shuns food and drink, with resultant exhaustion and dehydration

The cardinal feature of hypomania and mania is the elevated mood and this ranges from infectious jollity to wild and uncontrollable hilarity. There is excessive psychomotor activity and the patient spares no thought for food and drink; not suprisingly, exhaustion and dehydration may be complications of the psychiatric illness. Incessant conversation is another typical feature and characteristically there is a "flight of ideas" in which the connection between one idea and the next is based on puns, similar sounds, chance associations etc. Whilst the conversation may become boastful or grandiose, delusions are not a feature of the condition.

7 - Incessant conversation and a "flight of ideas" based on puns, boastful, noisy behaviour and a jubilant mood

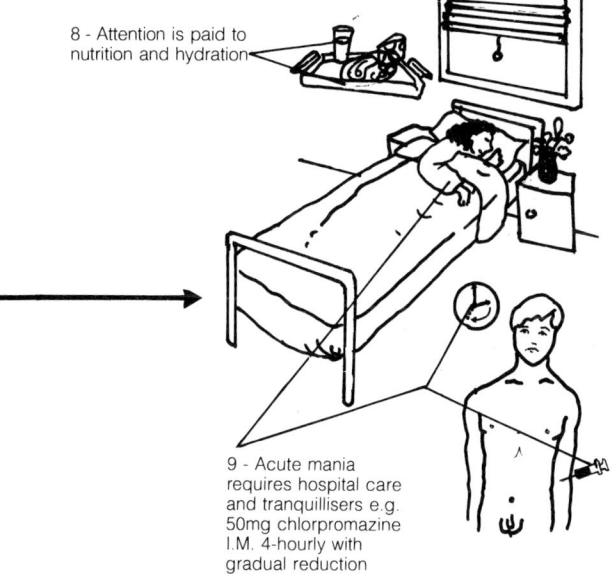

8 - Attention is paid to nutrition and hydration

Acute manic attacks require hospital admission (compulsory if necessary), and sedation by a major tranquilliser (eg. chlorpromazine 50 mg intramuscularly 4 hourly to start with – with later reducing frequency of administration). Attention is paid to nutrition and hydration.

9 - Acute mania requires hospital care and tranquillisers e.g. 50mg chlorpromazine I.M. 4-hourly with gradual reduction

Lithium carbonate is important in the **therapy** of the acute attack and prophylaxis. However, lithium has toxicity close to the therapeutic range and its use should be supervised by experts and preferably with plasma lithium concentration monitoring. Toxic effects include gastrointestinal effects (nausea, diarrhoea), neuromuscular effects, (weakness, tremors, ataxia), CNS effects (dizziness, obtundation, fits) and cardiovascular effects, (dysrhythmias, circulatory collapse). A bottle of lithium tablets is not safe for unreliable patients.

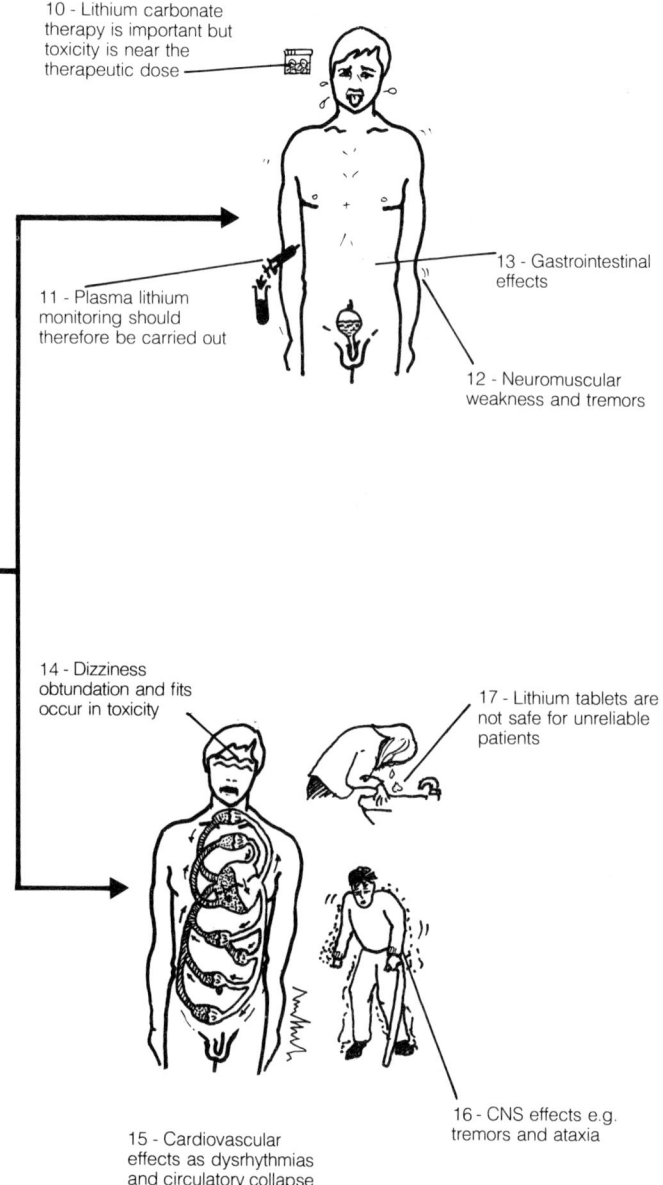

10 - Lithium carbonate therapy is important but toxicity is near the therapeutic dose

11 - Plasma lithium monitoring should therefore be carried out

12 - Neuromuscular weakness and tremors

13 - Gastrointestinal effects

14 - Dizziness obtundation and fits occur in toxicity

15 - Cardiovascular effects as dysrhythmias and circulatory collapse

16 - CNS effects e.g. tremors and ataxia

17 - Lithium tablets are not safe for unreliable patients

The **prognosis** for individual acute attacks is good and they usually remit within a few weeks. However, the attacks tend to recur. Hypomania and mania are more common in younger patients, and with increasing age depressive attacks become commoner than manic ones. Sometimes, attacks of manic-depressive disease consist of alternating mania and depression.

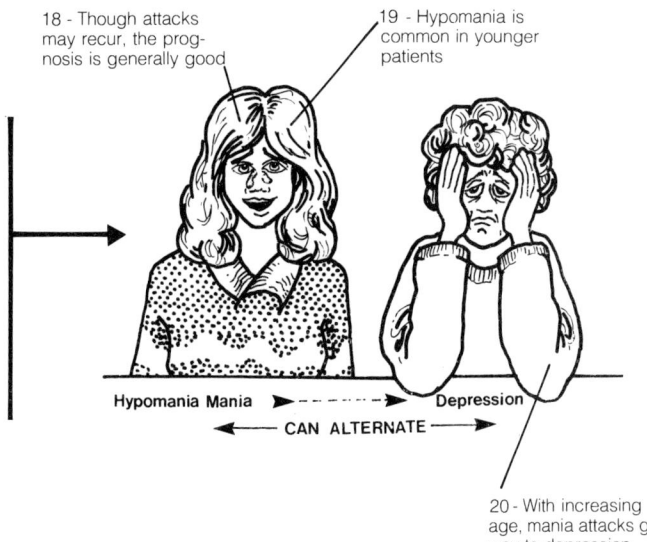

SCHIZOPHRENIA

The schizophrenic appears "cut off" from the world, having an inner life dominated by bizarre and unreal perceptions or experiences. His thinking and behaviour are often absurd due to false perceptions. Schizophrenia is the foremost psychosis.

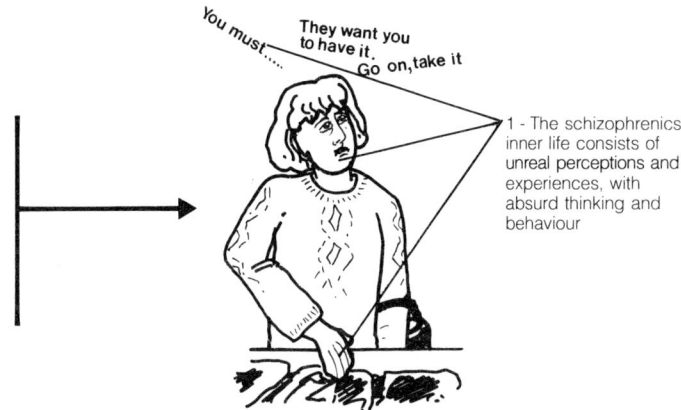

Schizophrenia is difficult to exactly define but is a syndrome including personality and thought disorders (with delusions) and disturbances in emotion, perception (with hallucinations) and behaviour.

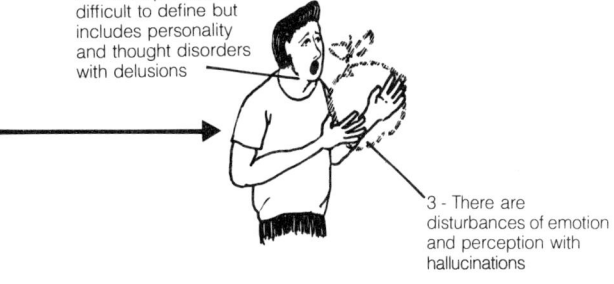

Schizophrenia

Schizophrenia occurs in 0.9% of the population and has a world-wide distribution. There is undoubtedly a familial basis to the disease, (but not by a simple mendelian inheritance), in many cases but in 60% of schizophrenics there is no family history.

Studies of biochemical disturbances, particularly studies of neurotransmitters and their catabolites have produced suggestive but not definite data on changes in schizophrenia. There is certainly a link between the pre-morbid personality: the schizoid personality, and schizophrenia itself. Childhood experiences may predispose to schizophrenia and persistent ambiguous commands and threats from parents is one of many factors in upbringing which so predispose.

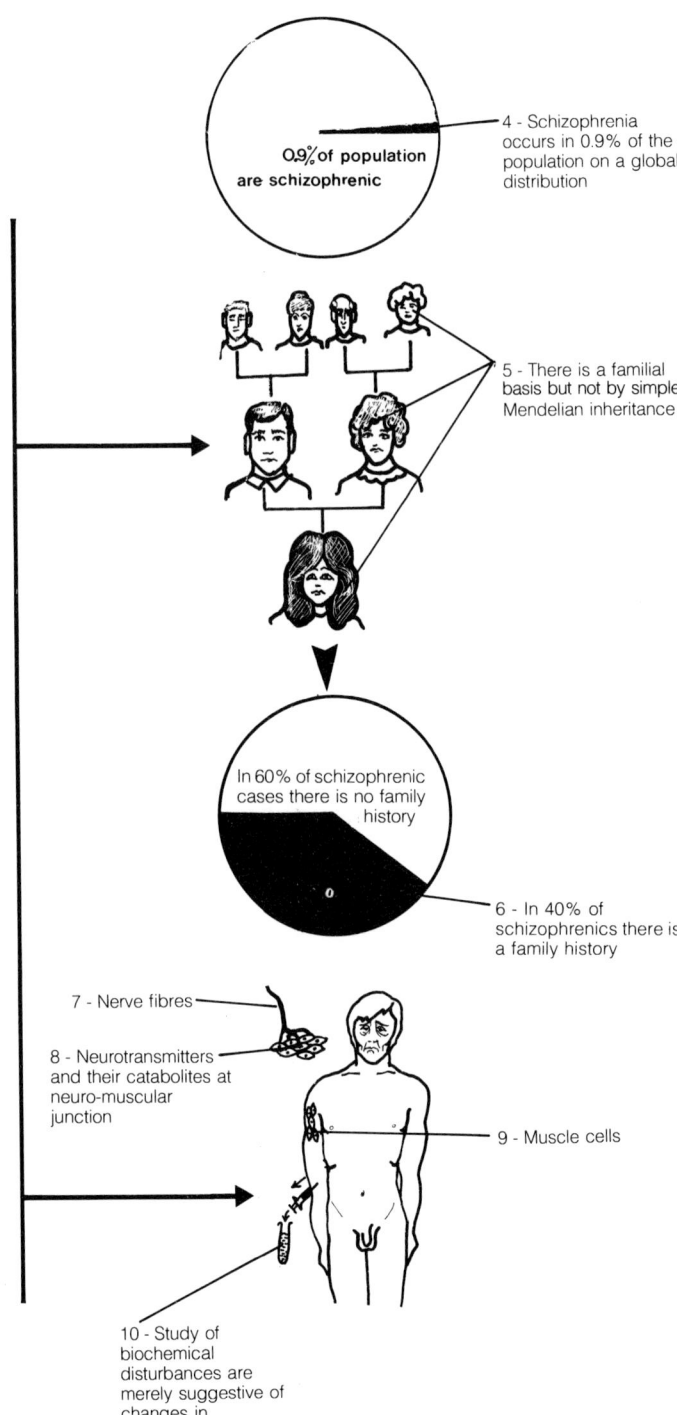

4 - Schizophrenia occurs in 0.9% of the population on a global distribution

5 - There is a familial basis but not by simple Mendelian inheritance

6 - In 40% of schizophrenics there is a family history

7 - Nerve fibres

8 - Neurotransmitters and their catabolites at neuro-muscular junction

9 - Muscle cells

10 - Study of biochemical disturbances are merely suggestive of changes in schizophrenics

Schizophrenia

An asthenic, (thin and lanky), body build has also been associated with schizophrenia, but of course this is not a cause of the disease.

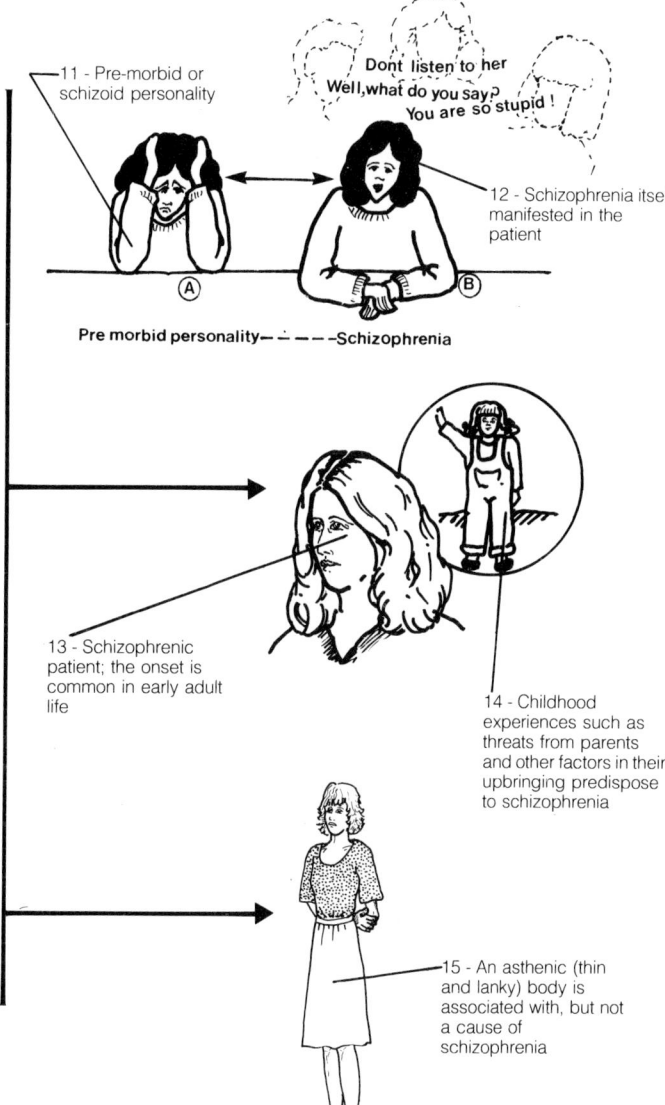

11 - Pre-morbid or schizoid personality

12 - Schizophrenia itself manifested in the patient

Pre morbid personality — — — Schizophrenia

13 - Schizophrenic patient; the onset is common in early adult life

14 - Childhood experiences such as threats from parents and other factors in their upbringing predispose to schizophrenia

15 - An asthenic (thin and lanky) body is associated with, but not a cause of schizophrenia

The **clinical onset** of schizophrenia is commonly in early adult life and the clinical manifestations may be discussed one by one:-

Schizophrenia

Thought disorder is a fundamental part of schizophrenia, the patient being at first unable to grasp the whole sequence of a logical succession of thoughts – grasping onto details which lead to tangential diversions in the train of thought, incoherent or jumbled thoughts or "completely missing the point" of a discussion. Later, completely different topics are mixed in the schizophrenics thoughts and then conversation – eg. "the politicians are always arguing about the economy but unless I hurry breakfast, I will miss that bus again". 'Thought blockade' is a term used when the patient's sequence of thoughts is suddenly interrupted and replaced by a new line of thought – it is manifest by gaps in his conversation, and may be provoked by some emotionally relevant subject. The 'knight's move in association', (a tribute to the curious movement of the knight in the game of chess), is a term used for a bizarre connection between concepts.

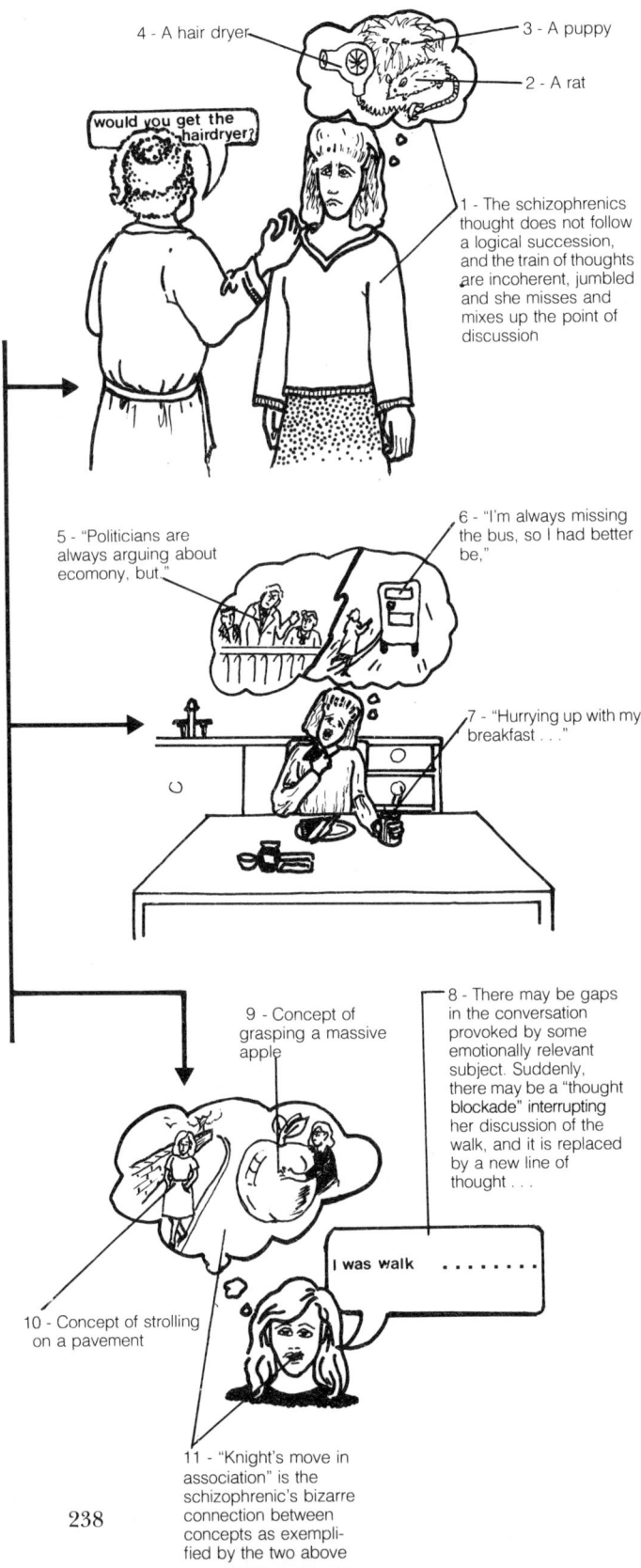

2 - A rat
3 - A puppy
4 - A hair dryer
1 - The schizophrenics thought does not follow a logical succession, and the train of thoughts are incoherent, jumbled and she misses and mixes up the point of discussion

5 - "Politicians are always arguing about ecomony, but."
6 - "I'm always missing the bus, so I had better be,"
7 - "Hurrying up with my breakfast..."

8 - There may be gaps in the conversation provoked by some emotionally relevant subject. Suddenly, there may be a "thought blockade" interrupting her discussion of the walk, and it is replaced by a new line of thought...

9 - Concept of grasping a massive apple
10 - Concept of strolling on a pavement
11 - "Knight's move in association" is the schizophrenic's bizarre connection between concepts as exemplified by the two above

Other thought disorders include: 'thought insertion', (where foreign thoughts 'appear' in the mind), 'thought withdrawal', (where thoughts are erased from the mind) and 'thought broadcasting', (where the patient believes all his thoughts are shared by others).

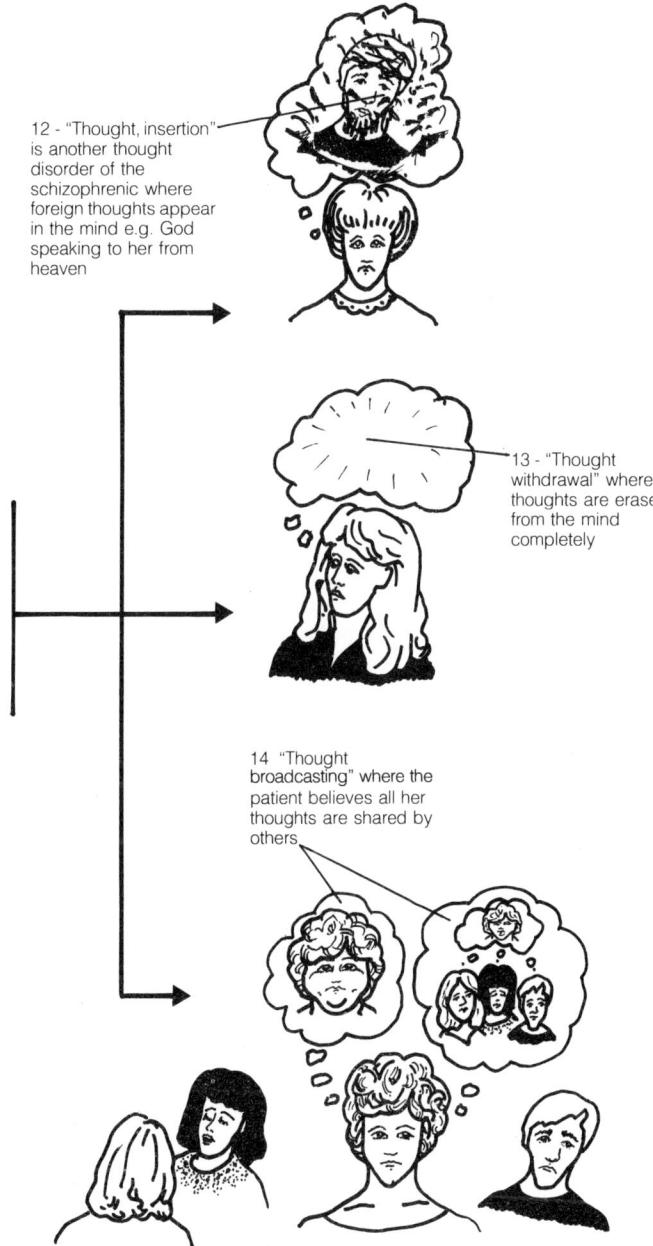

12 - "Thought, insertion" is another thought disorder of the schizophrenic where foreign thoughts appear in the mind e.g. God speaking to her from heaven

13 - "Thought withdrawal" where thoughts are erased from the mind completely

14 "Thought broadcasting" where the patient believes all her thoughts are shared by others

Schizophrenia

A **delusion** is defined as a false belief, quite inappropriate to an individual's socio-cultural background, and held in the face of logical argument. Delusions are frequently of grandeur, paranoia or relating to transformation of the body image or with disease – eg. the patient may believe that he is a prophet from God, eg. the patient may believe that his body is being controlled by other people – "they" or "them" in his conversation, ('passivity feelings'). Such passivity feelings are highly typical; examples would be objective newspaper reports or factual television news broadcasts having "special relevance" or "containing references about" or "messages to" the patient.

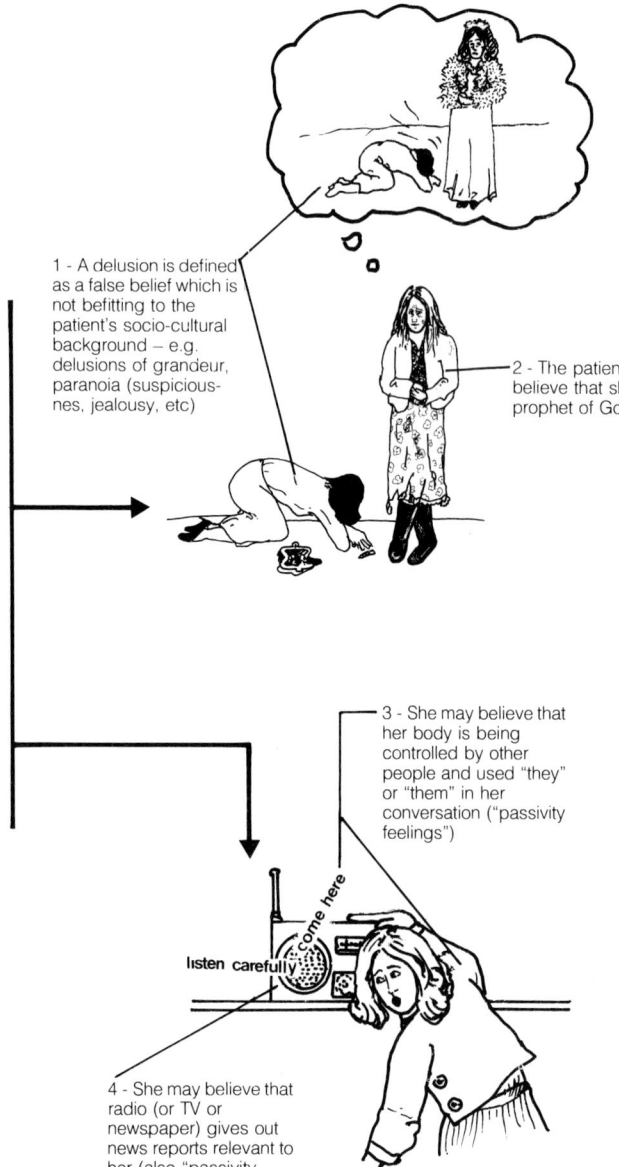

1 - A delusion is defined as a false belief which is not befitting to the patient's socio-cultural background – e.g. delusions of grandeur, paranoia (suspiciousness, jealousy, etc)

2 - The patient may believe that she is a prophet of God

3 - She may believe that her body is being controlled by other people and used "they" or "them" in her conversation ("passivity feelings")

4 - She may believe that radio (or TV or newspaper) gives out news reports relevant to her (also "passivity feelings")

Hallucinations are the hallmark of the perceptual disorder of schizophrenia. A hallucination is a perception occuring in the absence of an external stimulus. The commonest hallucination is the auditory hallucination; in particular, patients will hear voices commenting on their every action, criticising their life style, commanding them to do things, swearing at them etc. etc. Such auditory hallucinations are inextricably linked with thought disorders. Other hallucinations may be visual, olfactory, gustatory etc.

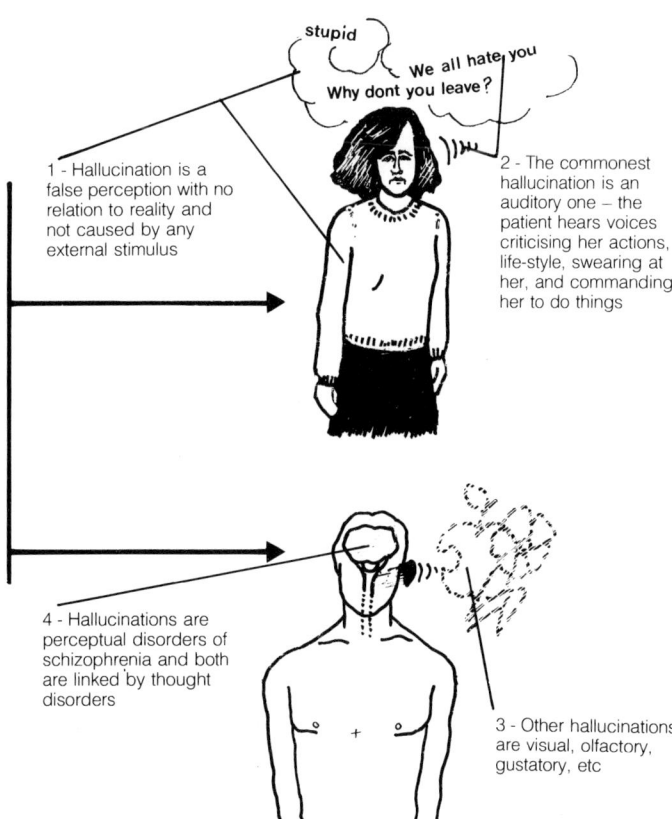

The **emotional disturbances** of schizophrenia may take many forms but in general the emotional display is detached and often quite inappropriate to the situation encountered. The schizophrenic seems so tied up with his inner world that he is cold, impartial or ambivalent to emotional situations and relationships. This also applies to the **behavioural disorder** of schizophrenia where the patient discards his friends to lead the life of a recluse.

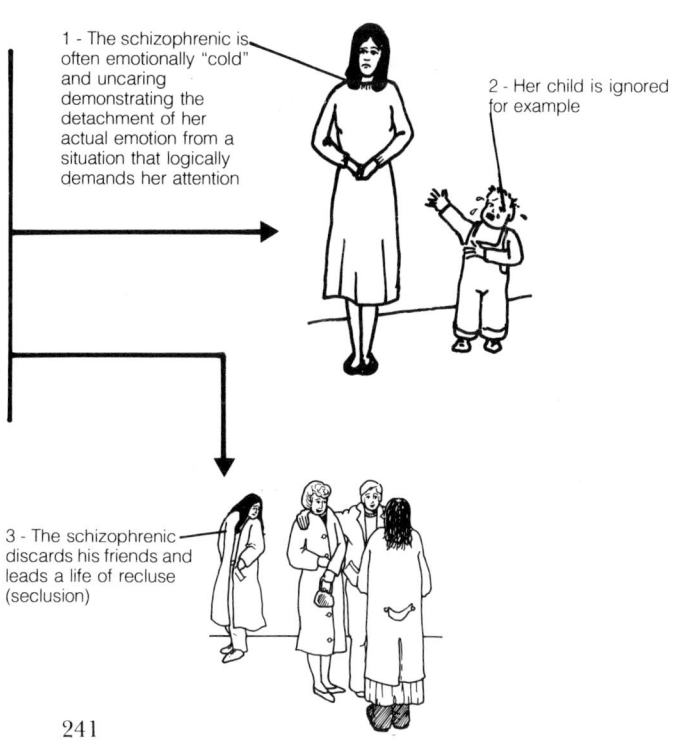

Schizophrenia

Other behaviour traits may appear odd with altered moral and social standards, a carelessness of personal hygiene and care, and a disintegrating personality. States of excitement, fanaticism and acts of impulse may occur but in general there is a deterioration in general activity, a lacking in drive, poor work performance etc. Motor disorders include strange movement patterns or postures and in catatonic epilepsy the patient may develop acute stupor, (acute catatonia).

Bleuler's original classification of schizophrenia into four main schizophrenic types is still useful today:-

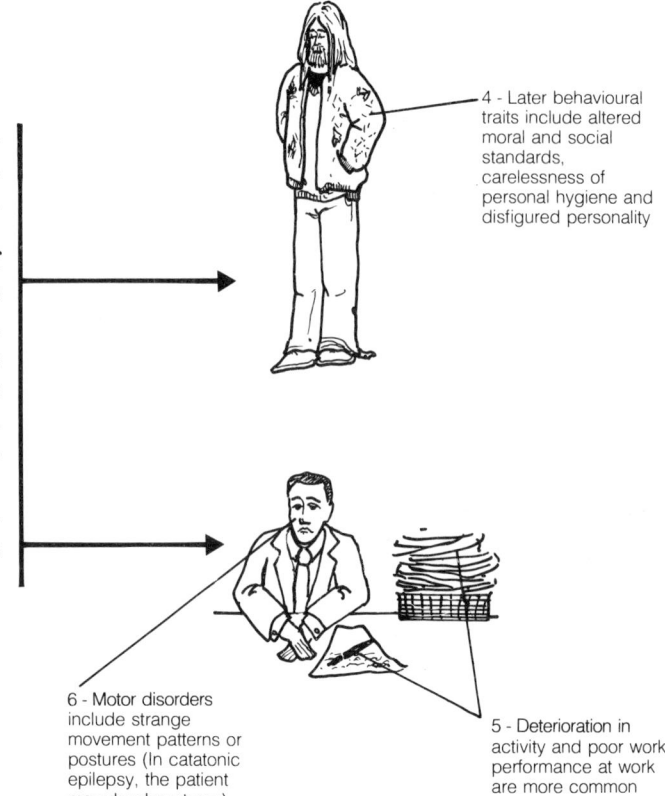

4 - Later behavioural traits include altered moral and social standards, carelessness of personal hygiene and disfigured personality

6 - Motor disorders include strange movement patterns or postures (In catatonic epilepsy, the patient may develop stupor)

5 - Deterioration in activity and poor work performance at work are more common

Simple Schizophrenia – Usually with an insidious onset, there is a general deterioration of the personality, level of normal activities and dynamism. There is blunting of the affect and thought disorder but delusions and hallucinations are not a feature. The patient is quite unaware of his problems as he lapses into a pathetic dullness and inability to cope in society.

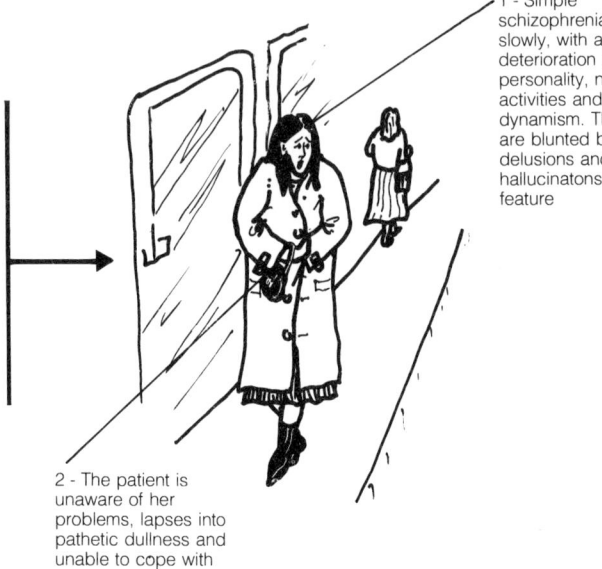

1 - Simple schizophrenia begins slowly, with a deterioration in personality, normal activities and dynamism. Thoughts are blunted but delusions and hallucinatons are not a feature

2 - The patient is unaware of her problems, lapses into pathetic dullness and unable to cope with society

Paranoid Schizophrenia – With an onset usually in middle age, complex paranoid delusions and hallucinations are usually dominant. The delusions are usually of persecution or less commonly of grandeur and the hallucinations usually auditory. Thought disorders may be mild and the personality is often well preserved such that, unless the delusions and hallucinations become marked and overbearing, survival in the community may be possible for years and it is this which governs the prognosis.

Hebephrenic Schizophrenia – This type of schizophrenia most commonly begins in late adolescence with behavioural manifestations which may at first be passed off by parents and friends as "silly", "mischievous" or "fatuous". Thought disorder becomes more marked, hallucinations occur and the personality fragments.

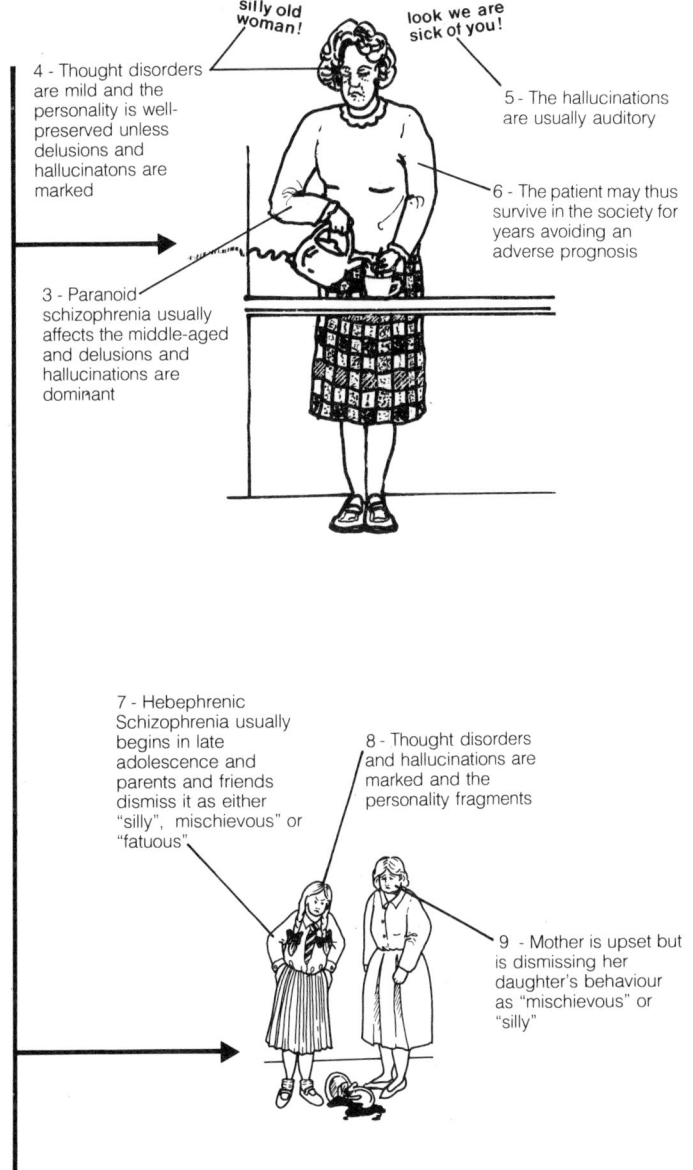

Schizophrenia

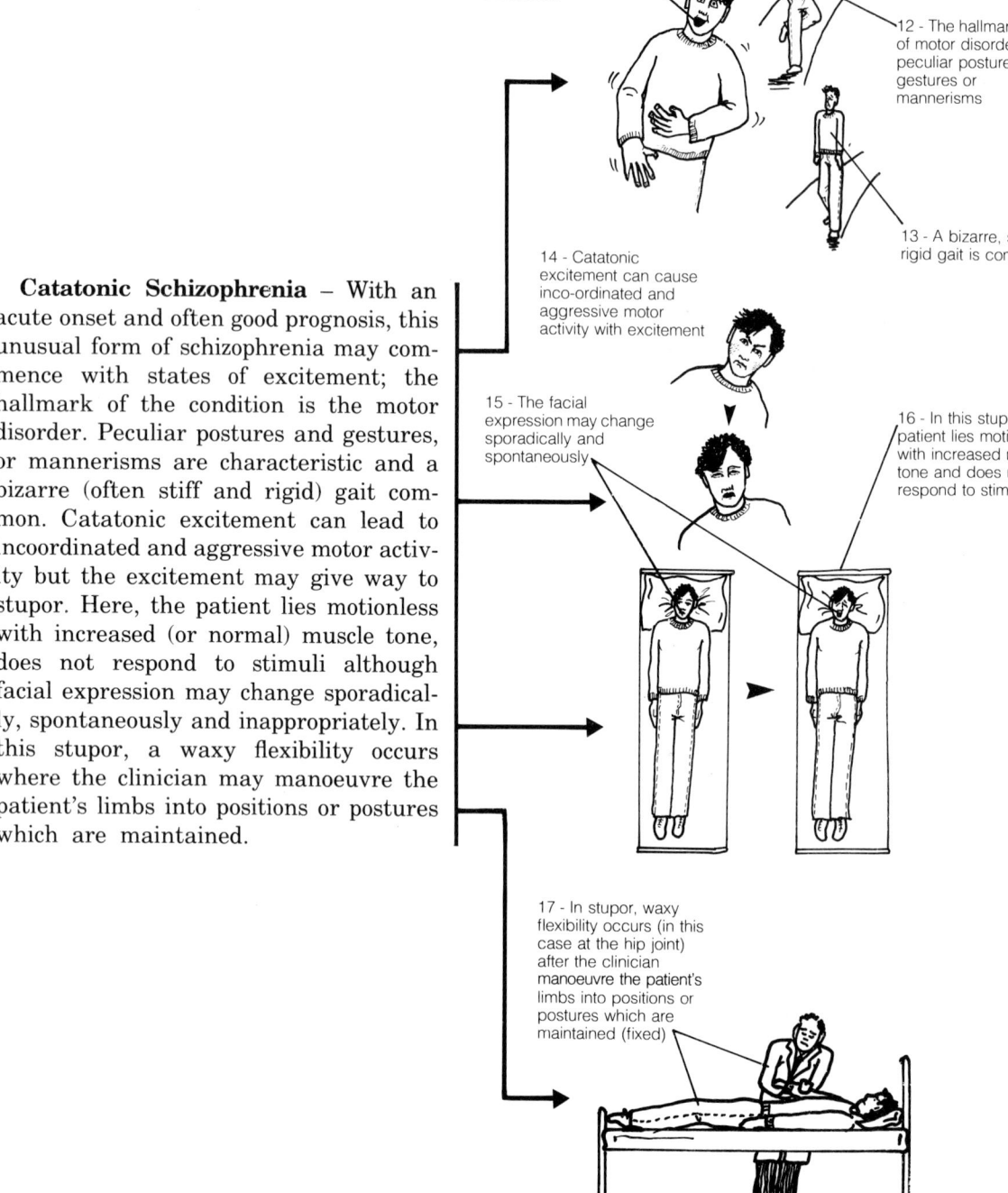

11 - Catatonic schizophrenia has a good prognosis and takes the form of excitement

12 - The hallmark is that of motor disorder with peculiar postures, gestures or mannerisms

13 - A bizarre, stiff and rigid gait is common

14 - Catatonic excitement can cause inco-ordinated and aggressive motor activity with excitement

15 - The facial expression may change sporadically and spontaneously

16 - In this stupor, the patient lies motionless, with increased muscle tone and does not respond to stimuli

17 - In stupor, waxy flexibility occurs (in this case at the hip joint) after the clinician manoeuvre the patient's limbs into positions or postures which are maintained (fixed)

Catatonic Schizophrenia – With an acute onset and often good prognosis, this unusual form of schizophrenia may commence with states of excitement; the hallmark of the condition is the motor disorder. Peculiar postures and gestures, or mannerisms are characteristic and a bizarre (often stiff and rigid) gait common. Catatonic excitement can lead to incoordinated and aggressive motor activity but the excitement may give way to stupor. Here, the patient lies motionless with increased (or normal) muscle tone, does not respond to stimuli although facial expression may change sporadically, spontaneously and inappropriately. In this stupor, a waxy flexibility occurs where the clinician may manoeuvre the patient's limbs into positions or postures which are maintained.

Another feature seen in the patients with catatonic schizophrenia is the tendancy to "echo" or copy patterns of behaviour (echopraxia) or words (echolalia), or even automatically obey all instructions (automatic obedience).

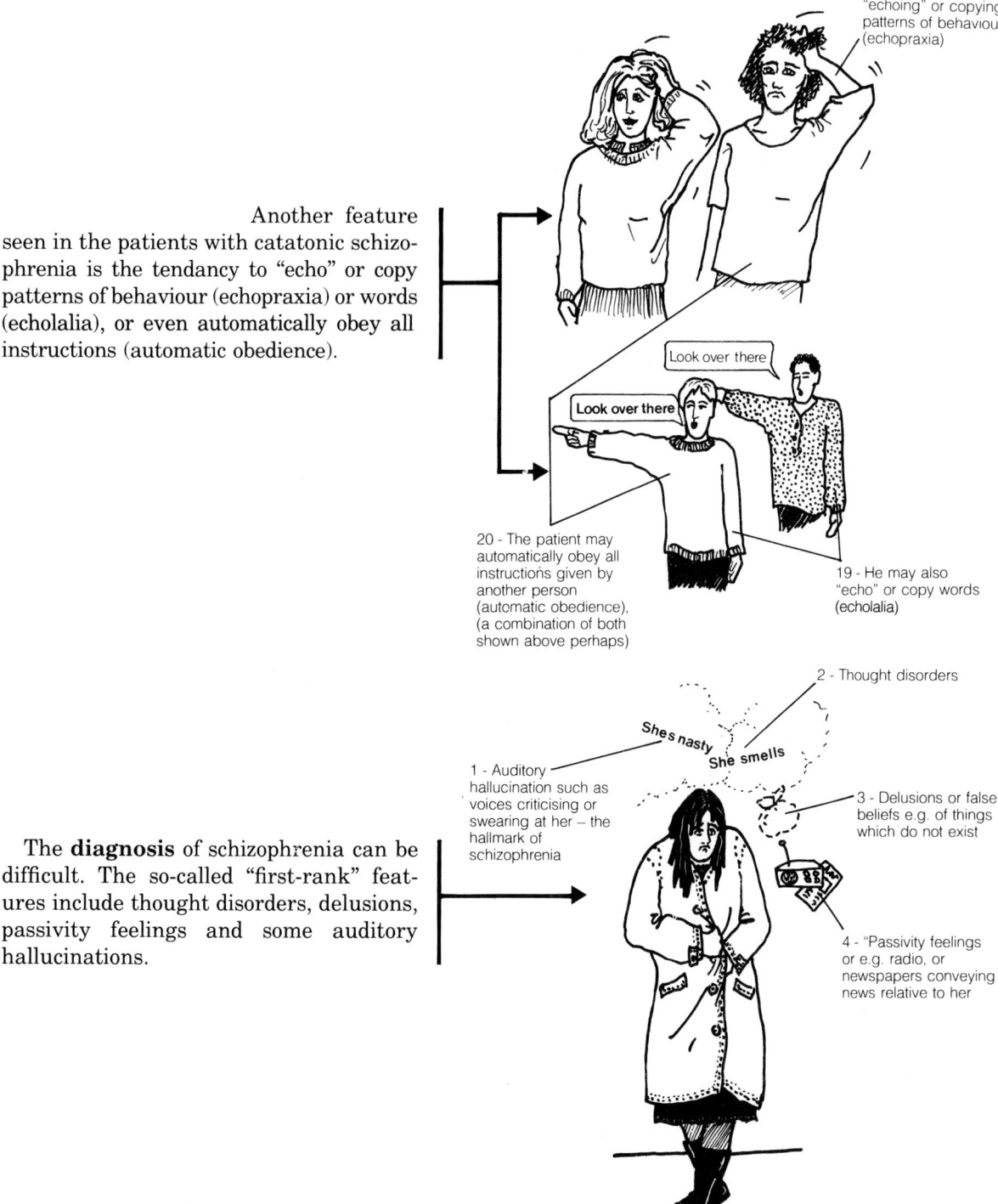

18 - Catatonic patient "echoing" or copying patterns of behaviour (echopraxia)

19 - He may also "echo" or copy words (echolalia)

20 - The patient may automatically obey all instructions given by another person (automatic obedience), (a combination of both shown above perhaps)

1 - Auditory hallucination such as voices criticising or swearing at her — the hallmark of schizophrenia

2 - Thought disorders

3 - Delusions or false beliefs e.g. of things which do not exist

4 - "Passivity feelings or e.g. radio, or newspapers conveying news relative to her

The **diagnosis** of schizophrenia can be difficult. The so-called "first-rank" features include thought disorders, delusions, passivity feelings and some auditory hallucinations.

Schizophrenia

However these are not pathognomonic of schizophrenia – all can occur in organic psychoses, (eg. temporal lobe epilepsy, severe physical illness, amphetamine or chronic bromide poisoning). Similarly, a paranoid reaction to a severe acute stress, or a hysterical disturbance can both give rise to apparently schizophrenic features. However, the mood disturbance or the relationship to acute stress or illness on top of a premorbid personality should make the clinician wary of the diagnosis of schizophrenia.

Treatment – The main thrust of treatment is to maintain the patient's contact with reality. Schizophrenics do badly if they are allowed to withdraw too completely from social contacts and practical activities; thus rehabilitation plays a major part in overall management. However, schizophrenics also do badly if involved in relationships or activities that are too demanding. Psychotherapy is not pushed to deep or analytical levels but largely plays a supportive role.

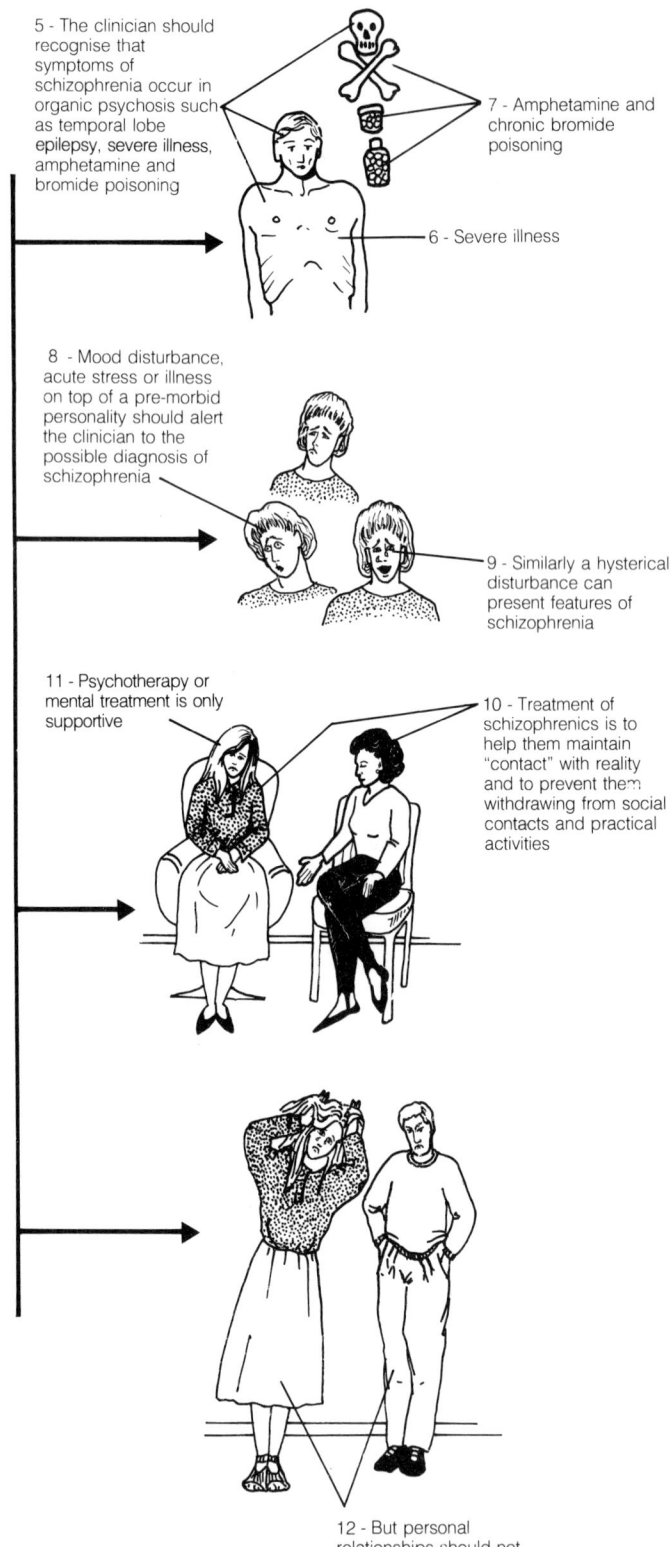

5 - The clinician should recognise that symptoms of schizophrenia occur in organic psychosis such as temporal lobe epilepsy, severe illness, amphetamine and bromide poisoning

7 - Amphetamine and chronic bromide poisoning

6 - Severe illness

8 - Mood disturbance, acute stress or illness on top of a pre-morbid personality should alert the clinician to the possible diagnosis of schizophrenia

9 - Similarly a hysterical disturbance can present features of schizophrenia

11 - Psychotherapy or mental treatment is only supportive

10 - Treatment of schizophrenics is to help them maintain "contact" with reality and to prevent them withdrawing from social contacts and practical activities

12 - But personal relationships should not be too demanding as they may worsen schizophrenia

Schizophrenia

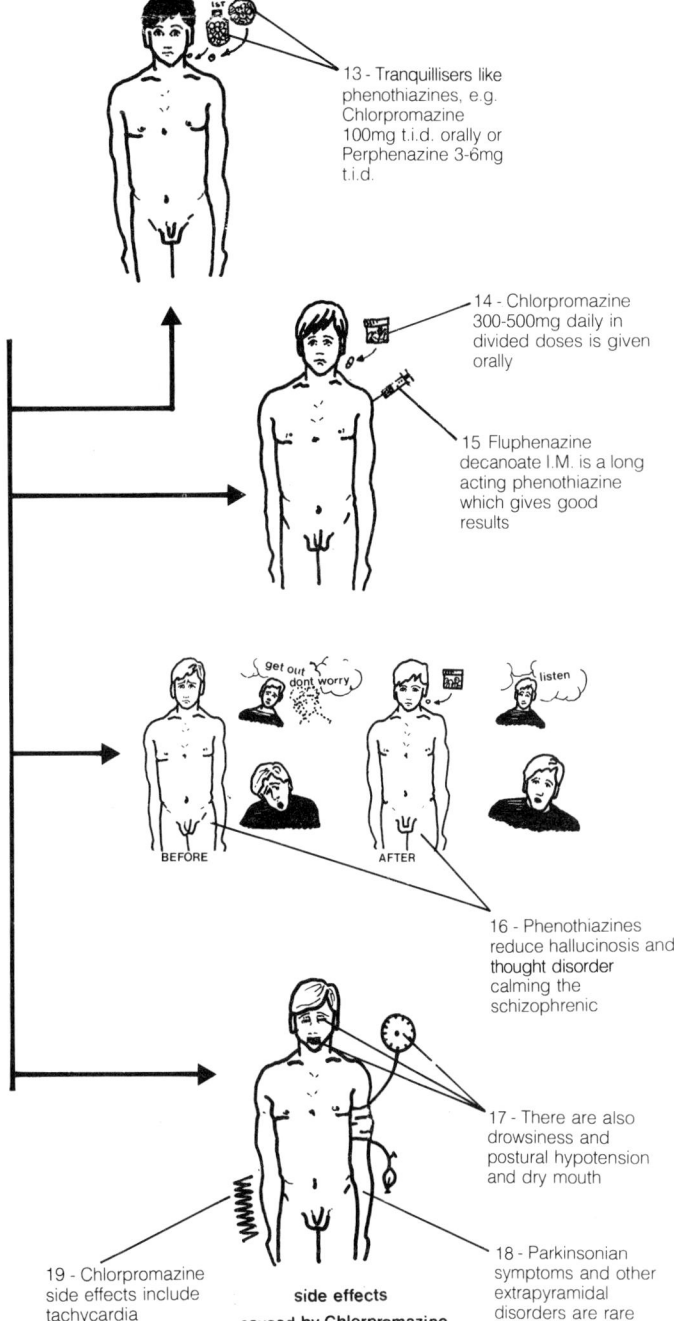

Neuroleptic drugs/the major tranquillisers are most useful and the phenothiazines are usually chosen first, the butyrophenones second. Chlorpromazine (300–500 mg daily in divided oral dosage) remains one of the most effective drugs but long acting intramuscular phenothiazine injections (eg. fluphenazine decanoate) have an important maintenance role in those responding to chlorpromazine induction. In general, the phenothiazines reduce hallucinosis and thought disorder and calm the agitated schizophrenic. The side effects of chlorpromazine include drowsiness, tachycardia and postural hypotension, (due to adrenergic blockade), dry mouth, parkinsonian symptoms and rarely other extrapyramidal disorders (eg. dystonias, akithesias). Skin rashes which may be photosensitive, blood dyscrasias notably agranulocytosis and obstructive jaundice due to intraphepatic cholestasis are rare but important idiosyncratic drug reactions.

Electroconvulsive therapy has a limited role in a schizophrenic illness of acute onset and where excitement and affective features are marked.

Most schizophrenics emerge from their acute illness with residual sequelae and re-integration into the community may need to be into a simpler occupation. Nevertheless re-employment is beneficial if possible and once again active rehabilitation is an important part of management. Indeed, approximately half of the schizophrenic population can be re-integrated into society. Acknowledged poor prognostic features include: insidious onset, low intelligence and those with simple or hebephrenic varieties of schizophrenia, more marked and persistent thought disorder.

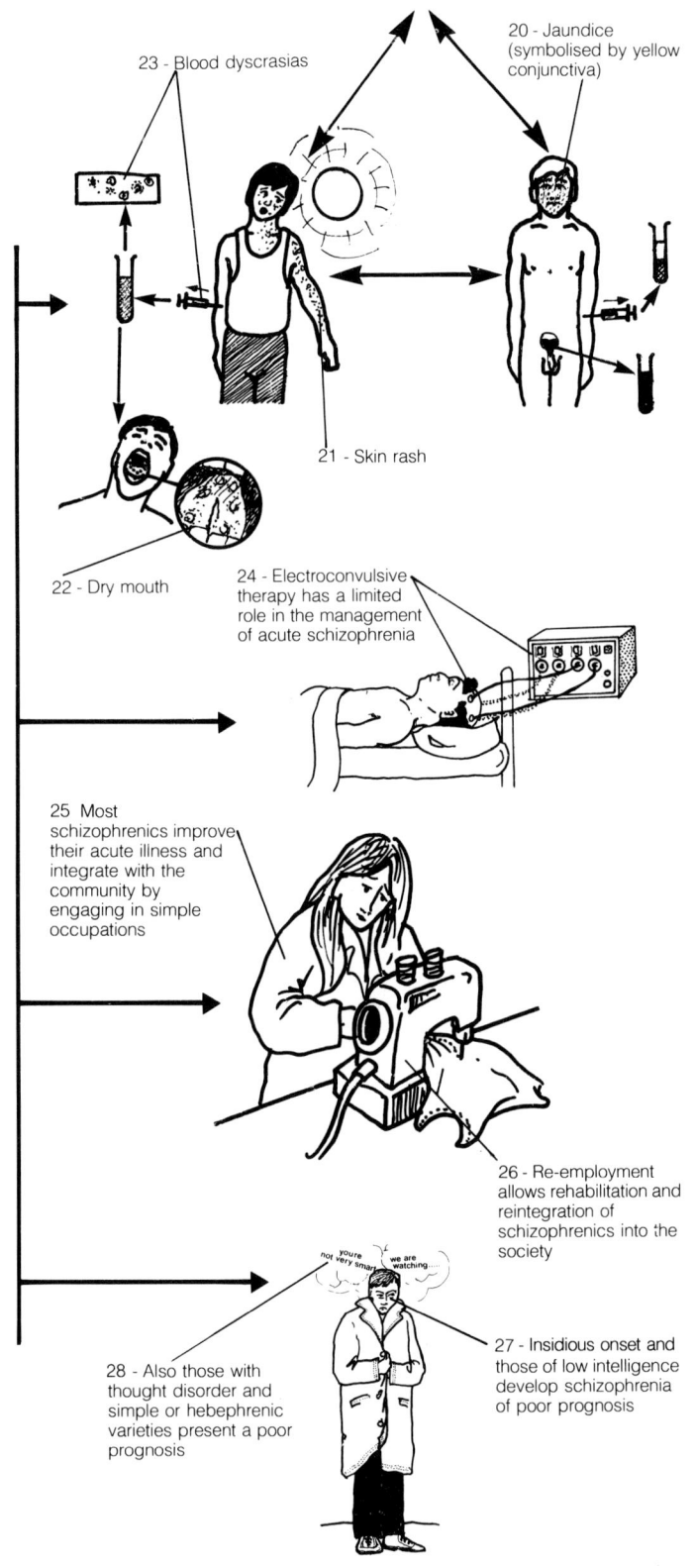

Organic Psychoses

ORGANIC PSYCHOSES

Although the term organic psychosis is considered outmoded by those believing in a biochemical basis to schizophrenia, nevertheless the term is useful to describe the psychoses occurring secondarily to other physical diseases. Let us first consider delirium and dementia before discussing toxic and metabolic disorders, endocrine disorders and disorders with organic brain disease.

DELIRIUM

Delirium is a state of impaired consciousness with disorientation in time and place, altered perception, (often with visual hallucinations and delusional ideas) and with emotional and motor disturbances. Thoughts are chaotic and motor activity often exaggerated. Delirium can be precipitated by acute febrile illness (eg. pneumococcal lobar pneumonia), drug intoxications (eg. alcohol or barbiturates) or other causes of acute cerebral disturbances (eg. acute dehydration, encephalitis, post head trauma, post-stroke etc.).

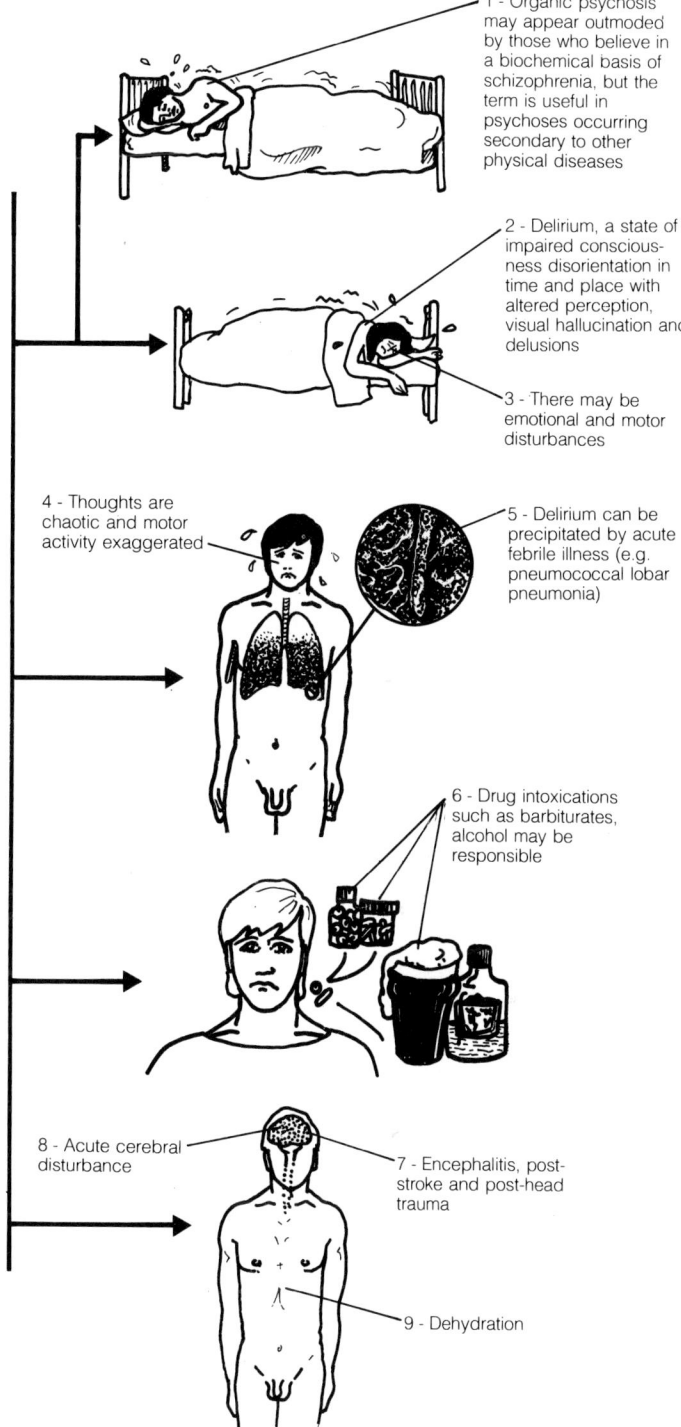

1 - Organic psychosis may appear outmoded by those who believe in a biochemical basis of schizophrenia, but the term is useful in psychoses occurring secondary to other physical diseases

2 - Delirium, a state of impaired consciousness disorientation in time and place with altered perception, visual hallucination and delusions

3 - There may be emotional and motor disturbances

4 - Thoughts are chaotic and motor activity exaggerated

5 - Delirium can be precipitated by acute febrile illness (e.g. pneumococcal lobar pneumonia)

6 - Drug intoxications such as barbiturates, alcohol may be responsible

7 - Encephalitis, post-stroke and post-head trauma

8 - Acute cerebral disturbance

9 - Dehydration

DEMENTIA

In dementia, there is a normal level of consciousness but an underlying cause of brain damage leads to progressive and irreversible intellectual decline. In particular, there is an impaired memory for recent events and a deterioration in the concentration span. The level of normal daily activity and energy declines and the state of apathy leads to a deterioration in social behaviour and self-care. Slowly, the personality fragments. The patient may be aware and distressed by his deteriorating performance, and this distress is exacerbated by the dementia itself, which often leads to distorted reasoning and large fluctuations in mood. For example, the discovery that a task is beyond his capability may lead to a state of great agitation and distress, (catastrophic reaction). Depression may be a feature of dementia.

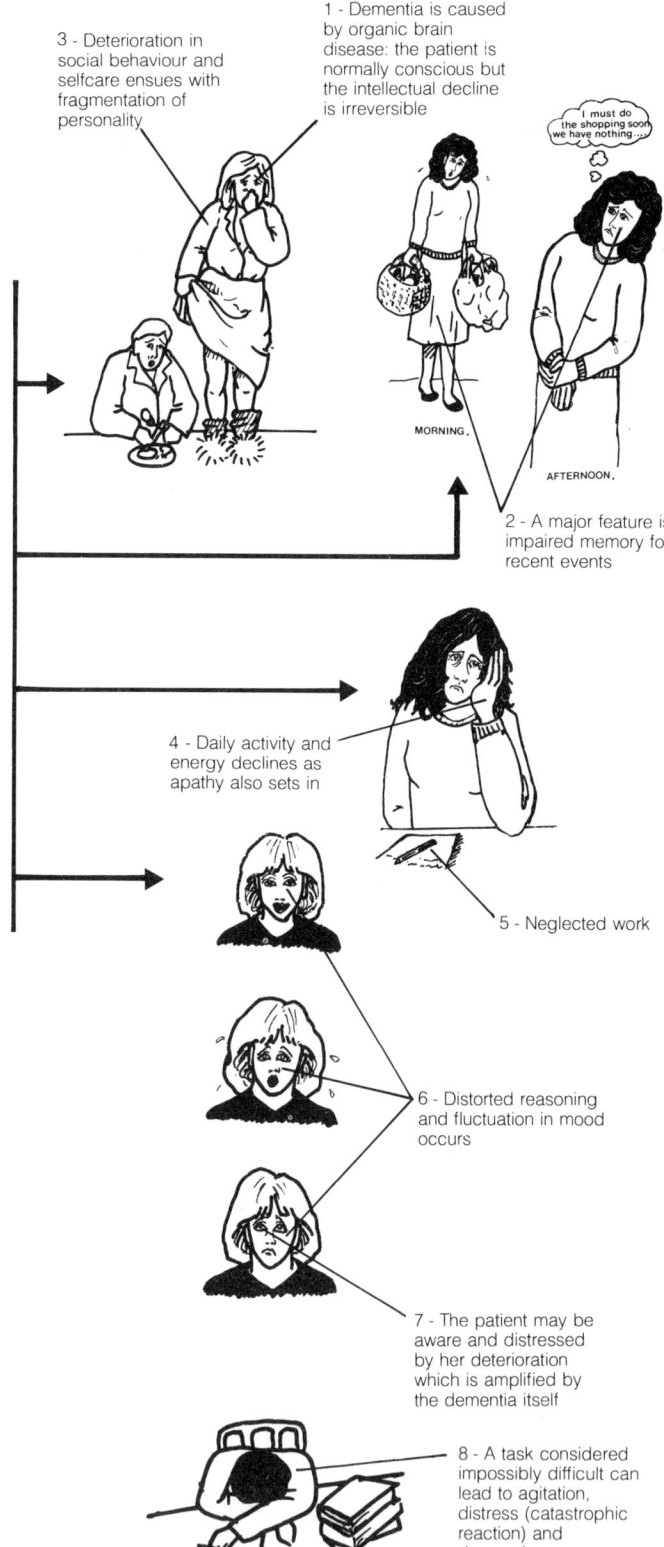

1 - Dementia is caused by organic brain disease: the patient is normally conscious but the intellectual decline is irreversible

2 - A major feature is impaired memory for recent events

3 - Deterioration in social behaviour and selfcare ensues with fragmentation of personality

4 - Daily activity and energy declines as apathy also sets in

5 - Neglected work

6 - Distorted reasoning and fluctuation in mood occurs

7 - The patient may be aware and distressed by her deterioration which is amplified by the dementia itself

8 - A task considered impossibly difficult can lead to agitation, distress (catastrophic reaction) and depression

Dementia

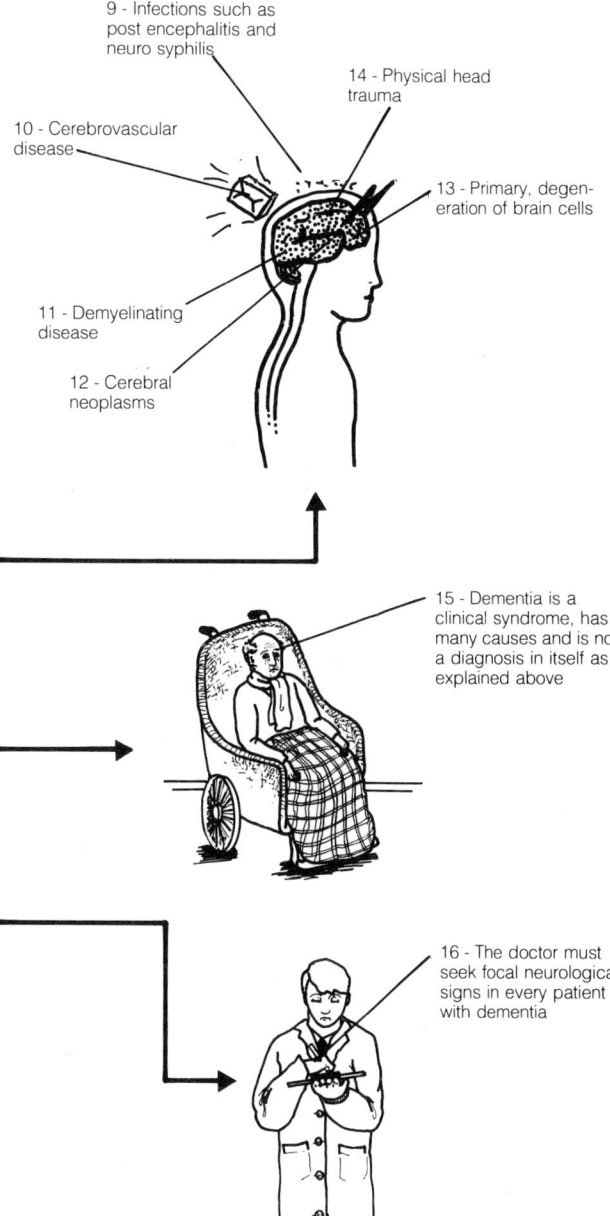

9 - Infections such as post encephalitis and neuro syphilis

10 - Cerebrovascular disease

11 - Demyelinating disease

12 - Cerebral neoplasms

13 - Primary, degeneration of brain cells

14 - Physical head trauma

15 - Dementia is a clinical syndrome, has many causes and is not a diagnosis in itself as explained above

16 - The doctor must seek focal neurological signs in every patient with dementia

Dementia, (like anaemia), is a clinical feature or syndrome rather than a specific diagnosis and the underlying cause must be sought:– In general, dementia may be caused by any severe and irreversible brain damage, (eg. infections – such as post-encephalitic and neurosyphilis, metabolic disorders, toxins, physical head trauma, cerebrovascular disease, primary degenerations of brain cells, demyelinating disease and cerebral neoplasms). It is obvious from the foregoing that focal neurological signs may accompany the signs of dementia and the clinician must record both.

Dementia

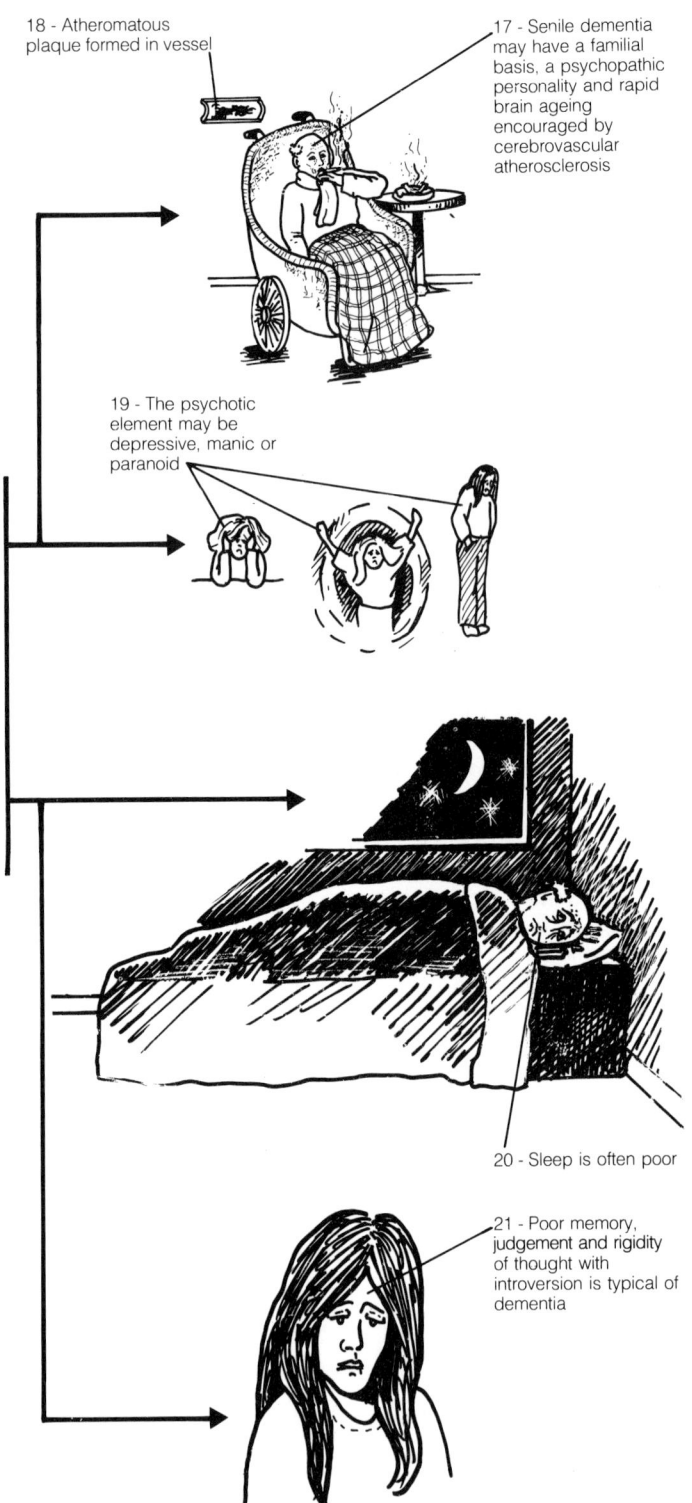

18 - Atheromatous plaque formed in vessel

17 - Senile dementia may have a familial basis, a psychopathic personality and rapid brain ageing encouraged by cerebrovascular atherosclerosis

19 - The psychotic element may be depressive, manic or paranoid

20 - Sleep is often poor

21 - Poor memory, judgement and rigidity of thought with introversion is typical of dementia

Senile dementia may have one or more of several aetiological bases including a familial basis, a psychopathic personality and rapid brain ageing, aided and abetted by cerebrovascular atherosclerosis. The psychotic element may be predominantly depressive, manic or paranoid whilst the poor memory and judgement together with rigidity of thought and progressive introversion are the main manifestations of the dementia. Sleep is poor and thought dwells incessantly on possessions and health.

Dementia

There are two well-recognised forms of pre-senile dementia, both of which afflict women more frequently than men. **Pick's disease** commences in middle age, usually in the 50–60's; there is a hereditary predisposition. There is progressive cerebral atrophy mainly affecting the frontal and temporal areas. Gradual behavioural disturbances and deteriorating judgement and activity level usually precede the disturbances in mood and memory. In **Alzheimer's disease** more scattered and focal cerebral lesions, (plaques and neurofibrillary changes), often lead to a more rapidly progressive dementia, not infrequently attended by disturbances in other higher functions (eg. dysphasia, dyspraxia, dysgraphia) and fits may occur.

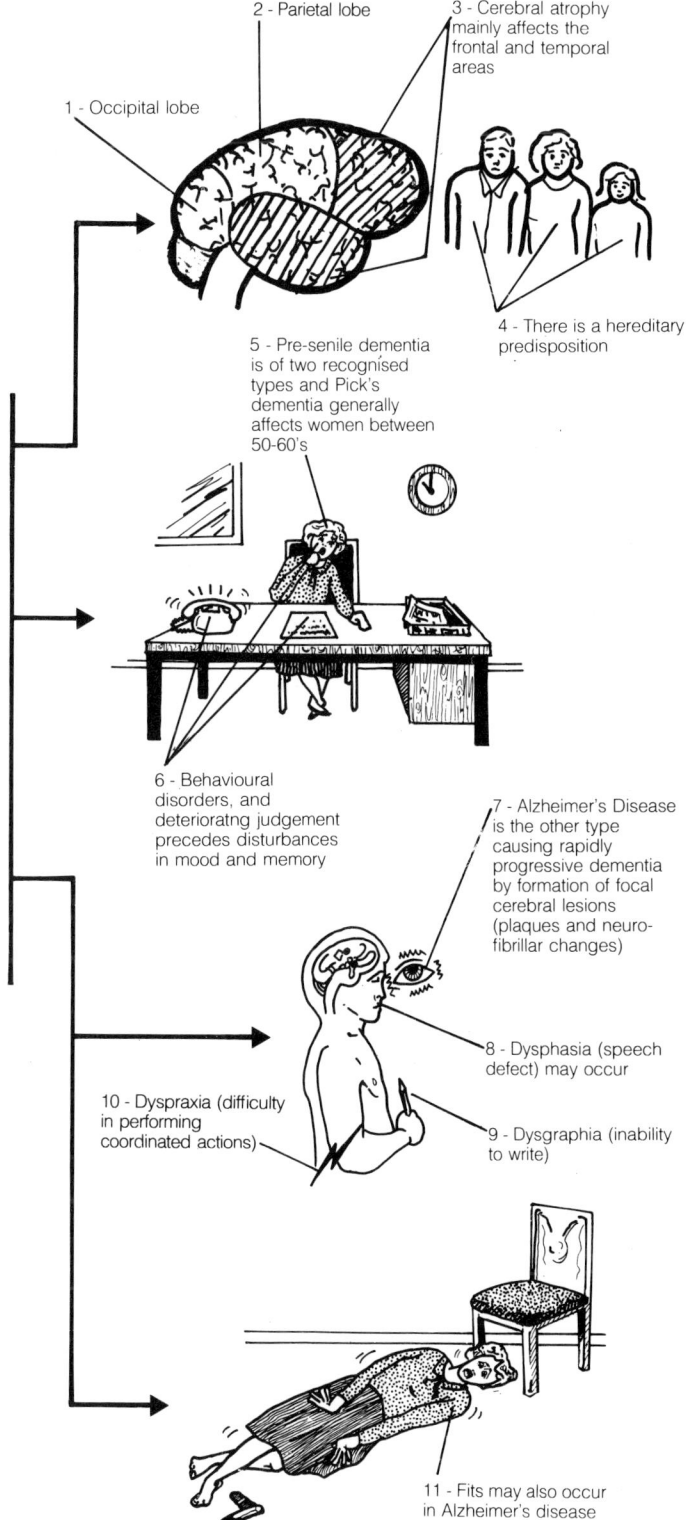

1 - Occipital lobe
2 - Parietal lobe
3 - Cerebral atrophy mainly affects the frontal and temporal areas
4 - There is a hereditary predisposition
5 - Pre-senile dementia is of two recognised types and Pick's dementia generally affects women between 50-60's
6 - Behavioural disorders, and deterioratng judgement precedes disturbances in mood and memory
7 - Alzheimer's Disease is the other type causing rapidly progressive dementia by formation of focal cerebral lesions (plaques and neurofibrillar changes)
8 - Dysphasia (speech defect) may occur
9 - Dysgraphia (inability to write)
10 - Dyspraxia (difficulty in performing coordinated actions)
11 - Fits may also occur in Alzheimer's disease

Dementia

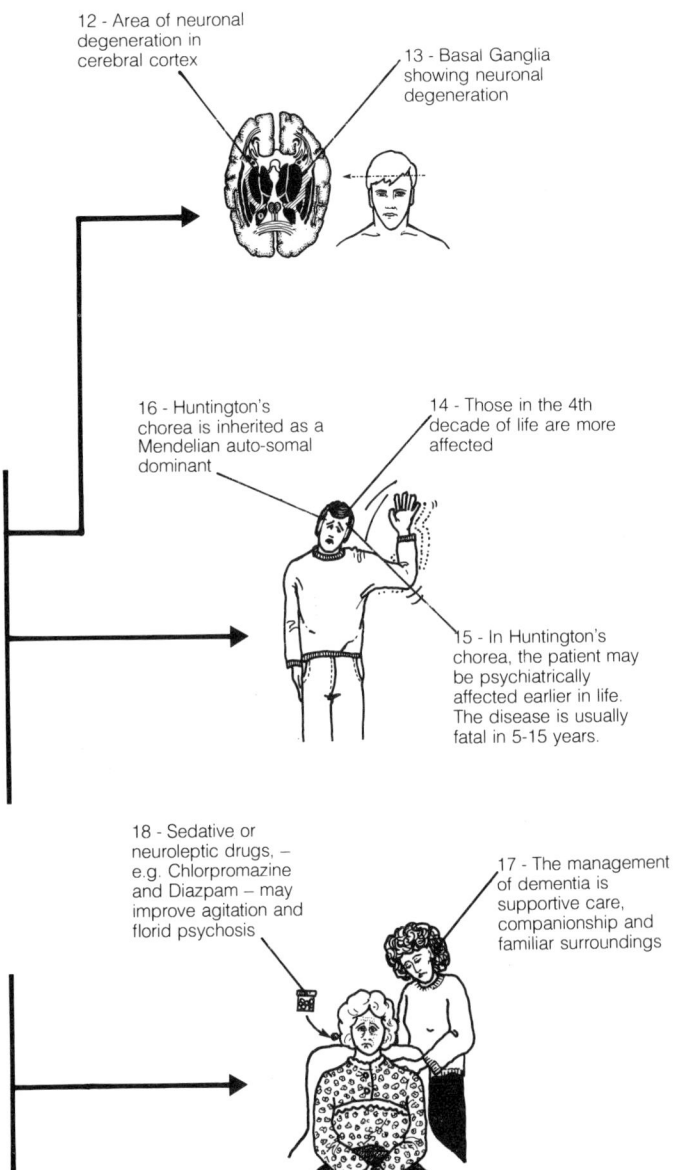

12 - Area of neuronal degeneration in cerebral cortex

13 - Basal Ganglia showing neuronal degeneration

16 - Huntington's chorea is inherited as a Mendelian auto-somal dominant

14 - Those in the 4th decade of life are more affected

15 - In Huntington's chorea, the patient may be psychiatrically affected earlier in life. The disease is usually fatal in 5-15 years.

18 - Sedative or neuroleptic drugs, – e.g. Chlorpromazine and Diazpam – may improve agitation and florid psychosis

17 - The management of dementia is supportive care, companionship and familiar surroundings

Huntington's chorea is also a specific form of pre-senile dementia. Inherited as a Mendelian autosomal dominant, there is neuronal degeneration particularly in the basal ganglia and cerebral cortex – usually manifesting clinically in the fourth decade of life. However, the patient may be psychiatrically disturbed much earlier in life than this. This disease is usually fatal within 5–15 years, (see also chorea).

The **management** of all these forms of dementia consists largely of supportive care, familiar surroundings and congenial companionship is advisable. Sedative or neuroleptic drugs are prescribed on an individual basis for agitation, florid psychosis etc.

The question now arises as to how far should a clinician investigate a seemingly obvious case of dementia to discover an underlying cause. It is suggested that a full history and examination precede a full blood count, tests for syphilis, skull X-ray series, EEG, C.T. scan of brain and perhaps arteriography to exclude a frontal lobe tumour.

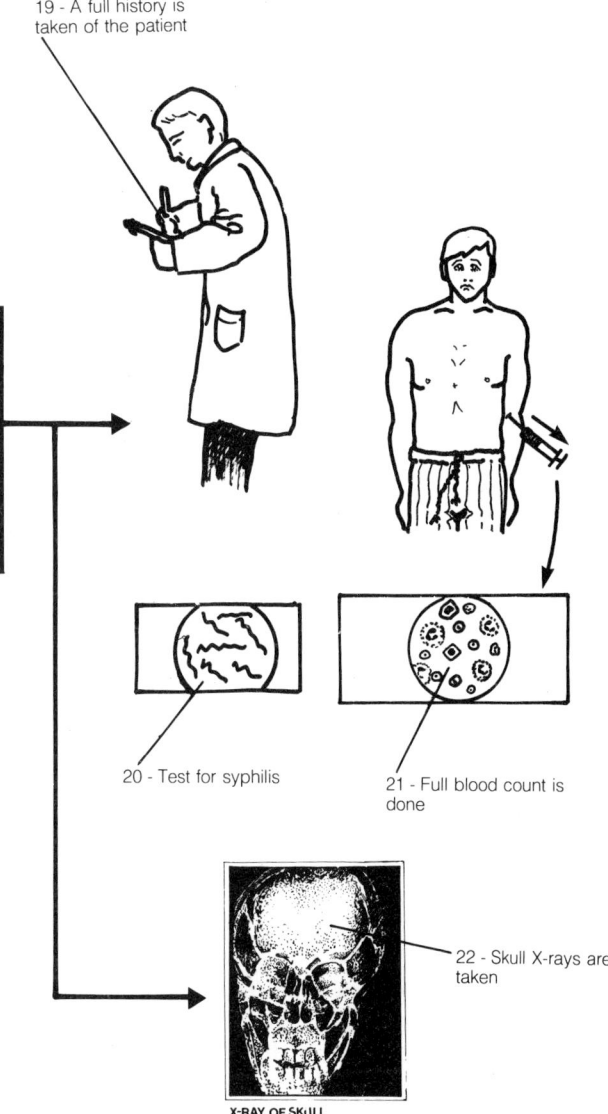

19 - A full history is taken of the patient

20 - Test for syphilis

21 - Full blood count is done

22 - Skull X-rays are taken

X-RAY OF SKULL

Cerebral tumours are a necessary inclusion in the differential diagnosis of many psychoses: Frontal lobe tumours may well present with memory disturbances and hallucinations.

ALCOHOLISM

In **alcoholics**, several organic psychoses may occur. A dementia is a feature of many chronic alcoholics whilst alcoholic hallucinosis is a more highly developed psychosis usually with auditory hallucinations and paranoid delusions. This psychosis may remit on alcohol withdrawal.

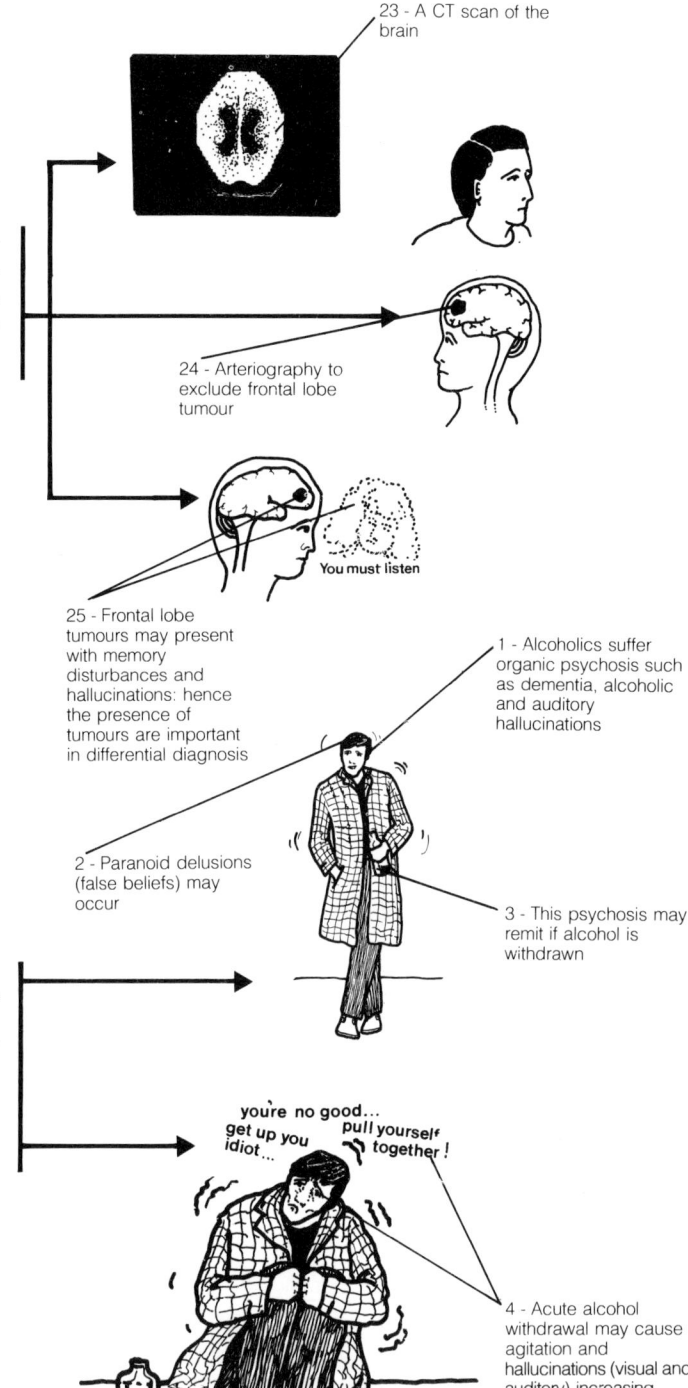

23 - A CT scan of the brain

24 - Arteriography to exclude frontal lobe tumour

25 - Frontal lobe tumours may present with memory disturbances and hallucinations: hence the presence of tumours are important in differential diagnosis

1 - Alcoholics suffer organic psychosis such as dementia, alcoholic and auditory hallucinations

2 - Paranoid delusions (false beliefs) may occur

3 - This psychosis may remit if alcohol is withdrawn

4 - Acute alcohol withdrawal may cause agitation and hallucinations (visual and auditory) increasing misinterpretation of surrounding events

Acute alcohol withdrawal from a chronic alcoholic may itself induce an acute syndrome of severe restlessness, agitation, hallucinations (visual and auditory), with worsening misinterpretation of surrounding events and perhaps wild excitation – even fitting. The condition usually occurs 24–48 hours after alcohol withdrawal and progresses to delirium (**delirium tremens**). **Management** involves the avoidance of complete and sudden withdrawal of alcohol from such individuals and where the symptoms occur, nursing under phenothiazine sedation and with vitamin and fluid supplementation.

The **Korsakoff's syndrome** is most commonly seen in alcoholics but vitamin B1 deficiency and other cerebral diseases may be associated with the syndrome. The clinical features are an amnesia often with an alcoholic polyneuritis. In alcoholic Korsakoff's syndrome, the deficiency in memory is often circumvented by confabulation – the patient fantasising to overcome the gap in memory. This memory gap is mainly for recent events and the possibility of reversibility with vitamin B supplementation both distinguish this condition from dementia.

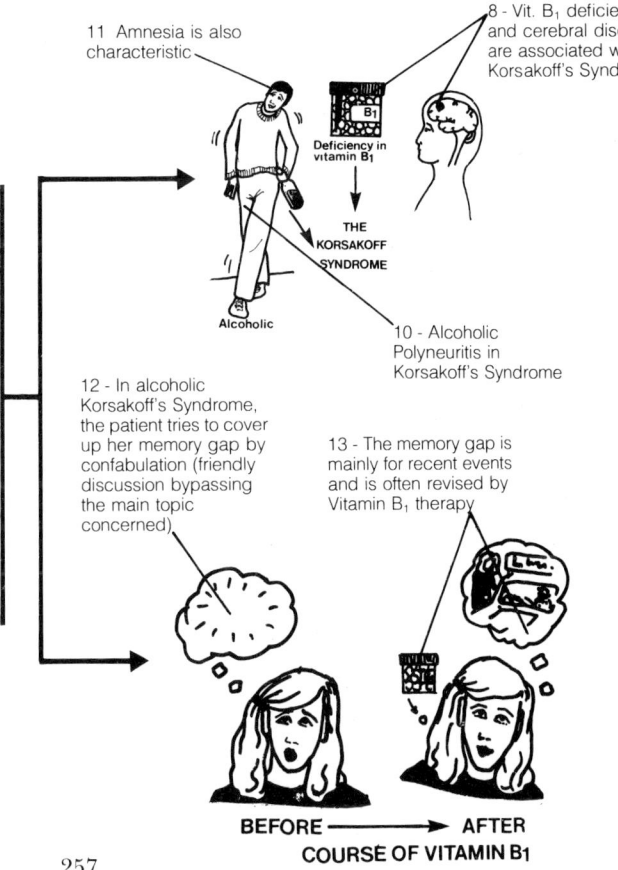

Alcoholism

Wernicke's encephalopathy occurs occasionally in chronic alcoholics suffering acute thiamine deprivation. Nystagmus and ophthalmoplegia precede ataxia anorexia and vomiting all of which lead to progressive apathy and then a coma which may prove fatal. The treatment involves the early administration of large doses of the vitamin B complex with supportive care.

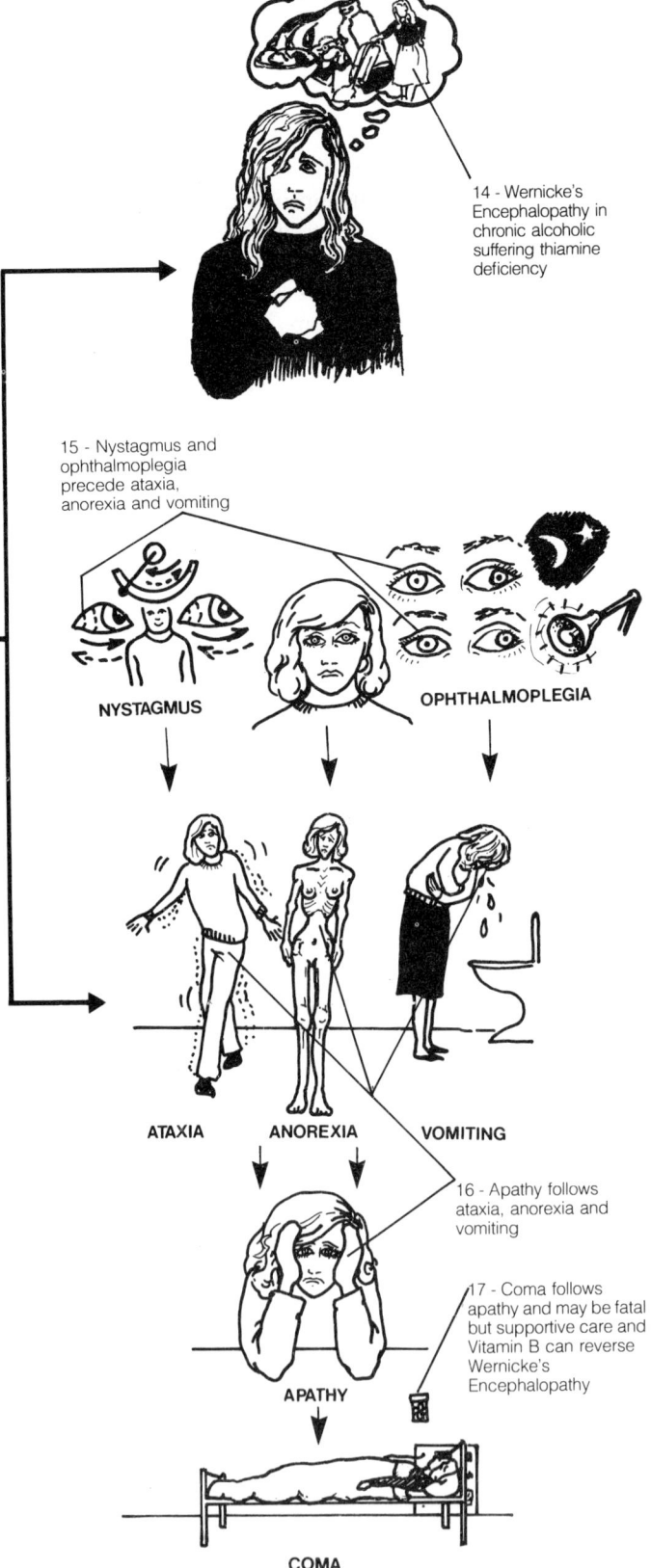

14 - Wernicke's Encephalopathy in chronic alcoholic suffering thiamine deficiency

15 - Nystagmus and ophthalmoplegia precede ataxia, anorexia and vomiting

16 - Apathy follows ataxia, anorexia and vomiting

17 - Coma follows apathy and may be fatal but supportive care and Vitamin B can reverse Wernicke's Encephalopathy

Pellagra results from nicotinamide deficiency and in the tropics it tends to occur in those living largely on maize. In Britain, it may occur in Malabsorptive states. Dermatitis and diarrhoea (2 × D's), are the main clinical manifestations, the rash being a photosensitive erythematous and later pigmented and scaly eruption. The mental condition usually begins as a subacute delirium; untreated, it progresses to dementia, (the third "D"). **Treatment** is with vitamin B complex.

Another vitamin deficiency associated with dementia is B12 deficiency, (see 'subacute combined degeneration of the cord'). Other metabolic causes of dementia include chronic cerebral hypoxia and hypoglycaemia.

Acute infections of the CNS may be accompanied by organic psychoses — usually delirium, and chronic infections, (notably neurosyphilis) may be associated with many organic psychiatric states and focal neurological signs.

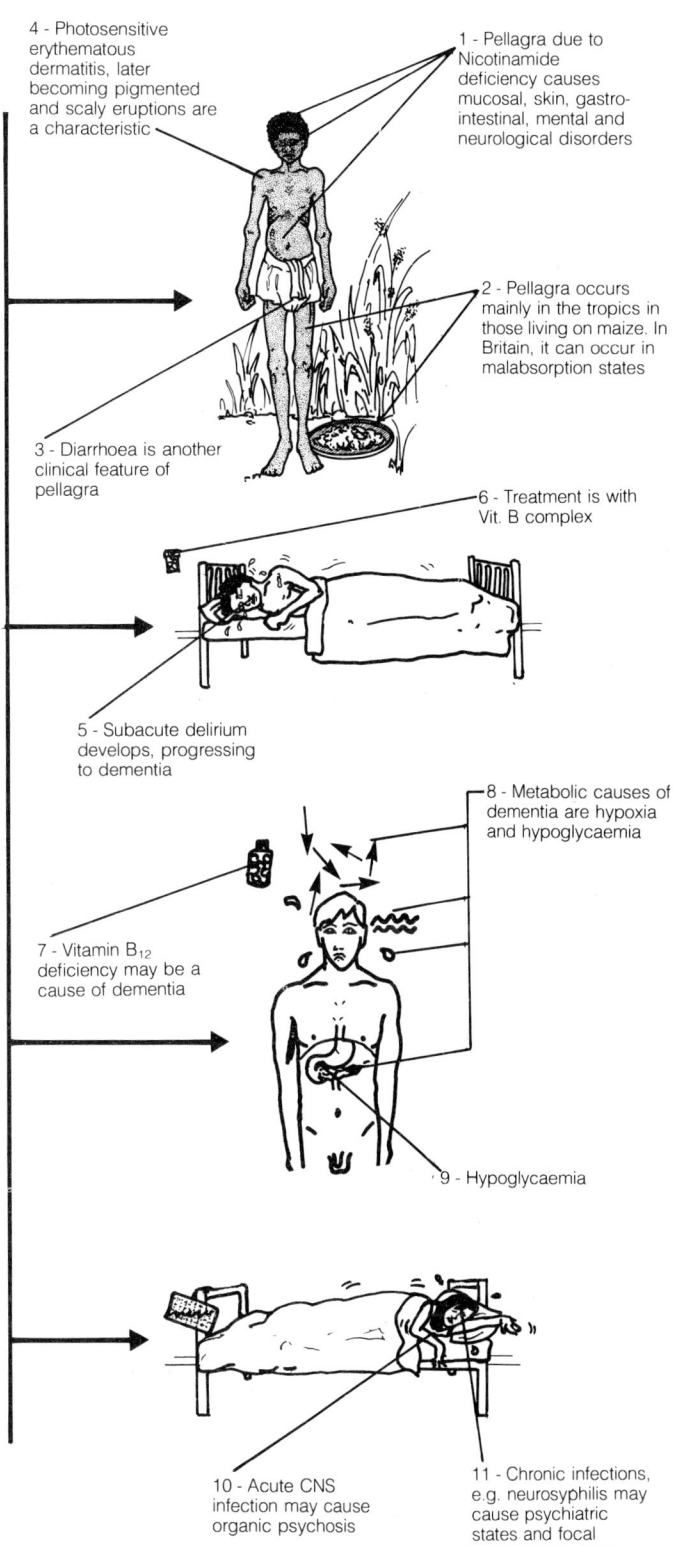

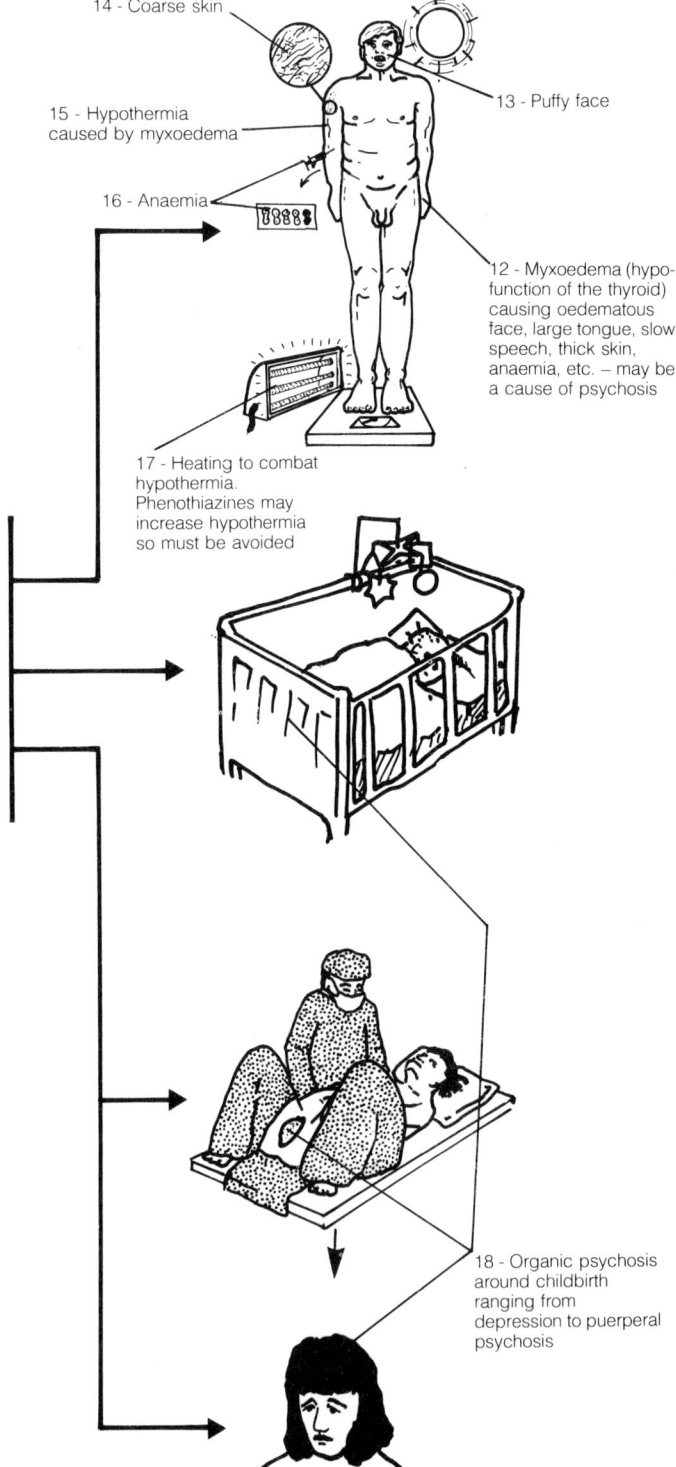

Various endocrine conditions may be associated with psychosis – for example, advanced myxoedema; (we might here note the potential danger of phenothiazines in precipitating severe hypothermia in this condition). Around the period of childbirth organic psychosis is well-recognised; the psychiatric illness may range from depression to florid psychosis, (eg. puerperal psychosis).

Index

Abdominal reflexes, superficial 66
Abnormal movement disorders 147-9
Abnormal personalities 201, 218-22
  antisocial (psychopath) 221
  cyclothymic 223
  hysterical 211, 219
  inadequate 222
  obsessional 219, 223
  paranoid 220
  schizoid 220
Acoustic neuroma 42, 45, 108
Acute infectious polyneuritis (Guillain-Barré syndrome) 177-8
Addisonian crisis 86
Agnosia 11
  visual 11
Agoraphobia 209
Alcohol
  acute withdrawal 257
  nystagmus due to 36
Alcoholism 257-9
  myopathy 193
  polyneuritis 257
Alzheimer's disease 253
Amnesia 12
Amphetamine poisoning 246
Amyloidosis 174
Amyotrophic lateral sclerosis 168
Angioma, cerebral 102
Anorexia nervosa 212-14
Anosmia 16
Anticholinesterase therapy 185
Anticonvulsants 133-7
  drug interactions 137
Antisocial personality (psychopath) 221
Anxiety 206
  morbid 207-8
Anxiolytic drugs 209
Aphasia
  nominal 6
  Wernicke's 12
Apraxia (dyspraxia) 9
  bilateral 9
  dressing 10
  ideomotor 6
Arboviruses 91

Argyll Robertson pupil 32, 97, 98
Arnold-Chiari malformation 164
Astrocytoma 100
Ataxia
  cerebellar 62, 63
  truncal 63
Athetosis 147
Automatic obedience 245
Autotopagnosia 11

Babinski sign 58, 66
Bell's palsy 46
Bell's phenomenon 44
Benedikt's syndrome 28
Beriberi 178
Berry aneurysm 112-14
Bjerrum screen 18
Brain abscess 94-5
Brain death 163
Brainstem, lesions causing oculomotor palsies 28-9
Brain tumours 99-108, 256
  calcification in 101
  clinical features 101-2
  investigation 102
  secondary 99
  treatment 103-4
Broca's area 6
Bromide poisoning, chronic 246
Bromocriptine 107
Bronchus, apical carcinoma of 34
Brown-Séquard lesion 71
Butyrophenones 247

Caloric test 49-50
Carbamazepine 135-6
Carcinomatous myopathy 193
Carotid nerve 30
Carpal tunnel syndrome 170
Catastrophic reaction 250
Catatonia, acute 242
Cerebral abscess 94-5
Cerebral embolus 123
Cerebral thrombosis 121-2
Cerebral tumours see Brain tumours
Cerebrospinal fluid 79-81
Cervical rib 171
Cervical spondylosis 156
Charcot's joints 97

Charcot's triad 63
Chiasmal lesions 17
Childbirth, psychoses associated 260
Chlorpromazine 247
Chorda tympani nerve 42
Chorea 147, 149
  Huntington's 149
  Sydenham's 149
Choroid, miliary tubercles in 20
Ciliary ganglion degeneration 33
Circumlocution 7
Clonazepam 136
Clonic facial spasm 46
Clonus 61
Coma 159-62
  causes 160
Common peroneal nerve palsy 169
Conduction deafness 48
Coordination testing 62
Corneal reflex 41
Cranial (temporal, giant cell) arteritis 122, 157
Cranial nerves
  I (olfactory nerve) 16
  II (optic nerve) 17-20
    atrophy 19-20
  III (oculomotor) 21-3
    palsy 23-5
  IV (trochlear) 21-3
    palsy 25-6
  V (trigeminal) 39-41
    long nuclei damage 41
    unilateral motor root lesion 40
  VI (abducent) 21-3
    palsy 26-7
  VII (facial) 42-3
    palsy 43-4; see also Bell's palsy
  VIII (vestibulocochlear) 47
    auditory (cochlear division) 47-8
    vestibular division 49-50
  IX (glossopharyngeal) 54-5
  X (vagus) 54-6
  XI (accessory) 56-7
  XII (hypoglossal) 57
Craniopharyngioma 102, 107
Cremasteric reflex 66

Index

Dandy-Walker malformation 164
Delirium 249
Delirium tremens 258
Delusions 240
Dementia 250-6
　frontal lobe tumour causing 255, 256
　investigations 255
　management 254
　myotonic dystrophy 191
　pellagra-induced 259
　presenile 253
　senile 253
Depression 216-18
　endogenous 216, 223-31
　　clinical presentation 224-6
　　differential diagnosis 229
　　suicide/attempted suicide 227-8
　　treatment 230-1
　involutional (peri-climacteric, menopausal) 218
　post-partum 218
　premenstrual 218
　reactive 216-17
Dermatomyositis 194
Devic's disease (neuromyelitis optica) 140
Dexamethasone 104
Diplopia 22, 26, 27
Dissociated sensory loss 164
Dopa (L−) 146
Drop attack 75
Dysarthria, spastic 58
Dyscalculia 8
Dysdiadokokinesis 63
Dysgraphia 8
Dyslexia 8
Dysphasia 6-8
　jargon 8
　motor (expressive) 7
　nominal 7-8
　sensory 8
Dysphonia 6
Dyspraxia *see* Apraxia

Eaton-Lambert syndrome 183
Echolalia 245
Echopraxia 245
Edrophonium chloride (Tensilon) 184
Electro-convulsive therapy (ECT) 230, 248
Encephalitis, viral 90-1
Encephalitis lethargica 32
Entrapment mononeuropathies 169
Ependymoma 100
Epilepsy 124-7
　cerebral tumour-induced 101
　cerebrovascular disease-induced 101

fits arising in frontal lobe 5
generalised 128
grand mal 128-9
investigation 127
Jacksonian 130-1
partial (focal) 130-1
petit mal 130
symptomatic 125-6
temporal lobe 131-2
treatment 133-7
trigger factors 127
Ergotamine tartrate 154-5
Exophthalmic ophthalmoplegia 29
Extradural haemorrhage 109-10

Facio-scapulo-humeral muscular dystrophy 190
Familial hypertrophic neuropathy 174
Familial periodic paralyses 193
Flight of ideas 233
Fluphenazine decanoate 248
Friedreich's ataxia 63-4
Frontal lobe
　lesions 4-6
　non-dominant 6
　tumour 4-5, 256

Gag (pharyngeal) reflex 54
Gaze palsies 22-3
General paralysis of the insane (GPI) 98
Gerstmann's syndrome 9
Giant cell (temporal, cranial) arteritis 122, 157
Glial cells 99
Glioblastoma multiforme 100, 102, 103
Glioma 99
Gnosis disorders 11
Gradenigo's syndrome 41
Grasp reflex 4
Guillain-Barré syndrome (acute infectious polyneuritis) 177-8

Hallucinations 205, 241
　in depression 225
Headache 150-8
　causes 158
　raised intracranial pressure 158
　vascular 156
　tension (psychogenic) 151
　see also Migraine; Temporal arteritis
Head trauma with loss of consciousness 160
Hemiballismus 149
Hemichorea 149

Hemicrania 153
Hemiparesis 6
Herpes encephalitis 90
Herpes zoster, geniculate ganglion 45
Higher cerebral functions, examination/assessment 13-15
Holmes-Adie pupil 33
Homonymous hemianopia 10, 17
Horner's syndrome 30, 34
Huntington's chorea 149, 254
Hyperacusis 43
Hypertonicity (spasticity) 60
Hypochondriasis 226
Hypomania 232-5
　prognosis 235
Hypothermia 260
Hysteria 210-12
Hysterical personality 211, 219

Illusions 205
Immunosuppressed patient
　cerebral abscess 95
　meningitis 83, 95
　septicaemia 94
Inadequate personality 222
Intention tremor 63
Internal carotid artery occlusion 118-19
Intervertebral disc prolapse 72-4, 75-7
Intracerebral haemorrhage 114-16
Intracranial haemorrhage 109-16
　extradural 109-10
　intracerebral 114-16
　subarachnoid 112-14
　subdural 111-12

Jakob-Creutzfeldt disease 92, 94
Jaw jerk 40

Kernig's sign 82-3
Klippel-Feil deformity 164, 166
Knight's move 238
Korsakoff's psychosis 179, 257
Kuru 94

Labyrinth 49
Lasèque's sign (straight leg raising test) 77
Leprosy 174
Limb-girdle muscular dystrophy 190
Limbic lesions 229
Lithium carbonate 234
Lower motor neurone lesion 58
Lumbago 75-7

McArdle's disease 193
Malingering 210

262

Index

Mania 232-5
  prognosis 235
Manic depressive illness 222
Medulloblastoma, cerebellar 100
Menière's disease 38, 52-3
Meningioma 105
Meningism 113
Meningitis 81-3
  acute pyogenic 83-4
  immunosuppressed patient 83, 95
  meningococcal 86
  tuberculous 86-8
  viral 89-90
Meningo-encephalitis, viral 90
Meningovascular syphilis 96
Mental defect (subnormality) 200
Meralgia paraesthetica 171
Methysergide 155
Mianserin 231
Migraine 151-6
  aura 152
  brainstem (basilar) 152
  prophylaxis 155-6
  secondary 154
  treatment 154-5
Millard-Gubler syndrome 45
Monoamine oxidase inhibitors 231
Mononeuritis multiplex 171
Mononeuropathy 169
Motor aphasia/dysphasia 6
Motor neurone disease 167-8
Motor system examination 60-6
Multiple sclerosis 137-43
  aetiology 138
  ataxic nystagmus 38
  clinical features 138-41
  prognosis 143
  tests 141-2
  treatment 142
  trigeminal neuralgia in 42
Muscles
  fasciculation 60
  root innervation 78
  wasting 60
Muscular dystrophy 187-90
  Duchenne 188-9
  facio-scapulo-humeral 190
  limb girdle 190
  ocular 190
Mutism 6
Myasthenia gravis 29, 181-5
  medical treatment 185
  thymectomy 184
Myopathies 186
  acquired 192-3
  carcinomatous 193
Myotonia congenita (Thomsen's disease) 192
Myotonic dystrophy 191
Myxoedema 229, 260

Neglect phenomena 6
Neologism 7
Nervous system
  examination 4
  history 3
Neuromuscular disorders, differential diagnosis 183
Neuromyelitis optica (Devic's disease) 140
Neuroses 199, 200, 206-15
Neurosyphilis 95-8
  meningovascular 121-2
  treatment 98
Nicotinamide deficiency 259
Nitroso urea drugs 103
Nystagmus 35-8
  ataxic 38
  cerebellar 38
  congenital 37
  drugs causing 36
  horizontal 37, 38
  pendular 37
  vertical 38
  vestibular 37

Obsessional neurosis 214-15
Obsessional personality 215, 219, 223
Occipital lobe lesions 13
  blindness due to 31
Occlusive cerebrovascular disease 117-23
Ocular muscular dystrophy 190
Oculomotor palsies 22, 23-4, 25-7
  brainstem lesions causing 28
Oligodendroglioma 100, 102
Ophthalmoscopy 19
Oppenheim's reflex 66
Optic atrophy 19-20
  primary 20

Palatal reflex 54
Papilloedema 19, 101
Paralysis agitans 143-5
  treatment 146-7
Paranoid personality 220
Paraphasias 7
Parietal lobe lesions 9-10
Parinaud's syndrome 31
Parkinsonism 143-5, 229
  treatment 146-7
Passivity feelings 240
Pellagra 259
Percussion myotonia 191
Perimetry 18
Peripheral motor system 58-66
Peripheral nerve diseases 169-78
Peripheral sensory system 67-8
Phaeochromocytoma 208
Pharyngeal muscle paralysis 55
Pharyngeal (gag) reflex 54
Phenobarbitone 134-6

Phenothiazines 247, 260
Phenytoin sodium 133-4, 136
Phobias 209-10
Pick's disease 253
Pineal tumour 25
Pituitary apoplexy 106
Pituitary tumour 105-7
Polymyalgia rheumatica 157, 195
Plantar reflex 58, 66
Polymyositis 194-5
Polyneuropathy 172-6
  causes 174-6
Post-denervation hypersensitivity 34
Praxis disorders 9
Presenile dementia 254
Primidone 134, 136
Progressive bulbar palsy 167
Progressive multifocal leucoencephalitis 94
Progressive muscular atrophy 167
Pseudohypertrophic muscular dystrophy (Duchenne type) 188-9
Psychiatric disorders classification 200-2
Psychiatric examination 203-5
Psychiatric history 202
Psychogenic (tension) headache 151
Psychopath (antisocial personality) 221
Psychoses 201
  functional 201, 222-35
  organic 201, 249-56, 259
    acute CNS infection-induced 260
    childbirth-induced 260
    endocrine conditions-induced 261
  puerperal 260
Psychosurgery 231
Ptosis 24
Puerperal psychosis 260
Pupil 29-35
  Argyll Robertson 32, 97
  bilateral fixed 35
  fixed dilated 35
  Holmes-Adie 33
  inequality in comatose patient 35
  reflex activity 31
Pupillo-constrictor centre 29
Pyknic build 223

Quadrantanopsia 17

Radial nerve palsy 169
Ramsay Hunt syndrome 45
Recurrent laryngeal nerve 56
Red nucleus 28

Reflexes
 jaw 40
 plantar 58, 66
 righting 49
 superficial 66
  abdominal 66
 tendon 65-6
Retinitis pigmentosa 20
Retrobulbar neuritis 139-40
Righting reflexes 49
Rinne's test 47
Romberg's test 62

Schizoid personality 220
Schizophrenia 235-48
 behavioural disorders 241-2
 catatonic 244-5
 delusions 240
 diagnosis 245-6
 emotional disturbance 241
 hallucinations 241
 hebephrenic 243
 paranoid 243
 prognosis 248
 simple 242
 thought disorder 238-9
 treatment 246-8
Schwannoma, benign 108
Scotoma 17
Scrapie 94
Semicircular canals 49
 lesions 37
Senile dementia 253
Sensory testing 68
Slow virus infections 92-3
Snellen's types 18
Sodium valproate 135-6
Spasticity (hypertonicity) 60
Spastic tetraplegia, jaw jerk in 40
Speech disorders 6-8

Spinal cord compression 69-71
Spondylosis, cervical 75
Stevens-Johnson syndrome 134
Straight leg raising test (Lasèque's sign) 77
Stroke 114-16, 118-19
 cerebral thrombosis-induced 121-2
 management 120-1
Subacute combined degeneration of cord 180
Subacute sclerosing panencephalitis 93
Subarachnoid haemorrhage 112-13
Subdural haemorrhage 111-12
Subhyaloid haemorrhage 20
Suicide/attempted suicide 227-8
Superficial reflexes 66
 abdominal 66
Sydenham's chorea 149
Syncopal attack 124-5
Syringobulbia 163
Syringomyelia 162-6

Tabes dorsalis 96-7
Tabo-paresis 98
Temporal (cranial, giant cell) arteritis 122, 157
Temporal lobe lesions 12
Tendon reflexes 65-6
Tension (psychogenic) headache 151, 207
Tentorial pressure cone 35
Thiamine deficiency 178-9
Thomsen's disease (myotonia congenita) 192
Thought blockade 238
Thymoma 181
Tic 148
Tic douloureux (trigeminal neuralgia) 41-2

Todd's paresis 131
Torsion dystonia 147
Tranquillisers 247
Transient ischaemic attack 117, 118-19
 management 120
Transverse myelitis
 in multiple sclerosis 140
 syphilitic 96
Tremor 147, 148
 benign 148
 drug-induced 148
 extrapyramidal 148
Tricyclic antidepressants 230
Trigeminal neuralgia (tic douloureux) 41-2

Ulnar nerve palsy 169
Upper motor neurone lesion 58

Venous sinus thrombosis 123-4
Vertebral artery compression 75
Vertigo 50-1
Visual evoked response 141-2
Visual pathways examination 18
Vitamin B_1 deficiency 178-9
Vitamin B_{12} deficiency 179, 259

Waterhouse-Friderichsen syndrome 86
Waxy flexibility 244
Weber's syndrome 28
Weber's test 48
Wernicke's aphasia 12
Wernicke's encephalopathy 179, 258
Wilson's disease 148

Xanthochromia 80